Lung Cancer Therapy
Annual 7

Lung Cancer Therapy
Annual 7

Edited by

Rolf A. Stahel, MD
Senior Staff Physician at the Clinic and Policlinic of Oncology,
University Hospital of Zürich, Switzerland

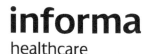

First published in 2012 by Informa Healthcare, 119 Farringdon Road, London EC1R 3DA, UK.

This edition published in 2012 by Informa Healthcare, 119 Farringdon Road, London EC1R 3DA, UK. Simultaneously published in the USA by Informa Healthcare, 52 Vanderbilt Avenue, 7th Floor, New York, NY 10017, USA.

Informa Healthcare is a trading division of Informa UK Ltd. Registered Office: Informa House, 30–32 Mortimer Street, London W1W 7RE, UK. Registered in England and Wales, number 1072954.

A CIP record for this book is available from the British Library.

ISBN-13: 978-1-8418-4865-5
eISBN: 978-184-1-84867-9

Orders may be sent to: Informa Healthcare, Sheepen Place, Colchester, Essex CO3 3LP, UK
Telephone: +44 (0)20 7017 6682
Email: Books@Informa.com
Website: http://informahealthcarebooks.com

For corporate sales please contact: CorporateBooksIHC@informa.com
For foreign rights please contact: RightsIHC@informa.com
For reprint permissions please contact: PermissionsIHC@informa.com

Typeset by Exeter Premedia Services Private Ltd., Chennai, India
Printed and bound in the United Kingdom

Dedication

Heine Hansen died in September 2011. He was the editor of the *Lung Cancer Therapy Annual* since its inception until he entrusted this task to me in 2011. The 7th edition of the *Lung Cancer Therapy Annual* is dedicated to his memory.

Heine Hansen was dedicated to the field of lung cancer and a mentor to many of us working in this field. After a productive stay in the USA, where he became assistant professor at the George Washington University, he returned home to Denmark, where he became professor at the Finsen Center. After his retirement he continued working at the Rigshospitalet in Copenhagen. He was the driving force behind the Danish Second Opinion System allowing cancer patients to explore the possibility of international treatment options.

Throughout his active life, he was committed to promote the fight against lung cancer by collaborative efforts. He was president of the International Association for the Study of Lung Cancer (IASLC) 1988–1991 and later became its first executive director. During this time he organized multidisciplinary workshops aimed at improving the diagnosis of treatment of lung cancer, interactive and friendly events that many of us keep in good memory. He also became editor in-chief of the journal *Lung Cancer*, at that time the official journal of the society until 2006, when this task passed to me.

Heine Hansen joined the European Society of Medical Oncology and became its president from 1995 until 1997 and subsequently became its executive director. Of his many visions and merits I would like to mention the promotion of medical oncology as a specialty, the activation of the Eastern European Task force, the initiation of the ESMO guidelines process, and the creation of a Global Core Curriculum for medical oncology.

Heine Hansen has been a spirited leader and a great mentor in the field. His visions and actions have shaped many organizations. He leaves behind many friends.

Rolf Stahel

Contents

Contributors

Paolo Boffetta
Professor of Medicine and Deputy Director, Tisch Cancer Institute, Mount Sinai School of Medicine, New York, NY, USA
Vice President for Research International Prevention Research Institute, Lyon, France

Menghua Tao
Institute for Translational Epidemiology, Mount Sinai School of Medicine, New York, NY, USA

Giulia Veronesi
Director, Lung Cancer Early Detection Unit, Division of Thoracic Surgery, European Institute of Oncology, Milan, Italy

Christophe Dooms
Respiratory Oncology Unit (Pulmonology), University Hospitals Leuven, Leuven, Belgium

Alex Soltermann
Institute of Surgical Pathology, University Hospital Zurich, Zurich, Switzerland

Solange Peters
Médecin Associé, Cancer Center, Centre Hospitalier Universitaire Vaudois (CHUV), Lausanne, Switzerland

Verena Tischler
Institute of Surgical Pathology, University Hospital Zurich, Zurich, Switzerland

Hiromichi Ebi
Assistant Professor, Division of Medical Oncology, Cancer Research Institute, Kanazawa University, Kanazawa, Japan

Tetsuya Mitsudomi
Professor, Department of Surgery, Division of Thoracic Surgery, Kinki University School of Medicine, Osaka, Japan

Cesare Gridelli
Division of Medical Oncology, S.G. Moscati Hospital, Avellino, Italy

Antonio Rossi
Division of Medical Oncology, S.G. Moscati Hospital, Avellino, Italy

Caicun Zhou
Department of Oncology, Shanghai Pulmonary Hospital, Cancer Institute of Medical School, Tongji University

David Heigener
Department of Thoracic Oncology, Hospital Grosshansdorf, Grosshansdorf, Germany

Sabine Bohnet
Department of Pulmonary Medicine, Medical University Luebeck, Luebeck, Germany

Martin Reck
Department of Thoracic Oncology, Hospital Grosshansdorf, Grosshansdorf, Germany

Enriqueta Felip
Oncology Department, Vall d'Hebron University Hospital, Barcelona, Spain

Alejandro Navarro Mendivil
Oncology Department, Vall d'Hebron University Hospital, Barcelona, Spain

Paul E. Van Schil
Department of Thoracic and Vascular Surgery, Antwerp University Hospital, Edegem (Antwerp), Belgium

Jeroen M. Hendriks
Department of Thoracic and Vascular Surgery, Antwerp University Hospital, Edegem (Antwerp), Belgium

Marjan Hertoghs
Department of Thoracic and Vascular Surgery, Antwerp University Hospital, Edegem (Antwerp), Belgium

Patrick Lauwers
Department of Thoracic and Vascular Surgery, Antwerp University Hospital, Edegem (Antwerp), Belgium

Cliff K. C. Choong
Associate Professor in Surgery, Monash Univeristy, Consultant Cardiothoracic Surgeon, Monash Medical Centre and Dandenong Hospital, Southern Health, Melbourne, Australia

Dirk K. M. De Ruysscher
Radiation Oncologist, Professor of Respiratory Oncology, Department of Radiation Oncology (Maastro Clinic), Maastricht University Medical Center, GROW School for Oncology and Developmental Biology, Maastricht, The Netherlands

José S.A. Belderbos
Radiation Oncologist, Department of Radiation Oncology, The Netherlands Cancer Institute/Antoni van Leeuwenhoek Hospital, Amsterdam, The Netherlands

Aleksandar Aleksic
Department of Medicine, Royal Marsden Hospital, London, UK

Sanjay Popat
Clinical Senior Lecturer, Imperial College, London Consultant Medical Oncologist, Royal Marsden Hospital, London, UK

Isabelle Opitz
Division of Thoracic Surgery, University Hospital Zurich, Switzerland

Emanuela Felley-Bosco
Laboratory of Molecular Oncology, Clinic of Oncology, University Hospital Zurich, Switzerland

Enrico Ruffini
Division of Thoracic Surgery, University of Torino, Torino, Italy

Pier Luigi Filosso
Division of Thoracic Surgery, University of Torino, Torino, Italy

Paolo Lausi
Division of Thoracic Surgery, University of Torino, Torino, Italy

Alberto Oliaro
Division of Thoracic Surgery, University of Torino, Torino, Italy

1 | Epidemiology of lung cancer

Menghua Tao and Paolo Boffetta

INTRODUCTION

The history of lung cancer epidemiology parallels the history of modern chronic disease epidemiology. Although an excess of lung cancer was first observed among miners and some other occupational groups in the 19th century, an epidemic increase in lung cancer began in the first half of the 20th century, with much speculation and controversy about its possible environmental causes. Later, lung cancer became a milestone in epidemiology when its predominant cause, tobacco smoking, was established in a series of landmark studies beginning in 1950. This chapter on the epidemiology of lung cancer will discuss the recent trends in lung cancer incidence and briefly review the current topics that have been widely discussed at meetings and in the literature: lung cancer in never-smokers, gender differences in the incidence of lung cancer, whether screening with low-dose computed tomography (CT) should be recommended, and the small but important improvements in survival among lung cancer patients. We also will present a summary of known risk factors of lung cancer.

INCIDENCE

Lung cancer has been the most common cancer in the world for several decades. According to the most recent statistics GLOBOCAN 2008, estimating the occurrence of cancer worldwide for the year 2008, 1,092,000 men and 516, 000 women were diagnosed with lung cancer, representing 12.7% of all new cancer cases.[1] There are now fewer lung cancer cases in more developed regions (Northern America, Japan, Europe, and Australia/ New Zealand) than in less developed regions of the world (rest of the world), corresponding to 16.2% or 479,000 of all cancers in males in the developed countries and 16.8% or 612,000 in developing countries.[1] Corresponding percentages for women were 9.4% and 7.9%. Worldwide, lung cancer is the leading cause of cancer death in men and the second leading cause of cancer death in women with about 1.38 million individuals dying from the disease in 2008, which equates to 18.2% of all cancer deaths.[1] Lung cancer incidence is generally higher in men than in women, the magnitude of the difference varies from two- to nine-fold. Worldwide, lung cancer is the fourth most frequent cancer in women, but the occurrence has recently shown a steeper increase among women over time than in men.

Among both women and men, the incidence of lung cancer is low in persons under age 40 and increases up to age 70 or 75. The decline in incidence in the older age groups can be explained, at least in part, by incomplete diagnosis or by a generation (birth-cohort) effect.

The main histological types of lung cancer are squamous cell carcinoma, small cell carcinoma, adenocarcinoma, and large cell carcinoma. Over the last 20 years, the distribution of histologic types of lung cancer has been changing. In North America, squamous cell carcinoma, formerly the predominant type, has declined by approximately 30%; small cell carcinoma rates have decreased less rapidly; however, adenocarcinoma has increased in both genders.[2,3] In Europe, similar changing patterns have been observed in men; however, both squamous cell carcinoma and adenocarcinoma rates are increasing among women.[3,4] In Japan, incidence rates of squamous cell carcinoma and small cell carcinoma decreased, while lung adenocarcinoma incidence rates have continuously increased in both men and women since 1990s.[5] The increased incidence of adenocarcinoma may be due, at least partially, to improvement of diagnostic techniques, while changes in composition and patterns of tobacco consumption (deeper inhalation of low-nicotine and tar tobacco smoke) are also possible explanations.[6]

GEOGRAPHICAL AND TEMPORAL VARIATIONS

The geographical and temporal variations in the incidence of lung cancer observed in both men and women reflect differences in the stage of the tobacco smoking epidemic.[7-9] In populations that are not exposed to tobacco smoke or industrial lung carcinogens, the age-adjusted incidence rate (standardized to the World Standard Population) of lung cancer is generally below 5 per 100,000 per year.[10,11] Among men, lung cancer is still the most common cancer in the world, with high incidence rates in central-eastern and southern Europe, northern America, and eastern Asia.[1] The highest incidence rates of lung cancer are reported in

African-American men (>80 per 100,000 per year) and in men in some Eastern European countries, and their lifetime risk for lung cancer was around 13%.[11,12] In females, the highest incidence rates, around 34 per 100,000 per year, are observed in North America and north-western Europe, the latter including women in Denmark, Iceland, and the United Kingdom.[1,11] In many developed countries, the age-standardized incidence of lung cancer has decreased in males compared with an increase in females over the past 33 years.[1]

Most developing countries have still not experienced the worst consequences of the tobacco epidemic, as cigarette smoking became widespread only during the last 30 years. In China, inhabited by one-fifth of the world population, and thus determining to a large scale the cancer burden at a global level, it was estimated that lung cancer incidence will increase by 27% in men and 38% in women from year 2000 to 2005, due mostly to changes in cancer risk (cigarette smoking), as well as to some degree to alterations of population size and age structure.[13] The total estimated number of lung cancer cases in China was 521,000 in 2008,[1] and it has been estimated that the new cases of lung cancer in China will increase to 693,727 by 2020.[14] The full effect of the increased tobacco consumption will be expected to occur in the next few decades; however, it has been estimated that worldwide smoking caused 3 million deaths out of a total of 30 million adult deaths from all causes in 1990,[15] while in around 2030, worldwide deaths from tobacco will most likely rise to approximately 10 million of 60 million all causes deaths, with majority of the increase taking place in Asia, Africa, and South America.[15]

GENDER

Since the early 1990s, it has been debated whether women are more susceptible to the carcinogenic effects of tobacco smoke than men as some case–control studies, comparing the risk of lung cancer dose by dose in men and women, have found up to 50% higher risk in women compared with men.[16,17] Results from screening studies also reported that women are more likely to be diagnosed with lung cancer than men when high-risk smokers are tested with low-dose computed tomographic (CT) scan,[18] suggesting that incidence of lung cancer may be higher in women than in men who reported past or active smoking. However, not all studies were able to confirm these risk estimates. Several recent large prospective studies in different populations have shown that women do not appear to have a higher relative risk than men for lung cancer associated with smoking.[19–24] Although relationship between gender and lung cancer incidence rates is complex and less convincing, the mortality rates of lung cancer are consistently found to be higher in men than women.[25–27] The difference in death rates may be partially due to cancer stage at diagnosis, cell type, treatment, as well as may indicate a less malignant disease in women when compared with men.[18]

NEVER SMOKERS

Although tobacco smoking is the predominant risk factor of lung cancer, there are a distinct proportion of patients who develop the disease without a history of tobacco smoking. Approximately 15% to 20% of all lung cancer cases arise in never smokers,[25] and lung cancer in never smokers has been an increasingly prominent public health issue.

There is a common perception that women who have never smoked are more often diagnosed with lung cancer compared with men. Using data from six large prospective cohort studies, Wakelee et al.[28] reported that age-adjusted incidence rates of lung cancer among never smokers aged 40–79 years ranged from 14.4 to 20.8 per 100,000 person-years in women and 4.8 to 13.7 per 100,000 person-years in men. Based on 13 cohort studies, Thun et al.[25] analyzed the lung cancer death rates in never smokers and found that never smoking men had higher death rates from lung cancer than women, with age-standardized mortality rates ranging from 32.3 to 13.8 per 100,000 in men and 16.5 to 10.5 per 100,000 in women. And the gender difference in mortality increases with age. The mortality rates from lung cancer among never-smoking African-Americans were higher than Caucasians for both men and women. In this study there was no evidence for statistically significant increasing of death rates in different racial groups over time.[25] The mortality rates have consistently reported to be higher in men who had never smoked than in women in two large American Cancer Society Cancer Prevention Study cohorts.[29] These findings suggested that more women than men have never smoked and have a greater longevity, leading to the above-mentioned perception, but never-smoking men have approximately 16% higher risk of dying from lung cancer than never-smoking women.

SCREENING

The prognosis of lung cancer patients is dismal. Although important progress has been made both in medical and surgical treatment of lung cancer, most patients still succumb to the disease. The main explanation is that patients are diagnosed at a late stage of the natural history of the disease, most patients have unresectable, metastatic disease; and even among patients considered resectable 60% eventually relapse.[30] There have been substantial efforts in developing and implementing screening strategies to detect early-stage lung cancers. Trials on the utility of chest X-ray and/or sputum cytology in detecting asymptomatic lung cancer have been conducted in many countries; however, a meta-analysis of seven trials found no difference in lung cancer mortality comparing screening with chest X-ray and sputum cytology to chest X-ray alone.[31] Recent results from a large clinical trial also showed that annual screening by chest X-ray did not reduce lung cancer mortality compared with usual care.[32]

The emergence of newer methods, such as low-dose CT scans and molecular markers in sputum, provides the possibility to detect lung cancer at earlier, more operable stages in high-risk populations. The CT technology has the potential to detect pulmonary nodules less than 5 mm, and the introduction of low-dose spiral CT has enabled examination of the entire lung in one breath-hold and increased the number of detected nodules.[33] Black et al.[34] systematically reviewed 12 studies conducted in the United States, Japan, and Europe with over 54,000 CT screening examinations for lung cancer. They reported that 70% to 100% of tumors detected after the first (baseline) screening round were found to be in stage I disease with survival rate of over 80%. However, some of the studies included were uncontrolled and most still have a limited follow-up and survival time in early detection studies can be biased in several ways, especially by lead-time and length-time bias. Recently, data from the National Lung Screening trial, a randomized trial to determine the effectiveness of lung cancer screening in high-risk individuals, revealed a 20% reduction in lung cancer-specific mortality with low-dose CT screening compared with standard chest X-ray group among current or former heavy smokers (≥30 pack-year history; <15 years since cessation for ex-smokers).[35] More results from the other ongoing randomized controlled trials are therefore eagerly awaited.[36,37] However, little is known how relevant the low-dose CT screening to individuals with a lesser smoking history. In addition, the potential risks associated with screening, such as accumulation of radiation exposures from multiple screening procedures, additional invasive procedures followed for false-positive patients, as well as the cost-effectiveness of screening are needed to be evaluated. More studies are also needed to determine optimal duration and frequency of CT screening in asymptomatic high-risk populations. It will take some time to develop guidelines based on careful evaluation of the benefits, limitations, and harms associated with low-dose CT screening.

SURVIVAL

Largely due to improvements in the diagnosis and treatment of lung cancer, the one-year relative survival of lung cancer has been improved in some countries. In the United States, the one-year lung cancer survival increased from 37% in 1975–1979 to 43% in 2003–2006.[38] However, lung cancer continues to have one of the lowest five-year survival rates among all malignancies. The EUROCARE project was set up in 1989 to measure and explain trends and variations in cancer survival in Europe. It is a collaborative study on the survival of cancer patients in Europe using information collected by population-based cancer registries; it currently includes data from 83 adult cancer registries on 2.7 million cancer patients.[39] The fourth reports showed age-adjusted five-year survival slightly improved from 9.2% in 1990–1994 to 10.2% in 1995–1999 for European adults.[39] Because the conventional cohort-based survival analyses provide information on patients diagnosed long before, they do not provide up-to-date information on the survival experience of current patients. To overcome this problem, the age-period-cohort analysis approach has been widely used, a method that restricts the analysis to the survival experience of cancer patients using only the most current information by left truncation of the data.[40] Using this approach, additional analyses were conducted for patients diagnosed in 2000–2002 from 47 European cancer registries, and the mean age-adjusted five-year survival of lung cancer was 10.9%.[41] Similarly, from the U.S. Surveillance, Epidemiology and End Results (SEER) Program dataset, the five-year relative survival of lung cancer patients diagnosed in 1998–2000 was 16.3%, unchanged from previous period.[42] Additionally, SEER data also showed that the five-year survival is 53% for patients diagnosed with localized lung cancer.[43] Data from these reports suggested the importance of early diagnosis and adequate treatment procedures for lung cancer survival and prognosis.

KNOWN RISK FACTORS OF LUNG CANCER
Tobacco
The carcinogenic effect of tobacco smoke on the lung was demonstrated in the 1950s and has been recognized by public health and regulatory authorities since the mid of 1960s.[7] Compared with never-smokers, the continuous smokers have 10- to 20-fold higher risk of development of lung cancer. The overall relative

risk reflects the contribution of the different aspects of tobacco smoking, including average consumption, duration of smoking, time since quitting, age at start, type of tobacco product, and inhalation pattern. Numerous epidemiological studies have consistently shown the relative contributions of duration and amount of cigarette smoking in excess lung cancer risk, and there is an exposure–response relationship between cigarette smoking and lung cancer risk.[7,44] Similar patterns of causal relationship have been shown for smoking of cigars, cigarillos, pipes, bidi, hookah, water pipe, khii yoo, and other types of tobacco products with lung cancer risk, indicating a carcinogenic effect of these products.[7,45,46]

An important aspect of tobacco-related lung carcinogenesis is the effect of cessation of smoking. The risk of lung cancer can sharply decline in former smokers starting approximately five years after quitting, and the effect is apparent even for cessation late in life.[7] However, compared with never smokers, a small excess risk of lung cancer likely persists even in long-term quitters throughout lifetime.[7,47]

Secondhand Hand Smoke

Secondhand hand smoke (SHS), also referred to as environmental tobacco smoke (ETS), is composed of side-stream smoke emitted by burning cigarette and mainstream smoke. The collective epidemiologic evidence and biological plausibility suggest that SHS is a lung cancer risk factor among never-smokers, after taking into account possible confounding effects of active smoking, diet, or other factors, and of possible reporting bias.[7,48] Never-smokers exposed to SHS have about 20% increased risk of lung cancer than those without history of SHS exposure.[7] The effect of SHS appears to be presented from both household exposure, mainly from the spouse, and workplace exposure,[7,48] while little evidence showed an association between childhood SHS exposure and lung cancer in adulthood.[49]

Diet and Obesity

There is limited evidence for the protective effects of vegetables and fruits consumption against lung cancer.[50,51] In particular, epidemiologic evidence suggests that intake of cruciferous vegetables may have weakly protective effect of lung cancer, possibly because of their rich content in isothiocyanates.[51,52] Although many studies have evaluated the associations of lung cancer with consumption of other foods, such as cereals, pulses, meat, fish, eggs, milk and dairy products, the evidence is limited and inconsistent to allow a judgment regarding the evidence of a carcinogenic or a protective effect.[51]

A large number of observational studies have shown decreased risk of lung cancer with increased dietary intake of carotenoids, especially β-carotene, and a clear dose–response relationship is apparent from cohort studies.[51,53] A similar relationship has also been reported between serum or plasma carotenoids concentrations and lung cancer.[51,53] In contrast to the observational studies, several large-scale randomized clinical trials designed to investigate the effects of β-carotene supplements failed to prove the protective association. In a large randomized prevention study with smokers, results suggest an increased lung cancer risk in the current smokers who were treated with β-carotene supplements,[54] while results from another trial with workers exposed to asbestos and heavy smokers showed no difference of risk between the treated and the control groups.[55] The difference in the results of observational studies and randomized clinic trials can be explained either by a confounding effect by other dietary components in observational studies, or by a paradox effect of -carotene at very high, non-physiological doses, in particular among smokers.

There is insufficient evidence of an excess risk of lung cancer from alcohol drinking, independent from tobacco smoking.[51,56,57] Both cohort and case–control studies have evaluated the association between body fatness, as measured by body mass index (BMI), and lung cancer risk,[51,58–61] and most of the results showed reduced risk associated with increased BMI. However, this association has high potential to be caused by inadequate adjustment of tobacco smoking, as smoking is strongly related with lower BMI, and by other residual confounding.[51] Similarly, results from certain studies suggested that physical activity may lower lung cancer risk,[51,62,63] but the potential residual confounding by tobacco smoking could not be eliminated for this inverse finding. Although the relationship between physical activity, BMI, and lung cancer makes the evidence difficult to explain, there is limited evidence of decreased lung cancer risk associated with either high BMI or physical activity.

Occupational Exposures

The risk of lung cancer is increased among workers employed in several industries and occupations. For several of these high-risk workplaces, the agent (or agents) responses for the increased risk have been identified. Of these, asbestos and combustion fumes are the most important occupational causes.[64] It has been established that occupational agents are responsible for an estimated 5–10% of lung cancers in industrialized countries.

There is conclusive evidence that exposure to ionizing radiation increases the risk of lung cancer.[65] Although atomic bomb survivors and patients treated with radiotherapy for ankylosing spondylitis or breast cancer have been reported to have moderately increased risk of lung cancer, studies of nuclear industry workers exposed to relatively low levels provided little evidence of an increased risk of lung cancer.[66] Underground miners exposed to radioactive radon and its decay products, which emit α-particles, have been consistently found to have increased risk for lung cancer.[67,68] In addition, several studies showed an increased risk of lung cancer in smoking miners compared with never-smoking miners, with both a possibly additive and a potentially synergistic and multiplicative interaction.[69,70] As radon exposure continues to be an occupational concern in underground work and mining around the world, more longitudinal evaluation of occupationally exposed individuals is needed to improve understanding of the carcinogenic effects of radon.

Environmental Air Pollution

Indoor air pollution has been thought to be responsible for the increased risk of lung cancer experienced by never-smoking women living in several regions of China and other Asian countries. The evidence is strongest not only for coal burning in poorly ventilated houses, but also burning of wood and other solid fuels, as well as for fumes from high-temperature cooking using unrefined vegetable oils such as rapeseed oil.[71] In other parts of the world, indoor exposure to radon and its decay products have been considered as the largest component of environmental radiation to general population. Several case–control studies conducted in North America have reported the significantly positive association between residential radon exposure and lung cancer.[72,73] Similarly, pool analysis of 13 European case–control studies found increased risk of lung cancer associated with high residential radon exposure, particular for smokers and recent ex-smokers.[74]

Outdoor air pollution has also been linked with elevated lung cancer risk.[75] However, it is still difficult to figure out the possible carcinogenic role played by single constituents of air pollution, including fine particles ($PM_{2.5}$), sulfur oxide-related pollution, and nitric oxide.

Inflammation

As an important factor of many types of cancer, the role of infection in lung carcinogenesis has been examined but remains much unknown. Some studies have reported that patients with pulmonary tuberculosis are at increased risk of lung cancer; it is not clear whether the excess risk is due to the chronic inflammatory status of the lung parenchyma or to the specific action of the Mycobacterium.[76,77] Chronic exposure to high levels of fibers and dusts might result in pulmonary fibrosis (e.g., silicosis and asbestosis),[64] a condition which entails an increase in the risk of lung cancer. Chronic bronchitis and emphysema have also been associated with lung cancer risk.

Some recent findings have suggested a potential role for infection of certain viruses, such as human papillomavirus (HPV), Epstein-Barr virus (EBV), BK virus, and JC virus, in the development of lung cancer. However, results from limited epidemiologic studies have remained inconclusive.[78]

Genetic Factors

There is a genetic component to the carcinogenesis of lung cancer, whether it is related with host susceptibility, with or without exposures to tobacco smoking and other potential risk factors, or to an individual's responsiveness to biologic therapies. A positive familial history of lung cancer has been found to be a risk factor in some studies. Gauderman et al.[79] suggested that inheritance of a major gene, in conjunction with tobacco smoking, might account for more than 50% of cases diagnosed below age 60. Using family linkage approaches, a pooled analysis of high-risk pedigrees identified a major susceptibility locus to chromosome 6q23-25.[80]

In addition to the possible effect of relatively rare genes with high penetrance, there have also been many studies on candidate low-penetrance susceptibility genes that are involved in the metabolism of tobacco or other carcinogens, DNA repair, and cell cycle control. For several genes (e.g., GSTM1 and GSTT1), the accumulated evidence suggests an increased risk of lung cancer among carriers of the rare variant.[81] However, for most genes, results have been mixed that do not allow conclusions on the presence or absence of an effect.[81] This may be due to methodological limitations in the available studies and low statistical power. With the availability of high-density genotyping and large sample size, recent genome-wide association studies (GWAS) have identified several susceptibility loci associated with the risk of lung cancer.[82] Although these results might shed light on mechanisms of lung carcinogenesis and may lead to novel therapies, their implications in terms of prevention remain modest.

CONCLUSION

As the most important cancer epidemic of the 20th century, lung cancer will likely continue to be a major public health problem in the current century. Considerable efforts are being made in the public and private domains to develop more effective therapeutic approaches. However, given the poor prognosis of lung cancer and the lack of effective screening procedures, primary prevention remains the main weapon against this neoplasm, and control of tobacco smoking remains the key strategy for the prevention of lung cancer. In some populations, the decreased incidence of the disease can be attributable to reduced consumption of tobacco. Much, however, remains to be done, in particular among women and the young, as well as in developing countries. Reduction in exposure to occupational and environmental carcinogens (in particular indoor pollution and radon), and increase in consumption of fruits and vegetables are additional preventive opportunities.

REFERENCES

1. The GLOBOCAN 2008 database. [Available from: http://globocan.iarc.fr]
2. Travis WD, Lubin J, Ries L, Devesa S. United States lung carcinoma incidence trends: declining for most histologic types among males, increasing among females. Cancer 1996; 77: 2464–70.
3. Devesa SS, Bray F, Vizcaino AP, Parkin DM. International lung cancer trends by histologic type: male:female differences diminishing and adenocarcinoma rates rising. Int J Cancer 2005; 117: 294–9.
4. Tyczynski JE, Bray F, Parkin DM. Lung cancer in Europe in 2000: epidemiology, prevention, and early detection. Lancet Oncol 2003; 4: 45–55.
5. Toyoda Y, Nakayama T, Ioka A, Tsukuma H. Trends in lung cancer incidence by histological type in Osaka, Japan. Jpn J Clin Oncol 2008; 38: 534–9.
6. Surgeon General's 2004 Report: The Health Consequences of Smoking. Rockville, MD: US Department of Health and Human Services, 2004.
7. International Agency for Research on Cancer. IARC monographs on the evaluation of carcinogenic risks of chemicals to humans. Tobacco Smoke and Involuntary Smoking, Vol. 83. Lyon: IARC Press, 2004.
8. Mackay J, Jemal A, Lee NC, Parkin DM. The Cancer Atlas. Atlanta: American Cancer Society, 2006.
9. Peto R, Lopez AD, Boreham J, Thun M. Mortality from Smoking in Developed Countries 1950–2000, 2nd edn. Oxford: Oxford University Press. [Available from: www.ctsu.ox.ac.uk/~tobacco]
10. American Cancer Society. Global Cancer Facts & Figures, 2nd edn. Atlanta: American Cancer Society, 2011.
11. Parkin DM. International variation. Oncogene 2004; 23: 6329–40.
12. Jemal A, Center MM, DeSantis C, Ward EM. Global patterns of cancer incidence and mortality rates and trends. Cancer Epidemiol Biomarkers Prev 2010; 19: 1893–907.
13. Yang L, Parkin DM, Ferlay J, Li L, Chen Y. Estimates of cancer incidence in China for 2000 and projections for 2005. Cancer Epidemiol Biomarkers Prev 2005; 14: 243–50.
14. Chen WQ, Zheng RS, Zeng HM. Bayesian age-period-cohort prediction of lung cancer incidence in China. Thorac Cancer 2011; 2: 149–55.
15. Peto R, Lopez AD, Boreham J, Thun M, Heath C Jr. Mortality from Smoking in Developed Countries 1950–2000. Oxford: Oxford University Press, 1994.
16. Khuder SA. Effect of cigarette smoking on major histological types of lung cancer: a meta-analysis. Lung Cancer 2001; 31: 139–48.
17. Zang EA, Wynder EL. Differences in lung cancer risk between men and women: examination of the evidence. J Natl Cancer Inst 1996; 88: 183–92.
18. Henschke CI, Yip R, Miettinen OS. Women's susceptibility to tobacco carcinogens and survival after diagnosis of lung cancer. JAMA 2006; 296: 180–4.
19. Bain C, Feskanich D, Speizer FE, et al. Lung cancer rates in men and women with comparable histories of smoking. J Natl Cancer Inst 2004; 96: 826–34.
20. Freedman ND, Leitzmann MF, Hollenbeck AR, Schatzkin A, Abnet CC. Cigarette smoking and subsequent risk of lung cancer in men and women: analysis of a prospective cohort study. Lancet Oncol 2008; 9: 649–56.
21. Vollset SE, Tverdal A, Gjessing HK. Smoking and deaths between 40 and 70 years of age in women and men. Ann Intern Med 2006; 44: 381–9.
22. Prescott E, Osler M, Hein HO, et al. Gender and smoking-related risk of lung cancer. The Copenhagen Center for Prospective Population Studies. Epidemiology 1998; 9: 79–83.
23. Bach PB, Kattan MW, Thornquist MD, et al. Variations in lung cancer risk among smokers. J Natl Cancer Inst 2003; 95: 470–8.
24. Nordlund LA, Carstensen JM, Pershagen G. Are male and female smokers at equal risk of smoking-related cancer: evidence from a Swedish prospective study. Scand J Public Health 1999; 27: 56–62.
25. Thun MJ, Hannan LM, Adams-Campbell LL, et al. Lung cancer occurrence in never-smokers: an analysis of 13 cohorts and 22 cancer registry studies. PLoS Med 2008; 5: e185.

26. Thun MJ, Henley SJ, Calle EE. Tobacco use and cancer: an epidemiologic perspective for geneticists. Oncogene 2002; 21: 7307–25.
27. Fu JB, Kau TY, Severson RK, Kalemkerian GP. Lung cancer in women: analysis of the national Surveillance, Epidemiology, and End Results database. Chest 2005; 127: 768–77.
28. Wakelee HA, Chang ET, Gomez SL, et al. Lung cancer incidence in never smokers. J Clin Oncol 2007; 25: 472–8.
29. Thun MJ, Henley SJ, Burns D, et al. Lung cancer death rates in lifelong nonsmokers. J Natl Cancer Inst 2006; 98: 691–9.
30. Mountain CF. Revisions in the international system for staging lung cancer. Chest 1997; 111: 1710–17.
31. Manser RL, Irving LB, Stone C, et al. Screening for lung cancer. Cochrane Database Syst Rev 2004; 1: CD001991.
32. Oken MM, Hocking WG, Kvale PA, et al. Screening by chest radiograph and lung cancer mortality: the Prostate, Lung, Colorectal, and Ovarian (PLCO) randomized trial. JAMA 2011; 306: 1865–73.
33. Diederich S, Wormanns D, Heindel W. Low-dose CT: new tool for screening lung cancer? Eur Radiol 2001; 11: 1916–24.
34. Black C, Bagust A, Boland A, et al. The clinical effectiveness and cost-effectiveness of computed tomography screening for lung cancer: systematic reviews. Health Technol Assess 2006; 10: 1–90.
35. Aberle DR, Adams AM, Berg CD, et al. National Lung Screening Trial Research Team. Reduced lung-cancer mortality with low-dose computed tomographic screening. N Engl J Med 2011; 365: 395–409.
36. Infante M, Cavuto S, Lutman FR, et al. A randomized study of lung cancer screening with spiral computed tomography: three-year results from the DANTE trial. Am J Respir Crit Care Med 2009; 180: 445–53.
37. van Iersel CA, de Koning HJ, Draisma G, et al. Risk-based selection from the general population in a screening trial: selection criteria, recruitment and power for the Dutch-Belgian randomised lung cancer multi-slice CT screening trial (NELSON). Int J Cancer 2007; 120: 868–74.
38. American Cancer Society. Cancer Facts & Figures 2012. Atlanta: American Cancer Society, 2012.
39. Berrino F, De Angelis R, Sant M, et al. Survival for eight major cancers and all cancers combined for European adults diagnosed in 1995-99: results of the EUROCARE-4 study. Lancet Oncol 2007; 8: 773–83.
40. Brenner H, Hakulinen T. Up-to-date and precise estimates of cancer patient survival: Model based period analysis. Am J Epidemiol 2006; 164: 689–96.
41. Verdecchia A, Francisci S, Brenner H, et al. Recent cancer survival in Europe: a 2000–02 period analysis of EUROCARE-4 data. Lancet Oncol 2007; 8: 784–96.
42. Brenner H, Gondos A, Arndt V. Recent major progress in long-term cancer patient survival disclosed by modeled period analysis. J Clin Oncol 2007; 25: 3274–80.
43. Altekruse SF, Kosary CL, Krapcho M, et al. (eds). SEER Cancer Statistics Review, 1975–2007, National Cancer Institute. Bethesda, MD, based on November 2009 SEER data submission, posted to the SEER web site, 2010. [Available from: http://seer.cancer.gov/csr/1975_2007/] [database on the Internet].
44. International Agency for Research on Cancer. IARC mongraphs on the evaluation of the carcinogenic risk of chemicals to human. Tobacco Smoking, Vol. 86. Lyon: IARC Press, 1986.
45. Akl EA, Gaddam S, Gunukula SK, et al. The effects of waterpipe tobacco smoking on health outcomes: a systematic review. Int J Epidemiol 2010; 39: 834–57.
46. Pednekar MS, Gupta PC, Yeole BB, Hébert JR. Association of tobacco habits, including bidi smoking, with overall and site-specific cancer incidence: results from the Mumbai cohort study. Cancer Causes Control 2011; 22: 859–68.
47. Nakamura K, Huxley R, Ansary-Moghaddam A, Woodward M. The hazards and benefits associated with smoking and smoking cessation in Asia: a meta-analysis of prospective studies. Tob Control 2009; 18: 345–52.
48. Samet JM, Avila-Tang E, Boffetta P, et al. Lung cancer in never smokers: clinical epidemiology and environmental risk factors. Clin Cancer Res 2009; 15: 5626–45.
49. Boffetta P, Tredaniel J, Grecco A. Risk of childhood cancer and adult lung cancer after childhood exposure to passive smoke: A meta-analysis. Environ Health Perspect 2002; 108: 73–82.
50. International Agency for Research on Cancer. IARC handbooks of cancer prevention. Fruit and Vegetables, Vol. 8. Lyon: IARC Press, 2003.
51. World Cancer Research Fund/American Institute for Cancer Research. Food, Nutrition, Physical Activity, and the Prevention of Cancer: a Global Perspective. Washington, DC: AICR, 2007.
52. Lam TK, Gallicchio L, Lindsley K, et al. Cruciferous vegetable consumption and lung cancer risk: a systematic review. Cancer Epidemiol Biomarkers Prev 2009; 18: 184–95.
53. Gallicchio L, Boyd K, Matanoski G, et al. Carotenoids and the risk of developing lung cancer: a systematic review. Am J Clin Nutr 2008; 88: 372–83.
54. Albanes D, Heinonen OP, Taylor PR, et al. Alpha-tocopherol and beta-carotene supplements and lung cancer incidence in the alpha-tocopherol, beta-carotene cancer prevention study: effects of base-line characteristics and study compliance. J Natl Cancer Inst 1996; 88: 1560–70.
55. Omenn GS, Goodman GE, Thornquist MD, et al. Risk factors for lung cancer and for intervention effects in CARET, the Beta-Carotene and Retinol Efficacy Trial. J Natl Cancer Inst 1996; 88: 1550–9.
56. Wakai K, Nagata C, Mizoue T, et al. Alcohol drinking and lung cancer risk: an evaluation based on a systematic review of epidemiologic evidence among the Japanese population. Jpn J Clin Oncol 2007; 37: 168–74.

57. Li Y, Yang H, Cao J. Association between alcohol consumption and cancers in the Chinese population–a systematic review and meta-analysis. PLoS One 2011; 6: e18776.
58. Renehan AG, Soerjomataram I, Leitzmann MF. Interpreting the epidemiological evidence linking obesity and cancer: a framework for population-attributable risk estimations in Europe. Eur J Cancer 2010; 46: 2581–92.
59. Koh WP, Yuan JM, Wang R, Lee HP, Yu MC. Body mass index and smoking-related lung cancer risk in the Singapore Chinese Health Study. Br J Cancer 2010; 102: 610–14.
60. Yang L, Yang G, Zhou M, et al. Body mass index and mortality from lung cancer in smokers and nonsmokers: a nationally representative prospective study of 220,000 men in China. Int J Cancer 2009; 125: 2136–43.
61. Kabat GC, Kim M, Hunt JR, Chlebowski RT, Rohan TE. Body mass index and waist circumference in relation to lung cancer risk in the Women's Health Initiative. Am J Epidemiol 2008; 168: 158–69.
62. Leitzmann MF, Koebnick C, Abnet CC, et al. Prospective study of physical activity and lung cancer by histologic type in current, former, and never smokers. Am J Epidemiol 2009; 169: 542–53.
63. Emaus A, Thune I. Physical activity and lung cancer prevention. Recent Results Cancer Res 2011; 186: 101–33.
64. Kamp DW. Asbestos-induced lung disease:an update. Transl Res 2009; 153: 143–52.
65. International Agency for Research on Cancer. IARC monographs on the evaluation of carcinogenic risks to humans. Ionizing radiation, Part 1: X- and Gama (γ)-Radiation, and Neutrons. Vol. 75. Lyon: IARC Press, 2000.
66. Wakeford R. Radiation in the workplace-a review of studies of the risks of occupational exposure to ionising radiation. J Radiol Prot 2009; 29: A61–79.
67. International Agency for Research on Cancer. IARC monographs on the evaluation of carcinogenic risks to humans. Ionizing Radiation, Part 2: Some Internally Deposited Radionuclides. Vol. 78. Lyon: IARC Press, 2001.
68. Field RW. Environmental factors in cancer: radon. Rev Environ Health 2010; 25: 23–31.
69. Leuraud K, Schnelzer M, Tomasek L, et al. Radon, smoking and lung cancer risk: results of a joint analysis of three European case-control studies among uranium miners. Radiat Res 2011; 176: 375–87.
70. Schnelzer M, Hammer GP, Kreuzer M, Tschense A, Grosche B. Accounting for smoking in the radon-related lung cancer risk among German uranium miners: results of a nested case-control study. Health Phys 2010; 98: 20–8.
71. International Agency for Research on Cancer. IARC monographs on the evaluation of carcinogenic risks to humans. Household Use of Solid Fuels and High-Temperature Frying. Vol. 95. Lyon: IARC Press, 2010.
72. Field RW, Krewski D, Lubin JH, et al. An overview of the North American residential radon and lung cancer case-control studies. J Toxicol Environ Health 2006; 69: 599–631.
73. Gray A, Read S, McGale P, Darby S. Lung cancer deaths from indoor radon and the cost effectiveness and potential of policies to reduce them. BMIJ 2009; 338: a3110.
74. Darby S, Hill D, Auvinen A, et al. Radon in homes and risk of lung cancer: collaborative analysis of individual data from 13 European case-control studies. BMJ 2005; 330: 223.
75. Boffetta P. Human cancer from environmental pollutants: the epidemiological evidence. Mutat Res 2006; 608: 157–62.
76. Liang HY, Li XL, Yu XS, et al. Facts and fiction of the relationship between preexisting tuberculosis and lung cancer risk: a systematic review. Int J Cancer 2009; 125: 2936–44.
77. Wu CY, Hu HY, Pu CY, et al. Pulmonary tuberculosis increases the risk of lung cancer: a population-based cohort study. Cancer 2011; 117: 618–24.
78. Rezazadeh A, Laber DA, Ghim SJ, Jenson AB, Kloecker G. The role of human papilloma virus in lung cancer: a review of the evidence. Am J Med Sci 2009; 338: 64–7.
79. Gauderman WJ, Morrison JL, Carpenter CL, Thomas DC. Analysis of gene-smoking interaction in lung cancer. Genet Epidemiol 1997; 14: 199–214.
80. Bailey-Wilson JE, Amos CI, Pinney SM, et al. A major lung cancer susceptibility locus maps to chromosome 6q23-25. Am J Hum Genet 2004; 75: 460–74.
81. Spitz MR, Wu X, Wilkinson A, Wei Q. Cancer of the lung. In: Schottenfeld J, ed. Cancer Epidemiology and Prevention, 3rd edn. New York: Oxford University Press; 2006.
82. Brennan P, Hainaut P, Boffetta P. Genetics of lung-cancer susceptibility. Lancet Oncol 2011; 12: 399–408.

2 | Prevention, early detection and screening

Giulia Veronesi

LUNG CANCER CHEMOPREVENTION

Numerous methods are available to help people to stop smoking. However smoking cessation programs have rather low success rates, and half of all lung cancers occur in people who have stopped smoking. Attention has therefore turned to chemoprevention as one potential means of reducing lung cancer incidence. According to field cancerization and multi-step carcinogenesis concepts, in at-risk individuals, the entire broncho-alveolar epithelium is continuously exposed to inhaled carcinogens. A chemopreventive agent is able to reverse, suppress or prevent the malignant transformation induced by carcinogens. Since chemoprevention has had some success in breast and prostate cancer, it is fast emerging as an area of research in lung cancer, and the hunt is still on for active compounds with a favorable toxicity profile that can be administered to persons who are at high risk of developing the disease. A number of compounds have been tested, but results so far have been disappointing: Beta-carotene and retinoids have even proven detrimental.[1] The paper by Omenn[2] comprehensively reviews past and ongoing lung caner chemoprevention trials.

Based on Omenn's data, the American College of Chest Physicians 2007 guidelines state that for individuals with a family history of the disease or individuals at risk for lung cancer, there are insufficient data to help recommend the use of any agent alone or in combination for primary, secondary, or tertiary chemoprevention outside the setting of a well-designed clinical trial.[3] However some interesting studies have been published more recently. One study examined effects of inhaled corticosteroids on lung cancer incidence in patients with chronic obstructive pulmonary disease (COPD).[4] Compared to controls, those receiving high-dose corticosteroids (>1,200 µg/day triamcinolone equivalents, n = 219) had reduced lung cancer risk (hazard ratio 0.39, 95% confidence interval 0.16–0.96). The limitations of the study were the relatively small number of subjects and incident lung cancer cases, and lack of confirmation of COPD diagnosis and of lung cancer histopathology.[5] A recent meta-analysis[6] of seven randomized trials analyzed the effect of inhaled corticosteroids on all-cause mortality in COPD patients treated for at least a year.[6] It was found that these agents significantly reduced all-cause mortality in COPD, but further studies were recommended to determine whether the benefits persisted beyond 2–3 years.

Van den Berg et al. investigated the effect of fluticasone (500 µg twice daily) on the number of pulmonary nodules detected on a single slice CT scan of the chest.[7] Compared to the placebo group, more nodules resolved and fewer had new nodules in the fluticasone group, although differences were not significant. Lam et al.[8] performed a randomized trial to investigate the effect of inhaled budesonide (800 mg twice daily) in people with bronchoscopy-identified bronchial dysplasia and peripheral lung nodules detected on low-dose CT (LDCT). Although there was no significant difference between the treated and the placebo arm for regression of bronchial dysplasia, a significant reduction of peripheral lung nodules was found in the treated arm. This preliminary finding was not confirmed in the second randomized trial performed by our group,[9] whose primary endpoint was the effect of inhaled budesonide on peripheral lung nodules. The trial, nested within a low-dose CT screening study, randomized 202 subjects with CT-detected peripheral lung nodules over 4 mm to receive either inhaled budesonide (800 mg twice daily) or placebo for a year. A trend toward regression of non-solid nodules after budesonide treatment was observed, but the effect was not significant.

Recent studies on selective cyclooxygenase-2 (COX-2) inhibitors as chemopreventive agents for lung cancer have also produced interesting findings.[10,11] In a case-control study, use of any selective COX-2 inhibitor for over a year resulted in a significant (60%) reduction in lung cancer risk (overall adjusted odds ratio 0.40; 95% CI, 0.19–0.81). Significant reductions of similar magnitude were also found for the non-selective COX-2 inhibitors, aspirin (325 mg) and ibuprofen (200 mg), taken at least three times a week. Low-dose aspirin (81 mg/day) produced a small risk reduction that did not reach significance, but acetaminophen (paracetamol)—without COX-2 activity—had no influence on risk. These results suggest COX-2 involvement in lung carcinogenesis, and show that COX-2 inhibitors hold promise as chemopreventive agents against lung cancer; however, further studies are required to find the most appropriate dose and intake frequency as well as duration of treatment. The same group also found 55%, 71%, 70%, and 79% reductions in the risk for prostate, breast, colon, and lung cancer, respectively, using COX-2 inhibitors.[11]

Mao et al.[12] conducted a randomized, double-blind, placebo-controlled trial of the selective COX-2 inhibitor, celecoxib (400 mg twice daily for six months), in former-smokers with no evidence of major cardiovascular, renal or hepatic abnormalities. Bronchial Ki-67 labeling index was the primary endpoint. The study found that celecoxib has a beneficial effect (P = 0.0006) on Ki-67 in a mixed-effects analysis, and that celecoxib significantly (P = 0.04, t-test) reduced Ki-67 by an average of 34%, whereas placebo increased Ki-67 by an average of 3.8%. The decrease in Ki-67 correlated with a reduction or resolution of lung nodules on CT. Celecoxib significantly reduced C-reactive protein and also interleukin-6 mRNA and protein levels in plasma, and increased 15(S)-hydroxy-eicosatetraenoic acid levels in bronchoalveolar lavage samples.

The results of a meta-analysis of randomized studies on the use of aspirin were published recently.[13] It concluded that daily dose of aspirin reduced deaths for several common cancers; that the benefit increased with treatment duration and was consistent across different study populations.

An interesting paper from Altorky et al.[14] investigated the use of the angiogenesis inhibitor pazotinib is a window-of-opportunity trial in lung cancer. The drug was given for 2–6 weeks preoperatively to non-small cell lung cancer (NSCLC) patients scheduled for surgical resection. A significant reduction in tumor size, documented by high-resolution CT, occurred in 30 of the 35 patients enrolled. The drug was fairly well-tolerated and was shown to dysregulate several target genes.

BIOMARKERS IN EARLY DETECTION

Biomarkers for lung cancer have several potential uses including risk stratification, detection of early disease, prognosis, prediction of treatment response, monitoring of response, and monitoring of recurrence. A simple test able to detect early lung cancer could, for example, be used as a first-line screening tool to select limited number of persons for further diagnostic investigation by low dose CT. Such a test would encourage the widespread implementation of lung cancer screening, as it has the potential to simplify participant recruitment, reduce the number of participants undergoing further diagnostic (including invasive) examinations, and thereby increase compliance and reduce costs compared to first-line low dose CT screening. Fairly recent advances in the identification and validation of biomarkers for lung cancer have been surveyed in the 2007 review by Greenberg and Lee.[15]

A growing number of reports describe a humoural immune response to lung cancer in the form of auto-antibodies against tumor-associated antigens (TAA).[16] Such autoantibodies can be detected a number of years before the appearance of clinical symptoms. Although it is possible to assay autoantibodies against a single TAA, sensitivity is low and the technique appears most promising when several autoantibodies are assayed together. Thus, when a panel of seven antibodies was employed on plasma from 82 NSCL cases, 22 small cell cases, and 50 controls, at least one raised antibody titer was found in 76% of all cases, with specificity 92%. Similar results were obtained when markers obtained from a training set were applied to 102 samples (cases and risk-matched controls) from the Mayo Clinic CT Screening trial. The five most predictive markers correctly predicted all six prevalence cancers, 32 of 40 cancers from samples taken 1–5 years before screening detection, and 49 of 56 risk-matched controls.[17]

Several studies have used proteomic methods to discover new lung cancer biomarkers.[18–20] Some of these were detected in plasma years before lung cancer deaths suggesting a relation to the early development of lung cancer.[20] Proteomic analysis has even been performed on exhaled breath condensate, although it is unclear whether condensate contains enough proteins to create profiles that differ significantly from those of normal controls, or those with other lung diseases.[21] Limitations of these studies are lack of reproducibility, small size, and lack of between-study consistency in choice of controls.

Another approach is to identify DNA hypermethylation markers of lung cancer in sputum. DNA hypermethylation is an important mechanism for inactivating tumor suppressor genes.[22] Tsou et al. identified 22 loci in squamous cell lung cancers with significantly higher DNA methylation levels than adjacent non-tumor lung. Of these, eight were significantly more hypermethylated; this eight-locus panel showed sensitivity and specificity of 95.6%.[22]

Malignancy associated changes (MAC) in the chromatin distribution within cell nuclei can be identified by DNA cytometry. This technique has been used to detect cervical, colon, breast, and lung cancers. In one study[23] automated sputum cytometry was performed on 1,235 high risk persons, 370 of whom had lung cancer. Conventional cytology detected 16% of the cancers with 99% specificity; automated sputum cytometry detected 40% of the cancers with 91% specificity. Automated sputum cytometry is more sensitive than

The NELSON trial adopted volume: Nodules less than 50 mm^3 (4.6 mm diameter) were considered negative, those above 500 mm^3 (>9.8 mm diameter) were positive, and those in the 50–500 mm range were indeterminate.[65] Indeterminate nodules underwent repeat LDCT at three months, and volume doubling times were used to direct nodules to either further investigation or just follow-up. Using this two-step approach, 2.6% of baseline NELSON scans were positive, and a fairly high proportion of positive scans turned out to be lung cancer.

However ground glass nodules pose unique assessment problems, as volume growth may be subtle. A 2011 publication by a Danish group proposed that the best predictor of malignancy was a combination of VDT and PET findings.[66]

For the COSMOS study[59,67], we set up a standardized diagnostic protocol which was modified over time as we gained experience (Fig. 2.2). At the end of five years we had high overall compliance (82%) even though 8% underwent further examinations after screening CT—lower than in other non-randomized studies,[44,47] and lower also than the NLST, where 24% of the CT arm were recalled for further investigations.[60] Overall 34 of COSMOS participants (15% of those with suspicious lung nodules) underwent surgical or CT-guided biopsy for benign disease over the five study years. To put this in perspective, the proportion was higher among those receiving standard surgical practice in the Division running COSMOS (Fig. 2.3).

A total of 16 COSMOS cases were missed at one CT scan and picked up a year later (Fig. 2.4). Most of these were central lesions for which the LDCT scan has a recognized limitation; others had a very high growth rate (usually NSCLC) or were below the threshold size in the previous year. Some delayed diagnoses were due to human failure as they were not recognized by the radiologists. Ten percent of diagnoses were reported as delayed by NY-ELCAP[68], a proportion closely similar to that of COSMOS.

CT-PET may be useful for the further investigation of uncertain nodules detected at screening, particularly when they are solid and 10 mm or more in diameter (Fig. 2.2). In the COSMOS study, 157 subjects underwent CT-PET, 66 of whom underwent surgical biopsy. Of the 58 lung cancers found on surgical biopsy, 51 were PET positive (standard uptake value >2.0) and 7 were negative. Sensitivity was 88% overall, and 100% in those with solid nodules of 10 mm or more. Among the eight patients with benign disease at surgical biopsy, CT-PET was positive in six and negative in two. We suggested that CT-PET was a promising alternative to invasive procedures for the further investigation of uncertain nodules in the screening setting and that the standard uptake value threshold for positivity could usefully be lowered to >1.5 for nodules <10 mm. However, in our experience of CT-PET for nodules detected after baseline, sensitivity was much lower, in relation to the increased proportions of small size lesions and ground glass nodules, and the utility of CT-PET was called into question (unpublished work).[67]

The IASLC Screening Workshop[69] guidelines suggest CT-guided biopsy for suspicious nodules, not least because in many cases it facilitates the surgical decision process. The NY-ELCAP group reported good diagnostic performance for CT-guided biopsy (sensitivity 82%; diagnostic accuracy 88% overall) although results were less good for nodules <8 mm.[68] However it must not be forgotten that the results of CT-guided biopsy are highly operator dependent, and other techniques, such as endobronchial ultrasound (EBUS),

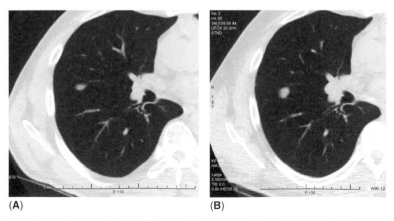

(A)   **(B)**

Figure 2.3 The picture shows a false positive screening case. The low dose CT scans (Computed Tomography) of this patient show a nodule of the right upper lobe that increased in size after one-year follow-up. The patient was submitted to surgical biopsy and a benign parenchimal lymph node was diagnosed.

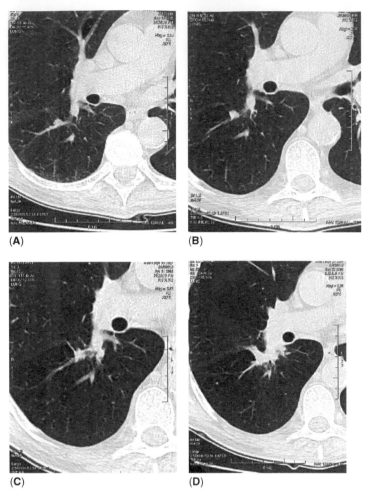

Figure 2.4 A case of delayed diagnosis in which a centrally located lung nodule in the right lower lobe was diagnosed as malignant after four CT scans (Computed Tomography) performed over a period of 16 months. A negative PET (Positron Emission Tomography) scan was done after the first two CT scans and favored the misdiagnosis of the cancer. The final stage was T2N1M0, the patient was operated with favorable outcome and long survival.

electromagnetic navigation (EMN), and minimally invasive surgical biopsy should be developed as alternatives to increase diagnostic yield of screening-detected lesions.

Treatment of Screening-Detected Cancers

The IASLC recommends that surgeons play an active role in defining diagnostic and treatment protocols for screening-detected cancers.[69] In view of the possibility of high rates of false positives in the screening setting, the IASLC urged maximum effort to limit inappropriate surgical interventions,[69] and strongly recommended that surgery be performed in centers that make full use of minimally invasive surgical procedures such as VATS and robotic surgical systems (Fig. 2.5).

The normal surgical approach to removing suspicious nodules for diagnosis should be a minimally invasive wedge resection, but the exact approach depends on the location and size of the lesion. For lesions below 10 mm or ground glass opacity lesions, a localization technique may be necessary. Preoperative CT-guided injection of radiolabeled particles and intraoperative use of a gamma ray detecting probe seems particularly effective.[70] More traditional options include marking with methylene blue, wire hooks, and metallic coils.

As regards treatment, anatomical resection by minimally invasive lobectomy with systematic lymph node dissection is the standard procedure. For small (<2 cm) peripheral lung cancers, more limited surgical approaches are being investigated in two ongoing randomized clinical trials: the U.S. CALBG trial revealed the presence of some barriers to the successful implementation of mass screening, especially in current smokers; however, the population surveyed was not a representative sample of the population (47% of eligible subjects declined to participate).

REFERENCES

1. Blumberg J, Block G. The Alpha-Tocopherol, Beta- Carotene Cancer Prevention Study in Finland. Nutr Rev 1994; 52: 242–5.
2. Omenn GS. Chemoprevention of lung caners: lessons from CARET, the beta-carotene and retinol efficacy trial, and prospects for the future. Eur J Cancer Prev 2007; 16: 184–91.
3. Gray J, Mao JT, Kelley M, Kurie J, Bepler G. Lung cancer chemoprevention: ACCP evidence-based clinical practice guidelines. 2nd edn. Chest 2007; 132: 56–8.
4. Parimon T, Chien JW, Bryson CL, et al. Inhaled corticosteroids and risk of lung cancer among patients with chronic obstructive pulmonary disease. Am J Respir Crit Care Med 2007; 175: 712–19.
5. Miller YE, Keith RL. Inhaled corticosteroids and lung cancer chemoprevention. Am J Respir Crit Care Med 2007; 175: 636–7.
6. Sin DD, Wu L, Anderson JA, et al. Inhaled corticosteroids and mortality in chronic obstructive pulmonary disease. Thorax 2005; 60: 992–7.
7. van den Berg RM, Teertstra HJ, van Zandwijk N, et al. CT detected indeterminate pulmonary nodules in a chemo-prevention trial of fluticasone. Lung Cancer 2008; 60: 57–61.
8. Lam S, leRiche JC, McWilliams A, et al. A randomized phase IIb trial of pulmicort turbuhaler (budesonide) in people with dysplasia of the bronchial epithelium. Clin Cancer Res 2004; 10: 6502–11.
9. Veronesi G, Szabo E, Decensi A, et al. Randomized phase II trial of inhaled budesonide versus placebo in high-risk individuals with CT screen-detected lung nodules. Cancer Prev Res (Phila) 2011; 4: 34–42.
10. Harris RE, Beebe-Donk J, Alshafie GA. Reduced risk of human lung cancer by selective cyclooxygenase 2 (COX-2) blockade; results of a case control study. Int J Biol Sci 2007; 3: 328–34.
11. Harris RE, Beebe-Donk J, Alshafie GA. Cancer chemoprevention by cyclooxygenase 2 (COX-2) blockade: results from case control studies. Subcell Biochem 2007; 42: 193–212.
12. Mao JT, Roth MD, Fishbein MC, et al. Lung cancer chemoprevention with celecoxib in former smokers. Cancer Prev Res (Phila) 2011; 4: 984–93.
13. Rothwell PM, Fowkes FG, Belch JF, et al. Effect of daily aspirin on long-term risk of death due to cancer: analysis of individual patient data from randomised trials. Lancet 2011; 377: 31–41; 2011; 4: 984–93.
14. Altorki N, Lane ME, Bauer T, et al. Phase II proof-of-concept study of pazopanib monotherapy in treatment-naive patients with stage I/II resectable non-small-cell lung cancer. Clin Oncol 2010; 28: 3131–7.
15. Greenberg AK, Lee MS. Biomarkers for lung cancer: clinical uses. Curr Opin Pulm Med 2007; 13: 249–55.
16. Chapman CJ, Murray A, McElveen JE, et al. Autoantibodies in lung cancer-possibilities for early detection and subsequent cure. Thorax 2008; 63: 228–33.
17. Zhong L, Coe SP, Stromberg AJ, et al. Profiling tumor-associated antibodies for early detection of non-small cell lung cancer. J Thorac Oncol 2006; 1: 513–19.
18. Bharti A, Ma PC, Sigia R. Biomarker discovery in lung cancer–promises and challenges of clinical proteomics. Mass Spectrom Rev 2007; 26: 451–66.
19. Ostroff RM, Bigbee WL, Franklin W, et al. Unlocking biomarker discovery: large scale application of aptamer proteomic technology for early detection of lung cancer. PLoS One 2010; 5: e15003.
20. Massion PP, Caprioli RM. Proteomic strategies for the characterization and the early detection of lung cancer. J Thorac Oncol 2006; 1: 1027–39.
21. Conrad DH, Goyette J, Thomas PS. Proteomics as a method for early detection of cancer: a review of proteomics, exhaled breath condensate and lung cancer screening. J Gen Intern Med 2007; 23: 78–84.
22. Tsou JA, Galler JS, Siegmund KD, et al. Identification of a panel of sensitive and specific DNA methylation markers for lung cancer. Mol Cancer 2007; 6: 70–83.
23. Kemp RA, Reinders DM, Turic B. Detection of lung cancer by automated sputum cytometry. J Thorac Oncol 2007; 2: 993–1000.
24. Li R, Todd NW, Qui Q, et al. Genetic deletions in sputum as diagnostic markers for early detection of stage I non-small cell lung cancer. Clin Cancer Res 2007; 13: 482–7.
25. Yendamuri S, Kratzke R. MicroRNA biomarkers in lung cancer: MiRacle or quagMiRe? Transl Res 2011; 157: 209–15.
26. Krol J, Loedige I, Filipowicz W. The widespread regulation of microRNA biogenesis, function and decay. Nat Rev Genetics 2010; 11: 597.
27. Schwarzenbach H, Hoon DS, Pantel K. Cell-free nucleic acids as biomarkers in cancer patients. Nature Rev Cancer 2011; 11: 426.
28. Boeri M, Verri C, Conte D, et al. MicroRNA signatures in tissues and plasma predict development and prognosis of computed tomography detected lung cancer. Proc Natl Acad Sci USA 2011; 108: 3713–18.
29. Bianchi F, Nicassio F, Marzi M, et al. A serum circulating miRNA diagnostic test to identify asymptomatic high-risk individuals with early stage lung cancer. EMBO Mol Med 2011; 3: 495.

30. Jemal A, Bray F, Center MM, et al. Global cancer statistics. CA Cancer J Clin 2011; 61: 69–90.
31. NCI: SEER Cancer Statistics Review, 1996–2002.
32. Mountain CF. Revisions in the international system for staging lung cancer. Chest 1997; 111: 1710–17.
33. Alberg AJ, Samet JM. Epidemiology of lung cancer. Chest 2003; 123: 21–49.
34. Tockman M. Survival and mortality from lung cancer in a screened population: the John Hopkins study. Chest 1986; 89: 325s.
35. Fontana RS, Sanderson DR, Taylor WF, et al. Early lung cancer detection: results of the initial (prevalence) radiologic and cytologic screening in the Mayo Clinic study. Am Rev Respir Dis 1984; 130: 561–5.
36. Melamed MR, Flehinger BJ, Zaman MB, et al. Screening for early lung cancer. Results of the Memorial Sloan-Kettering study in New York. Chest 1984; 86: 44–53.
37. Fontana RS, Sanderson DR, Woolner LB, et al. Screening for lung cancer. A critique of the Mayo Lung Project. Cancer 1991; 67(4 Suppl): 1155–64.
38. Sobue T, Suzuki T, Naruke T. A case-control study for evaluating lung-cancer screening in Japan. Japanese Lung-Cancer-Screening Research Group. Int J Cancer 1992; 50: 230–7.
39. Flehinger BJ, Kimmel M, Melamed MR. The effect of surgical treatment on survival from early lung cancer. Implications for screening. Chest 1992; 101: 1013–18.
40. Belloni E, Veronesi G, Micucci C, et al. Genomic characterization of asymtpomatic CT-detected lung cancers. Oncogene 2010; 30: 1117–26.
41. Bianchi F, Hu J, Pelosi G, et al. Lung cancers detected by screening with spiral computed tomography have a malignant phenotype when analyzed by cDNA microarray. Clin Cancer Res 2004; 10(18 Pt 1): 6023–8.
42. Henschke CI, McCauley DI, Yankelevitz DF, et al. Early Lung Cancer Action Project: overall design and findings from baseline screening. Lancet 1999; 354: 99–105.
43. Diederich S, Thomas M, Semik M. Screening for early lung cancer with low dose spiral computed tomography: results of annual follow-up examinations in asymptomatic smokers. Eur Radiol 2004; 14: 691–702.
44. Sone S, Li F, Yang ZG, et al. Characteristics of small lung cancers invisible on conventional chest radiography and detected by population screening using spiral CT. Br J Radiol 2000; 73: 137–45.
45. Sone S, Nakayama T, Honda T, et al. Long-term follow-up study of a population-based 1996–1998 mass screening programme for lung cancer using mobile low-dose spiral computed tomography. Lung Cancer 2007; 58: 329–41.
46. Swensen SJ, Jett JR, Hartman TE, et al. Lung cancer screening with CT: Mayo clinic experience. Radiology 2003; 226: 756–61.
47. Henschke CI; for the International Early Lung Cancer Action Program Investigators. Survival of patients with clinical stage I lung cancer diagnosed by computed tomography screening for lung cancer. N Engl J Med 2006; 355: 1763–71.
48. Carter D, Vazquez M, Flieder DB, et al. Comparison of pathologic findings of baseline and annual repeat cancers diagnosed on CT screening. Lung Cancer 2007; 56: 193–9.
49. Sone S, Nakayama T, Honda T, et al. Long-term follow-up study of a population-based 1996–1998 mass screening programme for lung cancer using mobile low-dose spiral computed tomography. Lung Cancer 2007; 58: 329–41.
50. Bach PB, Jett JR, Pastorino U, et al. Computed tomography screening and lung cancer outcomes. JAMA 2007; 297: 953–61.
51. Spaggiari L, Veronesi G, Bellomi M, et al. Computed tomography screening for lung cancer. JAMA 2007; 298: 514.
52. Jett JR. Does CT screening reduce Lung Cancer Mortality? Controversies Around Cancer Screening, Special Session, 2008 ASCO Annual Meeting. [Available from: http://www.asco.org/ascov2/MultiMedia/Virtual+Meeting?&vmview=vm_session_presentations_view&confID=55&sessionID=2485]
53. McMahon PM, Kong CY, Johnson BE, et al. Estimating Long-term Effectiveness of Lung Cancer Screening in the Mayo CT Screening Study. Radiology 2008; 248: 278–87.
54. Chien CR, Chen TH. Mean sojourn time and effectiveness of mortality reduction for lung cancer screening with computed tomography. Int J Cancer 2008; 122: 2594–9.
55. Veronesi G, Maisonneuve P, Spaggiari L, et al. Long-term outcomes of a pilot CT screening for lung cancer. Ecancermedicalscience 2010; 4: 186.
56. Henschke CI, Boffetta P, Gorlova O, et al. Assessment of lung-cancer mortality reduction from CT Screening. Lung Cancer 2011; 71: 328–32.
57. Infante M, Cavuto S, Lutman FR, et al. A randomized study of lung cancer screening with spiral computed tomography: three-year results from the DANTE trial. Am J Respir Crit Care Med 2009; 1805: 445–53.
58. Veronesi G, Maisonneuve P, De Pas TM, et al. Does lung cancer screening with LDCT remain promising despite disappointing DANTE results? Am J Respir Crit Care Med 2010; 18: 720–1.
59. Veronesi G, Bellomi M, Mulshine JL, et al. Lung cancer screening with low-dose computed tomography: a non-invasive diagnostic protocol for baseline lung nodules. Lung Cancer 2008; 61: 340–9.
60. National Lung Screening Trial Research Team. Aberle DR, Adams AM, Berg CD, et al. Reduced lung-cancer mortality with low-dose computed tomographic screening. N Engl J Med 2011; 365: 395–409.
61. Swensen SJ, Jett JR, Hartman TE, et al. CT screening for lung cancer: five-year prospective experience. Radiology 2005; 235: 259–65.
62. Henschke CI, Yankelevitz DF, Naidich DP, et al. CT screening for lung cancer: suspiciousness of nodules according to size on baseline scans. Radiology 2004; 231: 164–8.

63. MacMahon H, Austin JHM, Gamsu G, et al. Guidelines for management of small pulmonary nodules detected on CT scans: a statement from the Fleischner Society. Radiology 2005; 237: 395–400.
64. Bellomi M, Veronesi G, Rampinelli C, et al. Evolution of lung nodules < or =5 mm detected with LDCT in asymptomatic smokers. Br J Radiol 2007; 80: 708–12.
65. van Klaveren RJ, Oudkerk M, Prokop M, et al. Management of lung nodules detected by volume CT scanning. N Engl J Med 2009; 361: 2221–9.
66. Ashraf H, Dirksen A, Loft A, et al. Combined use of positron emission tomography and volume doubling time in lung cancer screening with LDCT scanning. Thorax 2011; 66: 315–19.
67. Veronesi G, Bellomi M, Veronesi U. Role of positron emission tomography scanning in the management of lung nodules detected at baseline computed tomography screening. Ann Thorac Surg 2007; 84: 959–66.
68. New York Early Lung Cancer Action Project Investigators. CT screening for lung cancer: diagnoses resulting from the New York Lung Cancer Action project. Radiology 2007; 243: 239–49.
69. Field JK, Smith RA, Aberle DR, et al. International Association for the Study of Lung Cancer Computed Tomography Screening Workshop 2011 report. J Thorac Oncol 2012; 7: 10–19.
70. Bellomi M, Veronesi G, Trifirò G, et al. Computed tomography-guided preoperative radiotracer localization of non-palpable lung nodules. Ann Thorac Surg 2010; 90: 1759–64.
71. Nakamura K, Saji H, Nakajima R, et al. Phase III randomised trial of lobectomy versus limited resection for small size peripheral NSCLC (JCOG0802/WJOG4607L). JJCO 2010; 40: 271–4.
72. Veronesi G, Maisonneuve P, Pelosi G, et al. Screening-detected lung cancers: is systematic nodal dissection always essential? J Thorac Oncol 2011; 6: 525–30.
73. Van de Wiel JC, Wang Y, Xu DM, et al. Neglectable benefit of searching for incidental findings in the Dutch-Belgian lung cancer screening trial (NELSON) using low-dose multidetector CT. Eur Radiol 2007; 17: 1474–82.
74. Rampinelli C, Preda L, Maniglio M, et al. Extrapulmonary malignancies detected at lung cancer screening. Radiology 2011; 261: 293–9.
75. Cronin KA, Gail MH, Zou Z, et al. Validation of a model of lung cancer risk prediction among smokers. J Natl Cancer Inst 2006; 98: 637–40.
76. Spitz MR, Etzel CJ, Dong Q, et al. An expanded risk prediction model of lung cancer. Cancer Prev Res 2008; 1: 250–4.
77. Cassidy A, Myles JP, van Tongeren M, et al. The LLP risk model: an individual risk prediction model for lung cancer. Br J Cancer 2008; 98: 270–6.
78. Maisonneuve P, Bagnardi V, Bellomi M, et al. Lung cancer risk prediction to select smokers for screening CT–a model based on the Italian COSMOS trial. Cancer Prev Res (Phila) 2011; 4: 1778–89.
79. Brenner DJ, Hall EJ. Computed tomography - an increasing source of radiation exposure. N Engl J Med 2007; 357: 2277–84.
80. Berrington de González A, Kim KP, Berg CD. Low-dose lung computed tomography screening before age 55: estimates of the mortality reduction required to outweigh the radiation-induced cancer risk. J Med Screen 2008; 15: 153–8.
81. Ashraf H, Tønnesen P, Holst Pedersen J, et al. Effect of CT screening on smoking habits at 1-year follow-up in the Danish Lung Cancer Screening Trial (DLCST). Thorax 2009; 64: 388–92.
82. Silvestri GA, Nietert PJ, Zoller J, et al. Attitudes towards screening for lung cancer among smokers and their non-smoking counterparts. Thorax 2007; 62: 126–30.
83. McMahon PM, Kong CY, Bouzan C, et al. Cost-effectiveness of computed tomography screening for lung cancer in the United States. J Thorac Oncol 2011; 6: 1841–8.

3 | Staging

Christophe Dooms

INTRODUCTION

Clinical TNM staging comprises accurate assessment of the extent of the primary tumor (T), the spread to locoregional lymph nodes (N), and the presence or absence of distant metastases (M), and is based on evidence acquired before treatment. The clinical TNM stage (or cTNM) is essential to select and evaluate treatment. Patients with distant metastasis (advanced stage), or stage IV, will be treated with cytotoxic and/or targeted agents. Patients with metastatic mediastinal lymph nodes, or stage III, will usually have a combined modality therapy including a systemic (chemotherapy) and locoregional (surgery and/or radiotherapy) component. Patients without metastatic lymph nodes or with hilar metastatic lymph nodes only (early stages I and II) are—also depending on their cardiopulmonary and general medical condition—candidates for upfront surgical resection often followed by postoperative chemotherapy. As such, the TNM stage determines the choice of treatment, and is also the most important prognostic factor in non-small cell lung cancer (NSCLC) to date. Staging nowadays is a truly multidisciplinary process—involving physical examination, imaging techniques, endoscopic techniques, and surgical techniques—to determine the most accurate clinical TNM stage.

THE MOST RECENT TNM STAGING SYSTEM (VERSION 7, TNM7)

The previous TNM, published in 1997, was based on a rather small (n = 5319) dataset of predominantly surgical patients treated in the era before the advent of combined modality therapy.[1] Many of these deficiencies are addressed in TNM7, which was based on a major effort by the Lung Cancer Staging Project of the International Association for the Study of Lung Cancer (IASLC).[2] Adequate data were sampled on 67,725 cases of NSCLC treated by all modalities between 1990 and 2000.[3] These recommendations were the basis for the now universally adopted TNM7.

In relation to early stage NSCLC, the changes are a reclassification of the T-factor according to size of the primary tumor[4]: T1 (<3 cm) is split into T1a (<2 cm) and T1b (2–3 cm), T2 is split into T2a (3–5 cm) and T2b (5–7 cm), and tumors larger than 7 cm are T3 now. Moreover, additional pulmonary nodules are reclassified as T3 (same lobe), T4 (other lobe same side), or M1a (other lung). Malignant pleural and/or pericardial effusions and/or nodules are reclassified as M1a. N-factors didn't change,[5] although a new lymph node map—solving the former discrepancies between the Western and Japanese maps—has been adopted (Fig. 3.1).[6] All distant metastases are reclassified as M1b. It is important to document all of the sites of (potential) distant metastatic disease and whether the metastases at each site are solitary or multiple. There is a change in the labeling of early stages (Table 3.1): T2bN0 cases move from stage IB to stage IIA, T2a N1 cases from stage IIB to stage IIA. Patients with tumors >7 cm move from IB to IIB if there are no lymph node metastases, and from IIB to IIIA if they have N1. Non-N3 patients with an additional nodule in the same lobe move from stage IIIB to stage IIIA if they have N1-2 and to stage IIB if they have N0. Patients with T3 (invasion) N1 move from IB to IIIA. There is also a change in the labeling of (locally) advanced stages (Table 3.1): T4 (extension) N0-1 cases move from stage IIIB to stage IIIA, and T4 (ipsilateral lung) N0-1 and N2-3, respectively, moves from stage IV to stage IIIA and stage IIIB. Finally, cases with malignant pleural or pericardial fluid or nodules moved from stage IIIB to stage IV.

IMAGING TECHNIQUES
Computed Tomography

Modern spiral contrast-enhanced multi-detector computed tomography (CT) offers great anatomic detail, and is the gold standard to assess the extent of the primary tumor (T-factor), e.g., anatomical extent or relationship of the tumor to the fissures (which may determine the type of resection), to mediastinal structures (which may determine resectability), or to the pleura and chest wall. Current generation multi-detector CT enables shorter acquisition time, less respiratory and cardiac artifacts, and improved image resolution. In addition, multiplanar reformatting from axial to coronal and sagittal images might allow a more accurate assessment of tumor extension or invasion into adjacent structures, but one should always be careful to lymph nodes on CT with a prevalence of malignant N2/3 disease of 68%.[31] A major drawback is that these non-randomized endosonography series sampled a mean of 1 to 1.8 mediastinal lymph nodes per patient, instead of a minimal requirement of at least three mediastinal nodal stations as stated in the ESTS guidelines.[32] Limited mediastinal sampling of two stations or less has the potential to understage patients. Block et al. demonstrated that the use of EBUS-TBNA alone to stage the mediastinum sampled ≥3 mediastinal nodal stations in 65% of patients.[33] Another important consideration is that EBUS-TBNA—just as EUS-FNA—has a suboptimal negative predictive value ranging from 70% to 80%, which requires a confirmatory surgical staging procedure in case of a non-malignant echo-endoscopic needle aspiration of a suspicious mediastinal lymph node.[34–36] No false positive mediastinal lymph node findings by EBUS-TBNA have been reported in the literature, and all but two authors reported no false positive needle aspirations for EUS-FNA.[34,37] A false positive finding can occur in case of (1) misclassification of activated/enlarged lymphocytes as suspicious epithelial cells by the cytopathologist, or (2) sampling of primary tumor tissue or hilar node in station 10R or 10L which is considered a mediastinal lymph node (N2 disease) by the endoscopist (Fig. 3.3).[34,37]

Randomized controlled data are needed in order to further evaluate the value of combined endosonography in terms of its NPV and its capability to adhere to the minimal requirements for mediastinal nodal mapping. So far only one large-scale randomized controlled clinical trial (ASTER trial) comparing surgical staging (mainly mediastinoscopy) to a combined endosonography for mediastinal staging of operable NSCLC has been published, while others are awaited.[38,39] ASTER demonstrated sensitivities for mediastinoscopy, combined endosonography, and endosonography followed by mediastinoscopy of 79%, 85%, and 94%, respectively.[38] In addition, ASTER demonstrated the feasibility to systematically sample at least three different mediastinal nodal stations at combined endosonography in the vast majority of patients.[38] A staging strategy commencing with combined endosonography detected significantly more mediastinal nodal N2/3 disease compared to mediastinoscopy alone. As a consequence, the implementation of endosonography for baseline mediastinal nodal staging clearly reduces the need for mediastinoscopy but does not replace it as a negative endosonography should still be followed by a mediastinoscopy. The number of cervical mediastinoscopies needed in order to detect one additional mediastinal nodal disease after a negative endosonography can be calculated from available studies in different patient settings. In ASTER including patients with clinical stage I–III lung cancer, 11 mediastinoscopies were needed in order to detect one additional mediastinal nodal disease after a negative combined endosonography.[38] In a large retrospective Mayo series including patients with clinical stage III lung cancer, five mediastinoscopies were needed in order to detect one additional mediastinal nodal disease after a negative EBUS staging.[40]

Patients with a centrally located primary tumor or patients with clinical N1 nodes on imaging, and normal sized FDG-negative mediastinal lymph nodes on CT and PET can have malignant involvement in their mediastinal nodes. Therefore, the ACCP and ESTS guidelines state that invasive preoperative mediastinal staging should be performed in these patients.[28,41] Non-randomized trials suggested the potential of EUS-FNA and/or EBUS-TBNA for mediastinal staging. However, the majority of these non-randomized trials studied the potential of echo-endoscopic techniques for the mediastinal staging of clinical N2/3 lung cancer. Clinical data focusing on the value of endoscopic ultrasonography for the mediastinal staging in patients

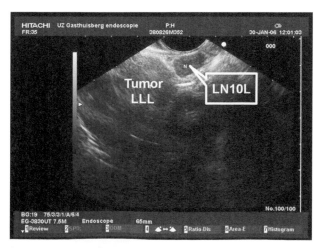

Figure 3.3 EUS showing the primary lung tumor in the LLL with adjacent hilar lymph node in level 10L.

with a normal mediastinum on CT and PET are scarce. Two non-randomized prospective studies reported on the test sensitivity and NPV of endosonography in patients with stage I–II lung cancer.[42,43] The prevalence of mediastinal nodal disease was 22% in the study by Szlubowski et al.; the sensitivity and NPV were 46% and 86% for EBUS-TBNA, and 68% and 91%, respectively, for combined EBUS-EUS.[42] As such, 11 surgical mediastinal staging procedures (using TEMLA) were needed in order to detect one additional mediastinal nodal disease after a negative combined endosonography.[42] The prevalence of mediastinal nodal disease was 6% in the study by Herth et al.; the sensitivity and NPV were 89% and 99% for EBUS-TBNA.[43] A post-hoc subanalysis of ASTER in patients with clinical stage I–II requiring invasive mediastinal nodal staging reported on a sensitivity and NPV of 70% and 92% for combined endosonography; the prevalence of mediastinal nodal disease in this subgroup was 23%.[44] Finally, in a recently published prospective trial by Yasufuku et al. patients with clinical stage I–III (of whom 59% had clinical stage I–II disease) lung cancer requiring preoperative invasive mediastinal staging underwent EBUS-TBNA followed by mediastinoscopy under general anesthesia.[45] The overall prevalence of mediastinal nodal disease in the study was 35%; sensitivity and NPV of EBUS-TBNA and mediastinoscopy were 81%, 91% and 79%, 90%, respectively.[45] As such, based on Yasufuku et al. 28 mediastinoscopies were needed to detect one additional N2/3 disease after a negative mediastinal staging with EBUS-TBNA. In general, it can be concluded that in a setting with a low prevalence of mediastinal disease, mediastinoscopy may not add significant advantages after a negative endosonography.

Standard White-Light Bronchoscopy and Autofluorescence Bronchoscopy

Standard white-light bronchoscopy (WLB) is considered mandatory in patients with suspected lung cancer. In addition to pathological confirmation in many patients, it also permits an evaluation of the endobronchial extension of the tumor (endobronchial T stage), which can be decisive for the extent of resection or for radiotherapy planning.

Autofluorescence bronchoscopy (AFB) added to WLB has a role in the routine work-up of patients suspected of having operable lung cancer based on chest imaging or in patients with newly diagnosed lung cancer planned for resection.[46] Adding AFB to WLB may reveal synchronous multi-centricity of pre-invasive and radio-occult invasive lesions in 10% of the patients in whom a primary radiographically visible invasive lung cancer was detected.[47] Video-autofluorescence bronchoscopy systems are nowadays available, making an easy access to anatomic and functional information possible at the time of the first bronchoscopy without significantly increasing examination time.

PREOPERATIVE SURGICAL STAGING TECHNIQUES
Cervical Mediastinoscopy

Cervical mediastinoscopy still is a central tool for staging the upper mediastinal lymph nodes in patients with resectable clinical stage I–III lung cancer. It is a surgical biopsy technique under general anesthesia.[48] The mediastinoscope is inserted through a small suprasternal incision. Blunt dissection then gives access to the pretracheal, right and left paratracheal, and anterior subcarinal lymph nodes (Table 3.2). The average sensitivity of cervical mediastinoscopy to detect mediastinal lymph node involvement is approximately 80% with a high NPV of 89%.[42] The results of the suboptimal sensitivity are partly explained by the fact that some lymph node stations (5, 6, 7 posterior, 8, 9) are not accessible by cervical mediastinoscopy. Other advantages of cervical mediastinoscopy are that it allows a complete mapping of mediastinal lymph nodes, discrimination between extra- and intracapsular lymph node disease, and between nodal disease and direct invasion of the mediastinum by the tumor itself. More recently, the introduction of video-mediastinoscopes improved visualization, allowing recording of the findings, and leading to improved teaching possibilities.[49]

Transcervical Extended Mediastinal Lymphadenectomy

In 2005, Kuzdzal and Zielinski introduced transcervical extended mediastinal lymphadenectomy (TEMLA) as new surgical staging procedure for initial mediastinal evaluation.[50] TEMLA includes a collar incision in the neck, elevation of the sternal manubrium with a special retractor, providing a thorough mediastinal lymph node dissection of all mediastinal nodal stations except of the pulmonary ligament nodes (station 9).[5,51] Sensitivity, NPV, and accuracy for primary staging of the mediastinum are reported to be >94%, >97%, and 98%, respectively, which is beyond comparison with any other (non-)invasive technique.[52,53] Without any doubt, TEMLA provides the most thorough evaluation of the mediastinum at the cost of an acceptable morbidity of 6.6% and mortality of 0.3%, and can presently be considered the gold standard for primary staging when a minimally invasive technique is used to obtain a proof of mediastinal involvement.[54]

Anterior Mediastinotomy

Left upper lobe tumors are known to metastasize predominantly to the aortopulmonary window and para-aortic lymph nodes (stations 5 and 6). These lymph node stations cannot be reached by cervical mediastinoscopy, EBUS or EUS, and need either left anterior mediastinotomy or left thoracoscopy (see below). The mediastinotomy procedure is more demanding and has a higher morbidity than the cervical approach. When a cervical mediastinoscopy is negative, this procedure may be indicated in case of high suspicion of involvement of lymph node stations 5 or 6 (e.g., in case of enlarged or FDG-avid lymph nodes in that area).

Video-Assisted Thoracic Surgery

This technique can be a useful add-on to cervical mediastinoscopy, as it allows one to reach subcarinal nodes or inferior mediastinal nodes on the right side, and para-aortic nodes or inferior mediastinal nodes on the left side (Table 3.2). For VATS, the false negative rate was 15% both in enlarged and normal sized nodes with a sensitivity varying widely from 37% to 100%.[42] The advantage over left anterior mediastinotomy is that anatomical landmarks such as the vagal and phrenic nerve are more easily recognized.

CONCLUSION

Clinical TNM staging of lung cancer is a multidisciplinary process involving imaging, endoscopic, and surgical techniques. Accuracy is vital in order to avoid false positive interpretations leading to a false stage III or IV diagnosis in early stage patients, or false negative findings leading to a false early stage diagnosis in patients with mediastinal lymph node disease. Additionally, resectability needs to be estimated as precisely as possible. Contemporary non-invasive staging relies on combination of an integrated PET-CT scan and brain MRI. When tissue confirmation of the locoregional lymph node status is needed, the historical gold standard status of mediastinoscopy is nowadays complemented by endosonographic techniques (EBUS-TBNA and/or EUS-FNA). The practical ESTS guidelines developed in 2007 remain important in modern staging algorithms. Rational staging in clinical practice is based on an integrated PET-CT. The implementation of FDG-PET/CT reduced the number of mediastinoscopies. Due to the high NPV of mediastinal staging with PET-CT, invasive staging procedures can be omitted in patients with a peripheral clinical stage I NSCLC. Care should be taken in situations with a little FDG-avid primary tumor, presence of a central tumor, or centrally located N1 nodes. On the other hand, because false positive findings may occur, tissue confirmation remains warranted in case of positive mediastinal FDG-PET/CT findings. Here, an important evolution has occurred over recent years, as minimally invasive mediastinal nodal staging by EUS-FNA and/or EBUS-TBNA has become a valid alternative to mediastinoscopy. The implementation of endosonography for invasive mediastinal nodal staging clearly reduced the number of mediastinoscopies, but in case of negative endosonography finding in clinical stage III lung cancer, a confirmatory mediastinoscopy is still indicated.

REFERENCES

1. Mountain CF. Revisions in the international system for staging lung cancer. Chest 1997; 111: 1710–17.
2. Goldstraw P, Crowley JJ. IASLC International Staging Project. The International Association for the Study of Lung Cancer international staging project on lung cancer. J Thorac Oncol 2006; 1: 281–6.
3. Goldstraw P, Crowley J, Chansky K, et al. The IASLC Lung Cancer Staging Project: proposals for the revision of the TNM stage groupings in the forthcoming (seventh) edition of the TNM Classification of malignant tumours. J Thorac Oncol 2007; 2: 706–14.
4. Rami-Porta R, Ball D, Crowley J, et al. The IASLC Lung Cancer Staging Project: proposals for the revision of the T descriptors in the forthcoming (seventh) edition of the TNM classification for lung cancer. J Thorac Oncol 2007; 2: 593–602.
5. Rusch VW, Crowley J, Giroux DJ, et al. The IASLC Lung Cancer Staging Project: proposals for the revision of the N descriptors in the forthcoming seventh edition of the TNM classification for lung cancer. J Thorac Oncol 2007; 2: 603–12.
6. Rusch VW, Asamura H, Watanabe H, et al. The IASLC lung cancer staging project: a proposal for a new international lymph node map in the forthcoming seventh edition of the TNM classification for lung cancer. J Thorac Oncol 2009; 4: 679–83.
7. Silvestri GA, Gould MK, Margolis ML, et al. Noninvasive staging of non-small cell lung cancer: ACCP evidenced-based clinical practice guidelines (2nd edition). Chest 2007; 132(Suppl 3): 178S–201S.

8. De Leyn P, Vansteenkiste J, Cuypers P, et al. Role of cervical mediastinoscopy in staging of non-small cell lung cancer without enlarged mediastinal lymph nodes on CT scan. Eur J Cardiothorac Surg 1997; 12: 706–12.

9. De Wever W, Ceyssens S, Mortelmans L, et al. Additional value of PET-CT in the staging of lung cancer: comparison with CT alone, PET alone and visual correlation of PET and CT. Eur Radiol 2007; 17: 23–32.

10. Lardinois D, Weder W, Hany TF, et al. Staging of non-small cell lung cancer with integrated positron-emission tomography and computed tomography. N Engl J Med 2003; 348: 2500–7.

11. Fischer BM, Mortensen J, Hojgaard L. Positron emission tomography in the diagnosis and staging of lung cancer: a systematic, quantitative review. Lancet Oncol 2001; 2: 659–66.

12. Al-Sarraf N, Gately K, Lucey J, et al. Lymph node staging by means of positron emission tomography is less accurate in non-small cell lung cancer patients with enlarged lymph nodes: analysis of 1,145 lymph nodes. Lung Cancer 2008; 60: 62–8.

13. Fischer B, Mortensen J, Hansen E, et al. Multimodality approach to mediastinal staging in non-small cell lung cancer. Faults and benefits of PET-CT: a randomised trial. Thorax 2011; 66: 294–300.

14. Darling G, Maziak D, Inculet R, et al. Positron emission tomography-computed tomography compared with invasive mediastinal staging in non-small cell lung cancer: results of mediastinal staging in the early lung positron emission tomography trial. J Thorac Oncol 2011; 6: 1367–72.

15. Lv Y, Yuan D, Wang K, et al. Diagnostic performance of integrated positron emission tomography/computed tomography for mediastinal lymph node staging in non-small cell lung cancer: a bivariate systematic review and meta-analysis. J Thorac Oncol 2011; 6: 1350–8.

16. Stroobants S, Dhoore I, Dooms C, et al. Additional value of whole-body fluorodeoxyglucose positron emission tomography in the detection of distant metastases of non-small cell lung cancer. Clinical Lung Cancer 2003; 4: 242–7.

17. Pieterman RM, Van Putten JW, Meuzelaar JJ, et al. Preoperative staging of non-small cell lung cancer with positron emission tomography. N Engl J Med 2000; 343: 254–61.

18. Lu Y, Xie D, Huang W, et al. 18F-FDG PET/CT in the evaluation of adrenal masses in lung cancer patients. Neoplasma 2010; 57: 129–34.

19. Fischer B, Lassen U, Mortensen J, et al. Preoperative staging of lung cancer with combined PET-CT. N Engl J Med 2009; 361: 32–9.

20. Maziak D, Darling G, Inculet R, et al. Positron emission tomography in staging early lung cancer. A randomized trial. Ann Intern Med 2009; 151: 221–8.

21. Kolodziejczyk M, Kepka L, Dziuk M, et al. Impact of [18F]fluorodeoxyglucose PET-CT staging on treatment planning in radiotherapy incorporating elective nodal irradiation for non-small-cell lung cancer: a prospective study. Int J Radiat Oncol Biol Phys 2011; 80: 1008–14.

22. Ung Y, Gu C, Cline A, et al. An Ontario Clinical Oncology Group randomized trial (PET START) of FDG PET/CT in patients with stage III non-small cell lung cancer: Predictors of overall survival. J Clin Oncol 2011; 29: 457s.

23. Hochhegger B, Marchiori E, Sedlaczek O, et al. MRI in lung cancer: a pictorial essay. Br J Radiol 2011; 84: 661–8.

24. Suzuki K, Yamamoto M, Hasegawa Y, et al. Magnetic resonance imaging and computed tomography in the diagnoses of brain metastases of lung cancer. Lung Cancer 2004; 46: 357–60.

25. Ohno Y, Koyama H, Nogami M, et al. STIR turbo SE MR imaging vs. coregistered PET/CT: quantitative and qualitative assessment of N-stage in non-small cell lung cancer patients. J Magn Reson Imaging 2007; 26: 1071–80.

26. Ohno Y, Koyama H, Yoshikawa T, et al. N stage disease in patients with non-small cell lung cancer: efficacy of quantitative and qualitative assessment with STIR turbo spin-echo imaging, diffusion-weighted MR imaging and fluorodeoxyglucose PET/CT. Radiology 2011; [Epub ahead of print].

27. Usuda K, Zhao X, Sagawa M, et al. Diffusion-weighted imaging is superior to positron emission tomography in the detection and nodal assessment of lung cancers. Ann Thorac Surg 2011; 91: 1689–95.

28. De Leyn P, Lardinois D, Van Schil P, et al. ESTS guidelines for preoperative lymph node staging for non-small cell lung cancer. Eur J Cardiothorac Surg 2007; 32: 1–8.

29. Piet AH, Lagerwaard FJ, Kunst PW, et al. Can mediastinal nodal mobility explain the low yield rates for transbronchial needle aspiration without real-time imaging? Chest 2007; 131: 1783–7.

30. Micames CG, McCrory DC, Pavey DA, et al. Endoscopic ultrasound-guided fine-needle aspiration for non-small cell lung cancer staging: a systematic review and meta-analysis. Chest 2007; 131: 539–48.

31. Gu P, Zhao YZ, Jiang LY, et al. Endobronchial ultrasound-guided transbronchial needle aspiration for staging of lung cancer: A systematic review and meta-analysis. Eur J Cancer 2009; 45: 1389–96.

32. Tournoy KG, De Ryck F, Vanwalleghem LR, et al. Endoscopic ultrasound reduces surgical mediastinal staging in lung cancer: a randomized trial. Am J Respir Crit Care Med 2008; 177: 531–5.

33. Block M. Endobronchial ultrasound for lung cancer staging: how many stations should be sampled? Ann Thorac Surg 2010; 89: 1582–7.

34. Annema JT, Versteegh MI, Veselic M, et al. Endoscopic ultrasound added to mediastinoscopy for preoperative staging of patients with lung cancer. JAMA 2005; 294: 931–6.

35. Cerfolio RJ, Bryant AS, Eloubeidi MA, et al. The true false negative rates of esophageal and endobronchial ultrasound in the staging of mediastinal lymph nodes in patients with non-small cell lung cancer. Ann Thorac Surg 2010; 90: 427–34.

36. Szlubowski A, Kuzdzał J, Kołodziej M, et al. Endobronchial ultrasound-guided needle aspiration in the non-small cell lung cancer staging. Eur J Cardiothorac Surg 2009; 35: 332–5.

37. Dooms C, Vansteenkiste J, Van Renterghem D, et al. Esophageal ultrasound-controlled fine needle aspiration for staging of mediastinal lymph nodes in patients with resectable lung cancer: do we always see the reality? J Thorac Oncol 2009; 4: 1043–5.

38. Annema J, van Meerbeeck J, Rintoul R, et al. Mediastinoscopy versus endosonography for mediastinal nodal staging of lung cancer: a randomized trial. JAMA 2010; 304: 2245–52.

39. http://www.clinicaltrial.gov/ct2/show/NCT00970645?term=EBUS+mediastinoscopy&rank=3

40. Defranchi S, Edell E, Daniels C, et al. Mediastinoscopy in patients with lung cancer and negative endobronchial ultrasound guided needle aspiration. Ann Thorac Surg 2010; 90: 1753–7.

41. Detterbeck FC, Jantz M, Wallace M, et al. Invasive mediastinal staging of lung cancer: ACCP evidence-based clinical practice guidelines (2nd edition). Chest 2007; 132(Suppl 3): 202S–20S.

42. Szlubowski A, Zieliński M, Soja J, et al. A combined approach of endobronchial and endoscopic ultrasound-guided needle aspiration in the radiologically normal mediastinum in non-small-cell lung cancer staging -a prospective trial. Eur J Cardiothorac Surg 2010; 37: 1175–9.

43. Herth FJ, Eberhardt R, Krasnik M, et al. Endobronchial ultrasound-guided transbronchial needle aspiration of lymph nodes in the radiologically and PET normal mediastinum in patients with lung cancer. Chest 2008; 133: 887–91.

44. Tournoy K, Dooms C, Rintoul R, et al. Mediastinoscopy after negative endosonography in lung cancer staging: sub-analysis of ASTER. J Thorac Oncol 2011; 6: s282–894.

45. Yasufuku K, Pierre A, Darling G, et al. A prospective controlled trial of endobronchial ultrasound-guided transbronchial needle aspiration compared with mediastinoscopy for mediastinal lymph node staging of lung cancer. J Thorac Cardiovasc Surg 2011; [Epub ahead of print].

46. Kennedy TC, McWilliams A, Edell E, et al. Bronchial intraepithelial neoplasia/early central airways lung cancer: ACCP evidence-based clinical practice guidelines (2nd edition). Chest 2007; 132(Suppl 3): 221S–33S.

47. Pierard P, Vermylen P, Bosschaerts T, et al. Synchronous roentgenographically occult lung carcinoma in patients with resectable primary lung cancer. Chest 2000; 117: 779–85.

48. De Leyn P, Lerut T. Conventional mediastinoscopy. Multimedia Manual of Cardiothoracic Surgery, 10.1510/mmcts.2004.000158 2004.

49. De Leyn P, Lerut T. Videomediastinoscopy. Multimedia Manual of Cardiothoracic Surgery, 10.1510/mmcts.2004.000166 2004.

50. Kuzdał J, Zieliński M, Papla B, et al. Transcervical extended mediastinal lymphadenectomy–the new operative technique and early results in lung cancer staging. Eur J Cardiothorac Surg 2005; 27: 384–90.

51. Kuzdzal J, Zielinski M, Papla B, et al. Transcervical extended mediastinal lymphadenectomy – the new operative technique and early results in lung cancer staging. Eur J Cardiothorac Surg 2005; 27: 384–90.

52. Zieliński M. Transcervical extended mediastinal lymphadenectomy: results of staging in two hundred fifty-six patients with non-small cell lung cancer. J Thorac Oncol 2007; 2: 370–2.

53. Zielinski M, Szlubowski A, Kolodziej M, et al. Comparison of diagnostic yield of endoscopic ultrasound staging of non-small cell lung cancer (NSCLC) performed with the use of endobronchial ultrasound(EBUS) and/or endo-esophageal ultrasound (EUS) with invasive staging of NSCLC performed with use of transcervical extended mediastinal lymphadenectomy (TEMLA). J Thorac Oncol 2011; 6: s282.

54. Van Schil PE, Hendriks JM, De Waele M, et al. Editorial comment: mediastinal restaging: has the Holy Grail been found? J Cardiothorac Surg 2010; 37: 780–1.

4 | Histo- and molecular pathology of lung cancer

A. Soltermann, S. Peters, and V. Tischler

INTRODUCTION

Lung cancer is a heterogeneous tumor entity. While in small cell lung cancer (SCLC) pathological classification and treatment were modified only marginally over the last decades, non-small cell lung cancer (NSCLC) is increasingly classified and treated by use of diverse molecular biomarkers in addition to traditional histologic subtyping. These biomarkers may have diagnostic, predictive, or prognostic relevance. At present no serum marker is available as a diagnostic or follow-up tool; however, this may become an important future topic—potentially involving circulating tumor cells, circulating DNA, serum microvesicles, or other serum proteomic marker, alone or in combination. Of note, how such a biomarker would be able to add to the promising results demonstrated by computer tomography screening in a high-risk smoker population will have to be determined.[1]

Currently, most relevant molecular biomarkers are genetic alterations which act as determinants of responsiveness to targeted therapy in the context of advanced NSCLC. Such predictors might be able to significantly reduce treatment costs and side effects. Predictive and prognostic biomarkers might also help in the future to guide the choice of chemotherapy regimens across all types of advanced lung cancer, as well as influence decisions on adjuvant chemotherapy for resected early stages of disease. Nevertheless, to date, no molecular biomarker regarding chemotherapy treatment for NSCLC was prospectively validated and none should therefore be used in clinical daily practice.

In the current setting, the histologic distinction of NSCLC into adeno- and squamous cell carcinoma has turned out to be crucial for further oncologic patient management. This is due to the fact that the prevalence of validated biomarkers is highly variable according to histology, in parallel to some clinical characteristics, including gender, smoking history, and ethnicity. For example, in a Caucasian population, only a subset of around 15% of adenocarcinomas (ADs) but next to no squamous cell carcinomas (SCCs) are characterized by an EGFR (epidermal growth factor receptor, HER1) activating mutation, rendering the tumor cells highly responsive to receptor tyrosine kinase inhibitors (RTKIs) such as erlotinib or gefitinib.

These new data have put lung pathologists in front row for adjustment of oncologic therapy. Particularly demanding is the issue of extensive molecular testing on small samples such as bronchial biopsies, because even if most patients present with extensive non-resectable disease at hospital entry they will all nowadays require some good quality tissue sample to guide therapy.[2]

NON-SMALL CELL LUNG CANCER HISTOPATHOLOGY

Staging

During the sixth to the current seventh 2010 edition of the UICC TNM classification of malignant tumors, several significant staging modifications were introduced. They are based on recommendations of the International Association for the Study of Lung Cancer (IASLC) staging committee which performed an analysis of >100,000 lung cancers worldwide.[3,4] In daily practice, most relevant are the following issues: small tumors ≤3 cm are further subdivided in T1a and T1b (≤2 cm and >2 but ≤3 cm); tumors of intermediate size >3 cm to ≤7 cm are also subdivided into T2a and T2b (>3 cm but ≤5 cm and >5 but ≤7 cm). These modifications resulted in a more accurate separation of prognostic subgroups and therefore discrimination of survival Kaplan–Meier curves. Tumoral infraction of the outmost elastica layer of the pleura visceralis (PL1) and consecutive superficial growth (PL2) both denote a pT2. Infiltration of the thoracic wall is classified PL3 = pT3, whereas growth just to the elastica layer or into it qualifies for PL0 = pT1. Assessment of this PL category necessitates an Elastica van Gieson (EVG) stain. Presence of separate tumor nodules of same histology in the same lobe is now T3, in another ipsilateral lobe T4 and only in case of controlateral manifestation M1a. Pleural nodules or malignant effusion is also M1a, but distant metastasis is M1b. Concerning nodal status, discrepancies in nomenclature among Asian and Western countries forced the development of a new lymph node map with precise anatomic definitions for all lymph node stations.[5] Implementing these modifications has ultimately led to an adapted stage grouping table (Table 4.1).

Potential correlation with particular subtypes such as papillary needs further investigation.[48] In recent years, research was highly focused on lung AC initially due to the presence of targeted drug sensitizing *EGFR* gene mutations found in more than 1–20% of them and in more than 50% of adenocarcinomas and tumors from East Asians, never smokers, and women.[44] These driver mutations occur in exons 18–21 of *EGFR*, modifying the active site of the EGFR kinase domain and favoring its activity. The biology of NSCLC harboring EGFR driver mutations is reviewed in chapter 5.

Wild-type *EGFR* is commonly overexpressed in NSCLC tumors (~30–80% of samples),[49] and this characteristic is correlated with a high EGFR gene copy number, as measured by fluorescence in situ hybridization found in 30–50% of NSCLC, encompassing true gene amplification and polysomy.[50] None of these characteristics were clearly shown to possess interesting prognostic or predictive value, and clinical relevance of their evaluation remains unclear.[50–52] SCCs express the EGFR protein at the plasma membrane to a higher degree than AC (p-value <0.001 on our Zurich NSCLC TMA cohort 1993–2002), according to the standard semi-quantitative IHC scale (score range 0–3). Thus, EGFR targeting in SCCs may be assumed to remain an interesting field of investigation in future prospective trials.[53] Interestingly, measurement of EGFR immunoreactivity has been refined by implementation of the so-called H-score (formerly known as IRS, immunoreactivity score). Retrospective analysis of a large phase III trial randomizing the addition of cetuximab—a monoclonal anti-EGFR antibody—to classical chemotherapy suggests that H-score might identify a patient subgroup benefiting in terms of survival from cetuximab, defined by an EGFR H-score of 200 or above (31% of the study population). The authors stated that these results warranted the possibility of offering cetuximab to patients with NSCLC and a high H-score.[54]

Rare Transforming Genetic Alterations

EML4-ALK, a targetable fusion gene between the echinoderm microtubule-associated protein-like 4 and the anaplastic lymphoma kinase, occurs in up to 5% of lung AD,[55] more frequently in young non-smoker patients. Together with *BRAF, HER2, MET,* and *PIK3CA* mutations, the whole group of rare genetic alterations with frequencies below 3% is reviewed in chapter 5. Of high future impact is also the recent discovery of frequent FGFR1 (fibroblast growth factor receptor 1) amplifications in around 20% of lung SCCs,[56] as well as the recent description of candidate driver mutation in this histologic subtype, including *DDR2* and *SOX2.*[57–59]

Other Quantitative Analysis of Biomarkers with Therapeutic Impact
c-MET Overexpression and Amplification

c-MET pathway is frequently activated in many human cancers. Its inappropriate activation can rely on specific genetic mutations, transcriptional upregulation, or ligand-dependent mechanisms. The most frequent cause of constitutive MET activation in human tumors is increased protein expression as a consequence of transcriptional upregulation, in the absence of gene amplification—demonstrating a prognostic value in many cancers including NSCLC.[60–63] In a recent trial using a MET-directed monoclonal antibody, only patients with tumors presenting significant expression of MET, as defined by more than 50% of the cells with a 2+ or 3+ IHC score (half of NSCLC patient trial population), seemed to benefit from the antibody in addition to erlotinib.[64] True amplification of the *MET* gene, with consequent protein overexpression and constitutive kinase activation is a rare event, and has been reported in a number of human primary tumors, including non-small-cell lung carcinoma (in 2–10%),[63] notably in the context of acquired resistance to EGFR inhibitors, found in about 25% of cases.[65] MET-targeted TKI might be of interest in the context of this rare group of patients.[66]

The true prevalence of MET overexpression and amplification in newly diagnosed NSCLC (not yet known accurately) and clinical correlations are emerging slowly. In addition, a standard definition for *MET* amplification is still lacking. Finally, if true *MET* amplification (as opposed to polysomy) seems to possess a transforming capacity, the role of *MET* mutations, mainly located in the extracellular SEMA and juxtamembrane domains in NSCLC, as being oncogenic drivers still remains somehow unsettled.

PIK3CA Amplification

The main catalytic subunit of PI3K proteins is the p110α isoform, which is encoded by *PIK3CA*. Mutations in this gene have been identified rarely in lung cancer (about 3% of NSCLC cases, as frequently found in squamous-cell carcinoma as in adenocarcinoma). NSCLC dependency on rare *PIK3CA* mutation remains to be proven in the context NSCLC patients.

However, increased copy number of the PIK3CA gene is a more frequent event in NSCLC being observed in 30% of squamous-cell carcinomas and 5–10% of adenocarcinomas,[67] maybe more often in males and smokers.[68] Amplification may play a role in EGFR TKI resistance. Even if literature remains elusive, tumors with *PIK3CA* mutations do not necessarily display amplification of the mutant allele. Again, oncogenic potential of PIK3CA amplification alone has not yet been shown biologically. Correlation of gene amplification and protein expression remains to be systematically analyzed and further described, besides their respective predictive or prognostic potential roles.

Several small-molecule inhibitors have been developed that target PI3K alone or in conjunction with mTOR proteins, and many dual inhibitors are in early clinical development.

Several other biomarkers are under clinical evaluation as potential targets in NSCLC,[69] including IGF1-R (a tyrosine kinase receptor), activated on binding of the insulin-like growth factor and often overexpressed, as well as its ligand in NSCLC. Several targeted IGF1-R TKIs and monoclonal antibodies are under evaluation in NSCLC.[70–72] LKB1, a serine/threonine kinase regulating fundamental metabolic, structural, and proliferative cell processes and fundamentally acting as a tumor suppressor gene was recently shown to harbor an inactivating mutation in 30–50% of lung adenocarcinoma,[65,73] predominantly in smokers and possibly more rarely in Asian patients. In mice models, LKB1 inactivation alone was insufficient for pulmonary neoplasia, but LKB1 inactivation in mutant *KRAS* tumors led to adenocarcinoma, squamous and large-cell carcinomas of the lung. However, molecular pathways involved remain poorly described and no specific therapeutic approach is to be expected in the near future to overcome LKB1 deficiency.

With upcoming implementation of all the further markers as described above and the possibility of multiplexing assays and deep or ultra-deep sequencing, it is somehow doubtful if complete molecular pathology work-up can be performed on small biopsies in future, taking into account the frequent tumor heterogeneity of NSCLC.

DNA Repair Enzymes

The above-mentioned markers are used for targeted therapy, but standard chemotherapy using platinum components is still widely administered and in all likelihood will be continued to be used. Cisplatin-DNA adducts are primarily removed by the NER system (nucleotide excision repair), where ERCC1 (excision repair cross complementing group 1 protein) plays the key role as a rate-limiting protein.[74] The so-called ERCC1 paradoxon was put forward, meaning that tumors which are ERCC1 negative respond better to platinum-containing chemotherapy due to less effective NER, whereas surgically resected NSCLC patients having not received adjuvant chemotherapy which are ERCC1 positive present a better survival due to higher general genomic stability.[74,75] ERCC1 is now used in clinical trials as a stratification parameter, but its technical assessment is under debate due to the presence of several antibodies with unclear specificity and remarkable outcome differences among studies, depending on type of tissue (frozen vs. fixed) or technology (mRNA vs. protein) used.[76–78] Importantly, it has not been formally prospectively validated and should not guide treatment decision at this point.[79]

NEUROENDOCRINE TUMORS OF THE LUNG
Histological Classification

In the 2004 WHO classification, the concept of pulmonary neuroendocrine tumors (lung NET) was introduced.[6,80,81] These lung NETs are viewed as a distinct subset of tumors that share certain morphologic, ultrastructural, and IHC characteristics. Four major categories are recognized: typical carcinoid (TC), atypical carcinoid (AC), large cell neuroendocrine carcinoma (LCNEC), and small cell lung carcinoma (SCLC). By deduction, one might assume that these tumors would develop from the diffuse neuroendocrine system of the lung, formerly called APUD-system. Yet, a comprehensive cancer stem cell (CSC) concept is still lacking and with regard to the huge difference in survival between TC/AC versus LCNEC/SCLC it is somewhat debatable if neuroendocrine differentiation is really the most adequate qualifier for creation of this subset.

From a clinical point of view, most important for the two low-grade lesions is the notion that TCs (= well-differentiated neuroendocrine tumor) metastasize in about 10% of cases with regional lymph nodes and ACs (= well-differentiated neuroendocrine carcinoma) in 30%, corroborating the historical finding of Oberndorfer in 1907 that carcinoids resemble adenocarcinomas but grow slower. The synonyms in brackets are widely used in GI-pathology but still not really accepted in the lung pathology world. For the two high-grade lesions, LCNEC are reported to have a worse prognosis than the NSCLC histotypes AD or SCC but a slightly better than SCLC. In brief, the current order of survival can be indicated as AC = SCC > LC/LC-NEC > SCLC.

Concerning neuroendocrine differentiation, the long lasting debate about the best IHC marker is still ongoing. Neuron-specific enolase (NSE) and argentaffin stains are nowadays rather abandoned and replaced by the three markers: synaptophysin (Syn), chromogranin A (CgA), and CD56. In terms of specificity for neuroendocrine differentiation, the order seems to be CgA > Syn > CD56. However, CgA is often weak and CD56 (neural cell adhesion molecule, NCAM) is critical, since this molecule has a widespread expression profile and many surgical pathologists do not rely on it.

For all four categories, precise definitions are indicated in the current classification, mostly based on presence of necrosis and mitotic count, but their implementation in reality is not an easy task. Frequently, typical carcinoids present an infiltrative growth at the tumor border to the surrounding lung parenchyma which is not taken in account since for the diagnosis of AC, only mitoses and necrosis are relevant. Next problem is the distinction of AC and SCLC on small biopsies which can only be solved by a Ki-67 labeling index using the Mib-1 antibody. Finally, the distinction between SCLC and LCNEC is clinically relevant, since SCLC patients will undergo primary chemotherapy whereas in case of LCNEC, many centers favor a strategy of surgical resection followed by adjuvant chemotherapy.[80] By definition, SCLC cells are smaller than the size of three resting lymphocytes. In reality, scarce interspersed larger elements with prominent nucleoli are often observed in SCLC but this does not justify a diagnosis of LCNEC.[82]

Staging and Treatment

According to the new consensus by Travis et al. broncho-pulmonary carcinoids were introduced into the seventh edition of the TNM classification.[83] The main problem of adaptation to the NSCLC data is normally the small size (<3 cm) of TC/AC; thus the question arises if cut-offs between 5 and 7 cm are meaningful for these tumors. Also, more than one carcinoid may be present or a main tumor may be surrounded by tumorlets. This issue of multicentricity needs to be addressed in future as well.

Biomarkers

Despite decades of research, no major progress has been achieved concerning prognosis and survival of SCLC. Thus, the paradigm of "cancer undefeated" as presented by Bailar and Gornik in 1997[84] can be applied for this lesion. Currently, apart from the diagnostic IHC antigens (CgA, Syn, and Mib-1), no predictive or prognostic biomarkers have been established in routine pathology. From a surgical point of view, limited disease SCLCs presenting with a so-called single pulmonary nodule (SPN) and/or combinations with LCNEC, AD, or SCC, called combined carcinomas, are candidates for resection. For metastasized carcinoids and LCNEC, IHC assessment of the somatostatin receptor 2 (SSTR-2) is sometimes requested before ^{90}Y-DOTA-Tyr-Octreotide (DOTATOC) therapy.

REFERENCES

1. Aberle DR, Adams AM, Berg CD, et al. Reduced lung-cancer mortality with low-dose computed tomographic screening. N Engl J Med 2011; 365: 395–409.
2. Thunnissen E, Kerr KM, Herth FJ, et al. The challenge of NSCLC diagnosis and predictive analysis on small samples. Practical approach of a working group. Lung Cancer 2012; 76: 1–18.
3. Goldstraw P, Crowley J, Chansky K, et al. The IASLC Lung Cancer Staging Project: proposals for the revision of the TNM stage groupings in the forthcoming (seventh) edition of the TNM Classification of malignant tumours. J Thorac Oncol 2007; 2: 706–14.
4. Travis WD. Reporting lung cancer pathology specimens. Impact of the anticipated 7th edn. TNM classification based on recommendations of the IASLC Staging Committee. Histopathology 2009; 54: 3–11.
5. Rusch VW, Asamura H, Watanabe H, et al. The IASLC lung cancer staging project: a proposal for a new international lymph node map in the forthcoming seventh edition of the TNM classification for lung cancer. J Thorac Oncol 2009; 4: 568–77.
6. 6. Travis WD, Brambilla E, Müller-Hermelink HK, Harris CC. Pathology and Genetics of Tumours of the Lung, Pleura, Thymus and Heart, 1st edn. In: Kleihues P, Sobin LH, eds. Lyon: IARC Press, 2004.
7. Righi L, Graziano P, Fornari A, et al. Immunohistochemical subtyping of nonsmall cell lung cancer not otherwise specified in fine-needle aspiration cytology: a retrospective study of 103 cases with surgical correlation. Cancer 2011; 117: 3416–23.
8. Chen Y, Cui T, Yang L, et al. The diagnostic value of cytokeratin 5/6, 14, 17, and 18 expression in human non-small cell lung cancer. Oncology 2011; 80: 333–40.
9. Ring BZ, Seitz RS, Beck RA, et al. A novel five-antibody immunohistochemical test for subclassification of lung carcinoma. Mod Pathol 2009; 22: 1032–43.
10. Travis WD, Brambilla E, Noguchi M, et al. International association for the study of lung cancer/american thoracic society/european respiratory society international multidisciplinary classification of lung adenocarcinoma. J Thorac Oncol 2011; 6: 244–85.

11. Soltermann A, Tischler V, Arbogast S, et al. Prognostic significance of epithelial-mesenchymal and mesenchymal-epithelial transition protein expression in non-small cell lung cancer. Clin Cancer Res 2008; 14: 7430–7.

12. Pedretti M, Soltermann A, Arni S, et al. Comparative immunohistochemistry of L19 and F16 in non-small cell lung cancer and mesothelioma: two human antibodies investigated in clinical trials in patients with cancer. Lung Cancer 2009; 64: 28–33.

13. Soltermann A, Kilgus-Hawelski S, Behnke S, et al. Automated ERCC1 immunochemistry on hybrid cytology/tissue microarray of malignant effusions: evaluation of antibodies 8F1 and D-10. J Clin Bioinforma 2011; 1: 25.

14. Husain AN, Colby TV, Ordonez NG, et al. Guidelines for pathologic diagnosis of malignant mesothelioma: a consensus statement from the International Mesothelioma Interest Group. Arch Pathol Lab Med 2009; 133: 1317–31.

15. Moch H, Oberholzer M, Dalquen P, Wegmann W, Gudat F. Diagnostic tools for differentiating between pleural mesothelioma and lung adenocarcinoma in paraffin embedded tissue. Part I: Immunohistochemical findings. Virchows Arch A Pathol Anat Histopathol 1993; 423: 19–27.

16. Kushitani K, Takeshima Y, Amatya VJ, et al. Immunohistochemical marker panels for distinguishing between epithelioid mesothelioma and lung adenocarcinoma. Pathol Int 2007; 57: 190–9.

17. Lau SK, Luthringer DJ, Eisen RN. Thyroid transcription factor-1: a review. Appl Immunohistochem Mol Morphol 2002; 10: 97–102.

18. Bakshi N, Kunju LP, Giordano T, Shah RB. Expression of renal cell carcinoma antigen (RCC) in renal epithelial and nonrenal tumors: diagnostic Implications. Appl Immunohistochem Mol Morphol 2007; 15: 310–15.

19. Saad RS, Cho P, Silverman JF, Liu Y. Usefulness of Cdx2 in separating mucinous bronchioloalveolar adenocarcinoma of the lung from metastatic mucinous colorectal adenocarcinoma. Am J Clin Pathol 2004; 122: 421–7.

20. Janku F, Garrido-Laguna I, Petruzelka LB, Stewart DJ, Kurzrock R. Novel therapeutic targets in non-small cell lung cancer. J Thorac Oncol 2011; 6: 1601–12.

21. Steeg PS. Metastasis suppressors alter the signal transduction of cancer cells. Nat Rev Cancer 2003; 3: 55–63.

22. Kim HJ, Bar-Sagi D. Modulation of signalling by Sprouty: a developing story. Nat Rev Mol Cell Biol 2004; 5: 441–50.

23. Wagner EF, Nebreda AR. Signal integration by JNK and p38 MAPK pathways in cancer development. Nat Rev Cancer 2009; 9: 537–49.

24. Hennessy BT, Smith DL, Ram PT, Lu Y, Mills GB. Exploiting the PI3K/AKT pathway for cancer drug discovery. Nat Rev Drug Discov 2005; 4: 988–1004.

25. Mahalingam D, Swords R, Carew JS, et al. Targeting HSP90 for cancer therapy. Br J Cancer 2009; 100: 1523–9.

26. Cox D, Brennan M, Moran N. Integrins as therapeutic targets: lessons and opportunities. Nat Rev Drug Discov 2010; 9: 804–20.

27. Mok TS. Personalized medicine in lung cancer: what we need to know. Nat Rev Clin Oncol 2011; 8: 661–8.

28. Pao W, Girard N. New driver mutations in non-small-cell lung cancer. Lancet Oncol 2011; 12: 175–80.

29. Kris MG, Johnson BE, Kwiatkowski DJ, et al. Identification of driver mutations in tumor specimens from 1,000 patients with lung adenocarcinoma: The NCI's Lung Cancer Mutation Consortium (LCMC). J Clin Oncol 2011; 29: CRA7506, ASCO Meeting abstract.

30. Krishnaswamy S, Kanteti R, Duke-Cohan JS, et al. Ethnic differences and functional analysis of MET mutations in lung cancer. Clin Cancer Res 2009; 15: 5714–23.

31. Tiseo M, Gelsomino F, Boggiani D, et al. EGFR and EML4-ALK gene mutations in NSCLC: a case report of erlotinib-resistant patient with both concomitant mutations. Lung Cancer 2011; 71: 241–3.

32. Popat S, Vieira de Araujo A, Min T, et al. Lung adenocarcinoma with concurrent exon 19 EGFR mutation and ALK rearrangement responding to erlotinib. J Thorac Oncol 2011; 6: 1962–3.

33. Chaft JE, Arcila ME, Paik PK, et al. Coexistence of PIK3CA and other oncogene mutations in lung adenocarcinoma - rationale for comprehensive mutation profiling. Mol Cancer Ther 2012; 11: 485–91.

34. Yano T, Haro A, Shikada Y, Maruyama R, Maehara Y. Non-small cell lung cancer in never smokers as a representative 'non-smoking-associated lung cancer': epidemiology and clinical features. Int J Clin Oncol 2011; 16: 287–93.

35. Lee YJ, Kim JH, Kim SK, et al. Lung cancer in never smokers: change of a mindset in the molecular era. Lung Cancer 2011; 72: 9–15.

36. Ren JH, He WS, Yan GL, et al. EGFR mutations in non-small-cell lung cancer among smokers and non-smokers: A meta-analysis. Environ Mol Mutagen 2012; 53: 78–82.

37. Sun Y, Ren Y, Fang Z, et al. Lung adenocarcinoma from East Asian never-smokers is a disease largely defined by targetable oncogenic mutant kinases. J Clin Oncol 2010; 28: 4616–20.

38. Mitsudomi T, Steinberg SM, Oie HK, et al. ras gene mutations in non-small cell lung cancers are associated with shortened survival irrespective of treatment intent. Cancer Res 1991; 51: 4999–5002.

39. Riely GJ, Marks J, Pao W. KRAS mutations in non-small cell lung cancer. Proc Am Thorac Soc 2009; 6: 201–5.

40. Mascaux C, Iannino N, Martin B, et al. The role of RAS oncogene in survival of patients with lung cancer: a systematic review of the literature with meta-analysis. Br J Cancer 2005; 92: 131–9.

41. Jackman DM, Miller VA, Cioffredi LA, et al. Impact of epidermal growth factor receptor and KRAS mutations on clinical outcomes in previously untreated non-small cell lung cancer patients: results of an online tumor registry of clinical trials. Clin Cancer Res 2009; 15: 5267–73.

42. Mao C, Qiu LX, Liao RY, et al. KRAS mutations and resistance to EGFR-TKIs treatment in patients with non-small cell lung cancer: a meta-analysis of 22 studies. Lung Cancer 2010; 69: 272–8.

43. Kim ES, Herbst RS, Wistuba II, et al. The BATTLE Trial: Personalizing Therapy for Lung Cancer. Cancer Discovery 2011; 1: 44–53.

44. Sharma SV, Bell DW, Settleman J, Haber DA. Epidermal growth factor receptor mutations in lung cancer. Nat Rev Cancer 2007; 7: 169–81.

45. Mok TS, Wu YL, Thongprasert S, et al. Gefitinib or carboplatin-paclitaxel in pulmonary adenocarcinoma. N Engl J Med 2009; 361: 947–57.

46. Eberhard DA, Johnson BE, Amler LC, et al. Mutations in the epidermal growth factor receptor and in KRAS are predictive and prognostic indicators in patients with non-small-cell lung cancer treated with chemotherapy alone and in combination with erlotinib. J Clin Oncol 2005; 23: 5900–9.

47. Soria JC, Mok TS, Cappuzzo F, Janne PA. EGFR-mutated oncogene-addicted non-small cell lung cancer: Current trends and future prospects. Cancer Treat Rev 2011; Nov 24.

48. Motoi N, Szoke J, Riely GJ, et al. Lung adenocarcinoma: modification of the 2004 WHO mixed subtype to include the major histologic subtype suggests correlations between papillary and micropapillary adenocarcinoma subtypes, EGFR mutations and gene expression analysis. Am J Surg Pathol 2008; 32: 810–27.

49. Liang Z, Zhang J, Zeng X, et al. Relationship between EGFR expression, copy number and mutation in lung adenocarcinomas. BMC Cancer 2010; 10: 376.

50. Cappuzzo F, Hirsch FR, Rossi E, et al. Epidermal growth factor receptor gene and protein and gefitinib sensitivity in non-small-cell lung cancer. J Natl Cancer Inst 2005; 97: 643–55.

51. Bunn PA Jr, Dziadziuszko R, Varella-Garcia M, et al. Biological markers for non-small cell lung cancer patient selection for epidermal growth factor receptor tyrosine kinase inhibitor therapy. Clin Cancer Res 2006; 12: 3652–6.

52. Cappuzzo F, Ligorio C, Janne PA, et al. Prospective study of gefitinib in epidermal growth factor receptor fluorescence in situ hybridization-positive/phospho-Akt-positive or never smoker patients with advanced non-small-cell lung cancer: the ONCOBELL trial. J Clin Oncol 2007; 25: 2248–55.

53. O'Byrne KJ, Gatzemeier U, Bondarenko I, et al. Molecular biomarkers in non-small-cell lung cancer: a retrospective analysis of data from the phase 3 FLEX study. Lancet Oncol 2011; 12: 795–805.

54. Pirker R, Paz AL, Eberhardt WEE. Epidermal growth factor receptor (EGFR) expression as a predictor of survival for first-line chemotherapy plus cetuximab in FLEX study patients with advanced non-small cell lung cancer (NSCLC) [Abstract]. Program and abstracts of the 14th World Conference on Lung Cancer. 3–7 July 2011, Amsterdam: The Netherlands, 2011. 00106.

55. Perner S, Wagner PL, Demichelis F, et al. EML4-ALK fusion lung cancer: a rare acquired event. Neoplasia 2008; 10: 298–302.

56. Weiss J, Sos ML, Seidel D, et al. Frequent and focal FGFR1 amplification associates with therapeutically tractable FGFR1 dependency in squamous cell lung cancer. Sci Transl Med 2010; 2: 62ra93.

57. Hammerman PS, Sos ML, Ramos AH, et al. Mutations in the DDR2 Kinase Gene Identify a Novel Therapeutic Target in Squamous Cell Lung Cancer Cancer Discovery. 2011; 1: 78–89.

58. Wilbertz T, Wagner P, Petersen K, et al. SOX2 gene amplification and protein overexpression are associated with better outcome in squamous cell lung cancer. Mod Pathol 2011; 24: 944–53.

59. Maier S, Wilbertz T, Braun M, et al. SOX2 amplification is a common event in squamous cell carcinomas of different organ sites. Hum Pathol 2011; 42: 1078–88.

60. Ichimura E, Maeshima A, Nakajima T, Nakamura T. Expression of c-met/HGF receptor in human non-small cell lung carcinomas in vitro and in vivo and its prognostic significance. Jpn J Cancer Res 1996; 87: 1063–9.

61. Park S, Choi YL, Sung CO, et al. High MET copy number and MET overexpression: Poor outcome in non-small cell lung cancer patients. Histol Histopathol 2012; 27: 197–207.

62. Go H, Jeon YK, Park HJ, et al. High MET gene copy number leads to shorter survival in patients with non-small cell lung cancer. J Thorac Oncol 2010; 5: 305–13.

63. Cappuzzo F, Marchetti A, Skokan M, et al. Increased MET gene copy number negatively affects survival of surgically resected non-small-cell lung cancer patients. J Clin Oncol 2009; 27: 1667–74.

64. Spigel DR, Ervin TJ, Ramlau R, et al. Final efficacy results from OAM4558g, a randomized phase II study evaluating Met-MAb or placebo in combination with erlotinib in advanced NSCLC. J Clin Oncol 2011; 29: 7505; ASCO meeting abstracts.

65. Engelman JA, Zejnullahu K, Mitsudomi T, et al. MET amplification leads to gefitinib resistance in lung cancer by activating ERBB3 signaling. Science 2007; 316: 1039–43.

66. Comoglio PM, Giordano S, Trusolino L. Drug development of MET inhibitors: targeting oncogene addiction and expedience. Nat Rev Drug Discov 2008; 7: 504–16.

67. Yamamoto H, Shigematsu H, Nomura M, et al. PIK3CA mutations and copy number gains in human lung cancers. Cancer Res 2008; 68: 6913–21.

68. Okudela K, Suzuki M, Kageyama S, et al. PIK3CA mutation and amplification in human lung cancer. Pathol Int 2007; 57: 664–71.

69. Sequist LV, Heist RS, Shaw AT, et al. Implementing multiplexed genotyping of non-small-cell lung cancers into routine clinical practice. Ann Oncol 2011; 22: 2616–24.

70. Dziadziuszko R, Merrick DT, Witta SE, et al. Insulin-like growth factor receptor 1 (IGF1R) gene copy number is associated with survival in operable non-small-cell lung cancer: a comparison between IGF1R fluorescent in situ hybridization, protein expression, and mRNA expression. J Clin Oncol 2010; 28: 2174–80.

71. Scagliotti GV, Novello S. The role of the insulin-like growth factor signaling pathway in non-small cell lung cancer and other solid tumors. Cancer Treat Rev 2011.
72. Gualberto A, Dolled-Filhart M, Gustavson M, et al. Molecular analysis of non-small cell lung cancer identifies subsets with different sensitivity to insulin-like growth factor I receptor inhibition. Clin Cancer Res 2010; 16: 4654–65.
73. Gill RK, Yang SH, Meerzaman D, et al. Frequent homozygous deletion of the LKB1/STK11 gene in non-small cell lung cancer. Oncogene 2011; 30: 3784–91.
74. Olaussen KA, Dunant A, Fouret P, et al. DNA repair by ERCC1 in non-small-cell lung cancer and cisplatin-based adjuvant chemotherapy. N Engl J Med 2006; 355: 983–91.
75. Friboulet L, Barrios-Gonzales D, Commo F, et al. Molecular Characteristics of ERCC1-Negative versus ERCC1-Positive Tumors in Resected NSCLC. Clin Cancer Res 2011; 17: 5562–72.
76. Arbogast S, Behnke S, Opitz I, et al. Automated ERCC1 immunohistochemistry in non-small cell lung cancer: Comparison of anti-ERCC1 antibodies 8F1, D-10 and FL-297. Appl Immunohistochem Mol Morphol 2011; 19: 99–105.
77. Bhagwat NR, Roginskaya VY, Acquafondata MB, et al. Immunodetection of DNA repair endonuclease ERCC1-XPF in human tissue. Cancer Res 2009; 69: 6831–8.
78. Booton R, Ward T, Ashcroft L, et al. ERCC1 mRNA expression is not associated with response and survival after platinum-based chemotherapy regimens in advanced non-small cell lung cancer. J Thorac Oncol 2007; 2: 902–6.
79. Cobo M, Isla D, Massuti B, et al. Customizing cisplatin based on quantitative excision repair cross-complementing 1 mRNA expression: a phase III trial in non-small-cell lung cancer. J Clin Oncol 2007; 25: 2747–54.
80. Travis WD. Advances in neuroendocrine lung tumors. Ann Oncol 2010; 21(Suppl 7): vii65–71.
81. Travis WD, Rush W, Flieder DB, et al. Survival analysis of 200 pulmonary neuroendocrine tumors with clarification of criteria for atypical carcinoid and its separation from typical carcinoid. Am J Surg Pathol 1998; 22: 934–44.
82. Nicholson SA, Beasley MB, Brambilla E, et al. Small cell lung carcinoma (SCLC): a clinicopathologic study of 100 cases with surgical specimens. Am J Surg Pathol 2002; 26: 1184–97.
83. Travis WD, Giroux DJ, Chansky K, et al. The IASLC Lung Cancer Staging Project: proposals for the inclusion of broncho-pulmonary carcinoid tumors in the forthcoming (seventh) edition of the TNM Classification for Lung Cancer. J Thorac Oncol 2008; 3: 1213–23.
84. Bailar JC 3rd, Gornik HL. Cancer undefeated. N Engl J Med 1997; 336: 1569–74.

5 | Oncogenic driver mutations

Hiromichi Ebi and Tetsuya Mitsudomi

INTRODUCTION
Oncogene Addiction and Driver Mutation

Human cancers usually evolve through multistep processes that can extend over a period of decades. This process is driven by the accumulation of genetic and epigenetic abnormalities in multiple genes that have highly diverse functions. In contrast to multistep tumorigenesis, the "oncogene addiction" model proposes that some cancers develop through genetic alternation, including mutation, of one gene.[1] These mutations induce and sustain tumorigenesis, and can be thus referred to as "driver mutations." These cancers are reliant upon the protein product of this gene for their malignant phenotype. In these tumors, targeting this protein, or "Achilles heel" of the cancer, can profoundly inhibit its growth and result in patient benefit. Support for this oncogene addiction model comes from the increasing number of examples of the therapeutic efficacy of drugs that target specific oncogenes in human cancers including epidermal growth factor receptor (EGFR) in *EGFR* mutant lung cancer.

While driver mutations have profound impact on the development and sustainability of a cancer, not all the somatic mutations present in a cancer genome have been involved in development of the cancer. Indeed, it is likely that most of them have made no contribution at all. These mutations, called "passenger mutations," have occurred during the growth of the cancer, but have not been selected, have not conferred clonal growth advantage and have therefore not contributed to cancer development. Since these passenger mutations often occur during cell division, a cell may have already biologically inert somatic mutations within its genome when the cell acquires a driver mutation.[2] These mutations are carried along in the clonal expansion that follows and therefore are observed in the mature cancer. A central goal of cancer research involves the discovery and characterization of the driver mutation conferring oncogene addiction, and delineating these mutations from those which merely accumulate passively during tumorigenesis. Therefore, a key challenge is to distinguish driver from passenger mutations.

Currently, we have no gold standard to fully assess the total circuitry that controls cell proliferation, differentiation, and apoptosis in cancer cells. Several empirical approaches can be used to help identify the driver mutations in specific types of human cancer. The methods frequently used to detect driver mutations and the results elucidated by using these methods are shown in Table 5.1. Some studies have unexpectedly pointed to a large percentage of potential driver mutations: for instance, a recent survey of somatic point mutations in a diverse set of human cancer genomes suggested that approximately 120 of the 518 protein kinase genes screened are estimated to carry potential driver mutations.[3] This large-scale sequencing study has also shown that the prevalence and signature of somatic mutations in human cancers are highly variable among patients and tumor origin. In a second study analyzing the whole genome in a lung adenocarcinoma patient, at least eight genes in the EGFR-RAS-RAF-MEK-ERK pathway were either mutated or amplified, and other cancer-related pathways also harbor multiple mutations.[4] Whereas this result might suggest that some tumors have functionally redundant mutations rather than being addicted to single oncogenes, it is likely that one of these mutations is the true driver mutation. Collectively, these studies highlight the need to clearly define driver mutations in cancers precisely because these are the genes that need to be targeted to treat patients successfully.

In this chapter, we will review the driver mutations that have been identified in lung cancer.

IDENTIFIED AND POTENTIAL DRIVER MUTATIONS IN LUNG CANCER
Aberrantly Activated Receptor Tyrosine Kinase Signaling
Activating Mutation of the EGFR Gene

EGFR and its three related proteins (the ERBB family) are receptor tyrosine kinases that play essential roles related to cell proliferation and survival in both physiologically normal and cancerous conditions (Fig. 5.1). Cells with *EGFR* driver mutations become highly dependent on the EGFR pathway, and cancer cells are vulnerable to inhibition of this pathway despite the presence of other "passenger" genetic alterations. *EGFR* mutations are almost exclusively present in adenocarcinoma and are predominantly observed in female

Table 5.1 Approaches to Define Driver Mutations in Lung Cancer

Author, Year	Samples	Method	Findings
Copy number analysis			
Weir BA et al. 2007[75]	371 lung adenocarcinoma	SNP arrays	31 recurrent focal events and NKX2-1 as a novel candidate proto-oncogene
Bass AJ et al. 2009[65]	47 lung SCC samples	SNP arrays	*SOX2* as a lineage-survival oncogene
Beroukim R et al. 2010[76]	3131 cancers including 733 lung cancers	SNP arrays	158 regions of somatic copy number alterations including BCL2 family proteins and NF-kB pathway proteins
Starczynowski DT et al. 2011[77]	261 lung tumors and 85 lung cancer cell lines	array CGH	TRAF6 is an amplified oncogene bridging the RAS and NF-κB pathways
Sanger re-sequencing			
Samuels Y et al. 2004[38]	35 colorectal cancers	sequencing predicted kinase domains of PI3K genes	p110α mutations in colorectal cancer. Validation set identified same mutations in lung cancer samples
Paez JG et al. 2004[78]	58 NSCLC tumors	sequenced the exons encoding the activation loops of 47 of 58 human receptor tyrosine kinase genes	EGFR mutations in gefitinib sensitive lung adenocarcinoma
Ding L et al. 2008[79]	188 lung adenocarcinoma	DNA sequencing of 623 genes that was combined with DNA copy number and gene expression	26 candidate driver mutations, identification of pathways significantly mutated in adenocarcinomas
Whole genome sequencing			
Campbell PJ et al. 2008[2]	a SCLC cell line and a neuroendocrine lung cancer cell line	somatically acquired rearrangements and copy number alterations	306 germline structural variants and 103 somatic rearrangements
Pleasance ED et al. 2010[59]	SCLC cell lines	somatic mutations, rearrangements, and copy number alterations	22,910 somatically acquired substitutions and CHD7 rearrangements in multiple SCLC cell lines
Lee W et al. 2010[4]	an adenocarcinoma patient	somatic mutations, rearrangements, and copy number alterations	530 somatic single nucleotide variants and 43 large scale structural variants

patients, never smokers, and those of Asian ethnicity.[5] In general, about 40% of East-Asian adenocarcinoma patients and 15% of Caucasian adenocarcinoma patients harbor *EGFR* gene mutation.

About 90% of these *EGFR* mutations consist of either short in-frame deletions in exon 19 (usually five amino acids) or point mutations that result in a substitution of leucine to arginine at amino acid 858 (L858R). To date, more than 20 variant types of deletions have been reported. In addition, about 3% of the mutations occur at codon 719, resulting in the substitution of glycine to cysteine, alanine or serine (G719X). Another 3% are in-frame insertion mutations in exon 20. It should be noted that these four types of mutations seldom occur simultaneously. Intriguingly, the tyrosine kinase domain mutations in *EGFR* occur almost specifically in lung cancers.[5,6] EGFR-targeted therapy can be classified into two types: small-molecule EGFR tyrosine kinase inhibitors (TKIs) and antibodies against the extracellular domain of the EGFR. The mutated version of the EGFR can have ~30 times higher affinity for EGFR-TKIs than does wild-type EGFR, which makes mutant EGFR particularly sensitive to EGFR tyrosine kinase inhibitors. Retrospective and prospective studies have shown that the response rate to EGFR-TKIs of patients with *EGFR* mutation is 70–80% and that, when treated with EGFR-TKIs, patients with *EGFR* mutation have a significantly longer survival than those with wild-type *EGFR*. However, it appears that not all patients with *EGFR* mutations respond well to EGFR TKI. For example, the exon 19 deletion and L858R are sensitive, while G719X shows

Early attempts to detect ALK rearrangement by IHC could not achieve satisfactory results because lung cancer expresses lower level of ALK in comparison to the expression levels in anaplastic large cell lymphoma. Since the initial efforts, sensitivity has been improved by utilizing a highly sensitive detection method. The advent of new antibodies to detect ALK by IHC has shown sufficient sensitivity (100%) and specificity (99%), although this mouse monoclonal antibody (D5F3) that was employed to obtain these impressive results is not yet commercially available.[18] Also, modified detection methods with currently available antibodies appear to achieve satisfactory results.[19] Lastly, IHC is a standard assay in the clinic for other purposes, and would be an easier assay to implement in cancer centers across the world. Therefore, IHC screening, however not yet approved in the United States, will likely eclipse FISH as the initial screening procedure to detect ALK overexpression in cancers, with the primary role of FISH most likely being confirmatory.

Clinical Data of ALK Kinase Inhibitor, Crizotinib

The identification of ALK rearrangement prompted researchers to investigate the efficacy of ALK inhibitors in clinic. Fortunately, crizotinib, which was originally designed to inhibit MET kinase activity and had already been assessed in clinic, was also shown to inhibit ALK kinase activity. Crizotinib, 250 mg, was administered orally twice daily to a total of 255 patients with locally advanced or metastatic ALK-positive NSCLC in two single arm trials, PROFILE (N = 136 patients) and Study 1001 (N = 119 patients).[20,21] The primary endpoint of both trials was objective response rate (ORR). In the PROFILE study, the ORR was 50% (95% CI: 42%, 59%) with a median response duration of 42 weeks. In the study 1001, the ORR was 61% (95% CI: 52%, 70%) with a median response duration of 48 weeks. Complete responses were observed in 1% of patients. Interestingly, no difference of response rate was observed in the number of prior chemotherapeutic regimens, or the percentage of cells found to have the ALK gene rearrangement. Transient and reversible vision disorders were characteristic side effects. Crizotinib has been associated with severe, life-threatening, or fatal treatment-related pneumonitis with a frequency of 1.6% in these clinical trials. All cases occurred within two months after the treatment initiation. Based on these results, the FDA granted accelerated approval to crizotinib (Crizotinib® Capsules, Pfizer Inc.) for the treatment of patients with locally advanced or metastatic ALK positive NSCLC in August 2011. Concurrently, the FDA approved the Vysis ALK Break-Apart FISH Probe Kit (Abbott Molecular, Inc.).

Resistant mechanisms of crizotinib have started to be identified. As has been reported in other targeted therapies, gatekeeper mutations within ALK gene (L1196) and other kinase domain mutations have been reported.[22] Resistant tumors harboring mutations within ALK kinase domain are expected to be sensitive to more potent ALK inhibitors such as AP26113 and CH5424802.[23] In addition, activation of an EGFR bypass tract confers resistance to ALK positive NSCLCs.[24]

HER2 Amplification and Point Mutations

HER2 (erbB-2/neu) is a member of the erbB receptor tyrosine kinase family. Whereas these family members usually dimerize upon ligand binding, HER2 has no known ligands. HER2 readily heterodimerizes with other erbB family members and activates downstream signaling including PI3K-AKT and MEK-ERK (Fig. 5.1). The frequencies of HER2 protein overexpression and HER2 gene amplification were reported to be present in 23–36% and in 20%, respectively, of NSCLC.[25] However, while addition of trastuzumab to chemotherapy conferred a survival advantage in breast and gastric cancer patients with HER2 protein expression or gene amplification, trastuzumab failed to show survival benefit in HER2-positive lung cancer.[26] HER2 mutations are also identified in about 2% of NSCLCs. Patients with HER2 mutations were predominantly observed in female, nonsmokers, and adenocarcinomas, featuring patient characteristics similar to those with EGFR mutations.[27] Most HER2 mutations were insertion mutations in a small stretch of exon 20 (codons 774–781 or 775–782) on the COOH-terminal side of the αC-helix. Mutations in similar domains are also observed in EGFR gene and such mutations alter the angle of the ATP binding cleft, resulting in greater activity of EGFR. Indeed, inducible expression of a HER2 mutant (HER2YVMA) in lung epithelium causes invasive adenosquamous carcinomas in mice model.[28] Furthermore, continuous expression of HER2YVMA is essential for tumor maintenance that suggests HER2 mutation is indeed a driver mutation in a subset of lung cancer. Intriguingly, combining dual-specific EGFR/HER2 inhibitor BIBW2992 with the mTORC1 inhibitor rapamycin caused significant reduction of tumor volume in mice xenografts and genetically engineered mice.[28] In addition, there are a small number of case reports of patients whose lung adenocarcinomas harbored a HER2 exon 20 mutation that responded to trastuzumab given with weekly paclitaxel or vinorelbine.[27,29] Single-arm trial of an EGFR/HER2 dual inhibitor BIBW 2992 (Afatinib) is currently ongoing in patients with adenocarcinoma or bronchoalveolar carcinoma harboring HER2 activating mutations.

MET Amplification and Mutation

MET (met proto-oncogene) is a receptor tyrosine kinase that phosphorylates several tyrosine residues after binding its specific ligand, hepatocyte growth factor. Activation of MET signaling leads to epithelial-mesenchymal transition, cell scattering, angiogenesis, proliferation, enhanced cell motility, invasion, and metastasis.[30]

MET amplification is detected in 3% of untreated NSCLC, most of which are adenocarcinomas.[31,32] Also, *MET* gene amplification could be detected in up to 20% of patients with adenocarcinomas who developed acquired resistance to EGFR-TKI.[33] Tumor cell lines with *MET* gene amplification have been shown to be highly sensitive to MET inhibitors in vitro and vivo. Short hairpin RNA-mediated MET knockdown induced significant growth inhibition, G1/S cell cycle arrest, and apoptosis in H1993 cells showing *MET* amplification, whereas it had little or no effect on cell lines not exhibiting *MET* amplification.[34]

In untreated NSCLC, *MET* mutations can be found in about 3% of all cases. These mutations in *MET* are splice mutations that results in deletion of exon 14 coding of the juxtamembrane domain, in contrast to *MET* mutations that occur within the tyrosine kinase domain in sporadic papillary-type renal cell carcinomas, childhood hepatocellular carcinomas, and head and neck squamous cell carcinomas.[31] The juxtamembrane domain is required for the binding with c-Cbl E3-ligase that leads to ubiquitination and receptor degradation. Similar to *MET* amplification, a lung cancer cell line (NCI-H596) harboring a splice variant of *MET* was sensitive to an anti-MET OA-5D5 antibody.[35] These results suggest that MET activation by either gene amplification or splice mutations are driver mutations for a subset of NSCLCs that is likely to respond to molecular therapies targeting MET.

Combination of MetMAb plus erlotinib in patients with previously treated advanced NSCLC was assessed in a randomized phase II trial.[36] MetMAb is a monovalent (1-armed) antibody directed against Met and acts by inhibiting the binding of hepatocyte growth factor to Met, thereby preventing activation of the Met signaling pathway. Whereas there was no benefit in either median PFS or median OS in the overall intent-to-treat population, patients in the MetMAb plus erlotinib arm achieved significant survival benefits (median PFS: 2.9 *vs.* 1.5 months; HR: 0.53; 95% CI: 0.28–0.99; P = 0.04 and median OS: 12.6 *vs.* 3.8 months; HR: 0.37; 95% CI: 0.19–0.72; P = 0.002) in the subset analysis of the patients with Met diagnostic–positive disease. The benefit in OS among the Met diagnostic–positive patient population was observed across patient subgroups regardless of *EGFR* mutations. Another study of a small molecule Met inhibitor, ARQ 197, also suggested that patients with *KRAS* mutations had a particularly robust PFS benefit with Met inhibition therapy.[37] Although these results suggest that the MET pathway itself is a potential therapeutic target, it is not clear that MET inhibitor can actually delay the emergence of resistance by inhibiting MET signaling especially in patient with *EGFR* mutation.

Activating Mutation in PI3K-AKT Signaling

PI3K-AKT signaling plays a significant role in cell growth and survival. Among three classes of PI3Ks grouped according to structure and function, class I$_A$ PI3K is the most clearly implicated in human cancer. Class I$_A$ PI3Ks consist of a regulatory subunit and a catalytic subunit. p110α, which is encoded by *PIK3CA*, is the main catalytic isoform and somatically mutated in cancers, and these mutations promote activation of the PI3K pathway. Class I$_A$ PI3Ks are activated by growth factor stimulation through receptor tyrosine kinases (RTKs). The regulatory subunit, p85, directly binds to phosphotyrosine residues on RTKs and/or adaptors that relieves the intermolecular inhibition of the p110 catalytic subunit by p85 and allows PI3K to localize to the plasma membrane where its substrate, phosphatidylinositol 4,5-bisphosphate (PI[4,5]P$_2$), resides. PI3K phosphorylates PIP$_2$ on the 3′OH position to produce PI(3,4,5)P$_3$ (PIP$_3$). PIP$_3$ propagates intracellular signaling by directly binding pleckstrin homology (PH) domains of various signaling proteins including phosphoinositide-dependent kinase 1 (PDK1) and AKT. PDK1 also activates AKT by phosphorylating AKT at threonine 308. AKT mediates many downstream signaling pathways which contribute to cell growth and survival (Fig. 5.1).

PIK3CA Mutations

The mutations of the *PIK3CA* gene usually occur within two "hotspot" areas, the helical domain (exon 9) and the kinase domain (exon 20).[38] The frequency of *PIK3CA* mutations in lung cancer is about 2%, which is much lower than what is observed in other cancers including colorectal and breast. Clinical characteristics of patients with *PIK3CA* mutant lung cancer remain to be elucidated. Mutational status of *PIK3CA* is not mutually exclusive to *EGFR* or *KRAS*.[39,40] Although *PIK3CA* copy number gains occur at much higher frequencies in lung cancers than activating mutations, the oncogenicity of *PIK3CA* amplification has not yet been proved biologically.[40] The evidence that *PIK3CA* mutations are driver mutations in lung cancer was provided in a series of eloquent experiments in which mice genetically engineered to express mutant *PIK3CA* developed lung adenocarcinoma and subsequent withdrawal of p110 expression in these mice led to rapid and dramatic tumor regression.[41] However, the coexistence of *PIK3CA* mutation with multiple PI3K pathway aberrations or *EGFR* mutation or *KRAS* mutations in a single tumor could suggest that *PIK3CA* mutation is a weak driver mutation.[42] A phase I clinical trial of PI3K inhibitors for lung cancer patients with *PIK3CA* mutation is undergoing.

AKT Mutations

A recurrent gain-of-function mutation E17K (Glu17lys) in the PH domain of the *AKT1* gene has been identified in breast, colon, and ovarian cancers. The E17K mutation results in constitutive activation of AKT1 serine/threonine kinase activity by localization of AKT1 to the plasma membrane in a PI3K dependent manner. Although the AKT1 E17K mutation was found in 2 of 36 patients (5.5%) in the initial report,[43] subsequent reports studying larger populations have suggested the frequency of *AKT* mutations in NSCLC to be about 1%.[44–46] Interestingly, all of the reported tumors harboring AKT1 K17E mutation had squamous cell carcinoma histology. It suggests that the *AKT1* mutation may contribute to the development of squamous cell carcinoma and the prevalence of the mutation might be higher in this histology. An AKT inhibitor, MK-2206, is under clinical trial for lung cancer patients with *AKT*, *PIK3CA*, or PTEN mutations.

Mutations Activating MEK-ERK Signaling

KRAS Mutations

Clinicopathological Characteristics of *KRAS* Mutation

RAS is a small protein with guanosine triphosphate (GTPase) activity. Oncogenic point mutations of RAS impair its intrinsic GTPase activity and confer resistance to GAPs, thereby causing RAS to accumulate in its active GTP-bound state, which sustains the activation of RAS signaling. GTP-bound active RAS binds to more than 20 effector proteins and stimulates downstream signaling cascades. Mutation of the *RAS* gene usually occurs in adenocarcinoma, rarely in squamous cell carcinoma, and never in small cell lung cancer. The frequency is higher in Caucasian patients (~30% of lung adenocarcinomas) versus Asian patients (~10% of lung adenocarcinomas). *KRAS* mutations in lung cancer usually occur at codon 12, occasionally at codon 13, and rarely at codon 61. *KRAS* mutations are associated more with mucinous bronchioloalveolar cell carcinoma (BAC) or lung cancer with goblet cell morphology rather than with non-mucinous BAC.

Recently, the intriguing possibility that not all cancers with *KRAS* mutations are addicted to mutant *KRAS* proteins has emerged.[47] To this point, shRNA targeting KRAS revealed that half of the lung cancer cell lines are resistant to KRAS knockdown. The comparison between these KRAS-dependent and -independent cancer cells showed epithelial mesenchymal transition (EMT) is a characteristic phenotype of KRAS independency.[47] These results may suggest that some unknown pathway(s) also play roles in KRAS-driven tumors since EMT is promoted by several pathways such as Wnt and TGF-β.

Current Approaches to Treat KRAS Mutant Cancers

Since targeting mutant KRAS is not sufficient to kill cancer cells, alternative therapeutic strategies have been developed. Although MEK-ERK signaling is an essential downstream of mutant KRAS, single treatment of MEK inhibitor exhibits variable responses and PI3K pathway activation strongly influences its sensitivity. Therefore, simultaneous downregulation of MEK-ERK and PI3K-AKT may have potential therapeutic value. Indeed, several laboratories have shown that direct concomitant downregulation of PI3K and ERK led to impressive regressions of *KRAS* mutant cancers in vivo.[41,48] The combination of PI3K inhibitor and MEK inhibitor is under phase I trials.

Another approach is compound screening coupled with large cohorts of cell lines harboring various driver mutations that enables the identification of the candidate compound targeting only *KRAS* mutant cell lines. In a pilot study, screening of 12 inhibitors in 84 genomically validated cell lines identified that *KRAS* mutant cells conferred enhanced heat shock protein (HSP) 90 dependency that was also confirmed in vivo.[49]

Synthetic Lethal Approach to Identify Targets for KRAS Mutant Cancers

Recently, a synthetic lethal approach has been applied to identify a strategy for the treatment of *KRAS* mutant cancers (results are summarized in Table 5.2). The concept of synthetic lethality is that loss of

Table 5.2 Genes of Synthetic Lethal Interaction with Mutant KRAS

Author, Year	Methods	Identified proteins
Luo J et al. 2009[50]	pooled shRNA screening	PLK1
Barbie DA et al. 2009[51]	one well shRNA screening	TBK1
Scholl C et al. 2009[52]	one well shRNA screening	STK33
Babij C et al. 2011[53]	siRNA library screening	Invalidated STK33
Vicent S et al. 2010[80]	Pooled shRNA screening	WT1
Puyol M et al. 2010[81]	non screening	Cdk4

function of one gene results in cell death only in the presence of genetic alteration of the other, in this case *KRAS* mutation, while loss of function of either gene alone does not affect viability.

Luo et al. used pooled screening to identify proteins showing synthetic lethality with KRAS. In this screen, *KRAS* wild-type and mutant cells are infected with an shRNA library.[50] Cells in both populations that are successfully infected with shRNA are sequenced to determine whether certain shRNAs are depleted only in *KRAS* mutant cells. This method has identified several genes with synthetic lethality in *KRAS* mutant models, including components of the anaphase promoting complex (APC/C) and PLK1, suggesting an increased dependency of *KRAS*-mutant cells on mitotic checkpoints and progression. Importantly, xenograft models in mice using these *KRAS*-mutant cell lines show regression upon treatment with a PLK1 inhibitor. PLK1 inhibitors are currently in clinical trials.

Concurrently, Barbie et al. performed a single-well shRNA screen in 19 different cell lines to identify synthetic genetic interactions with oncogenic KRAS.[51] In single-well arrays, shRNAs are transduced at 1 per well. Negative effect on growth and survival is evaluated individually by direct comparison of corresponding wells in different plates containing *KRAS* wild-type and mutant cells. They identified a synthetic lethal interaction between KRAS and TBK1, and were able to validate this interaction in an isogenic cell line panel and an independent panel of lung cancer cell lines. TBK1 activates NF-κB by inhibiting IκB, an inhibitor of NF-κB, and results in the activation of prosurvival proteins including Bcl-xl. In addition, inhibition of NF-κB by dominant-negative IκB remarkably decreased both the number and the size of lung tumors induced by mutant KRAS. These results suggest that while NF-κB and TBK1 do not have a direct genetic interaction with KRAS, they are linked to characteristics associated with the addiction to oncogenic KRAS signaling.

However, notwithstanding the potential power of RNAi screening, one should be cautious to interpret the data. The main problem, "off-target effect," describes the phenomenon of individual siRNAs (or shRNAs) that have been shown to downregulate tens or even hundreds of genes by binding in a micro RNA-like manner to the 3′ untranslated regions of off-target mRNAs. For example, the single-well shRNA screen led to the identification of STK33. The oncogenic KRAS-dependent effects were tested in a large panel of tumor cell lines from different origins and showed that the dependency on STK33 correlated with addiction to oncogenic KRAS expression.[52] However, a subsequent and comprehensive study from a pharmaceutical company could not reproduce these results, despite performing siRNA rescreening, dominant mutant overexpression, and employing small molecule inhibitors that targeted STK33.[53] Thus, validation of initial screening results is critical. Usually, multiple individual siRNA or shRNA sequences are used to cause the same phenotype, and rescue experiments are performed with cDNA sequences that are resistant to RNAi.

BRAF Mutations

BRAF lies downstream of KRAS, and directly phosphorylates MEK, which in turns phosphorylates ERK. The pathway culminates in the transcription of genes favoring proliferation and survival, as well as the translational alteration of the pro-apoptotic protein, BIM (Fig. 5.1). The frequency of *BRAF* mutation ranges from 1% to 4% in NSCLC, most of which are found in adenocarcinomas.[54–56] *BRAF* mutations were originally found in melanoma. The most common mutation in melanoma is a valine to glutamine substitution at codon 600 (V600E), which accounts for more than 90% of *BRAF* mutations in this cancer.[57] In contrast, the V600E substitution was observed in only half of NSCLC patients with *BRAF* mutation. Non-V600E mutations were distributed in two regions of the kinase domain: the activation segment in exon 15 (codon 594 to 606) and glycine rich loop in exon 11 (codon 446 to 449). Expression of the *BRAF* V600E mutation in lung epithelial cells is required for tumor maintenance in a model of mouse lung cancer suggesting at least *BRAF*

Table 5.3 Potential Driver Mutations in Squamous Cell Lung Cancer

Targets	Methods	Frequency (%)	Possible treatment	Reference
FGFR1 amplifications	SNP arrays	22	FGFR-TKIs	60
DDR2 mutations	Sanger sequencing of entire tyrosine kinome	3.2	Dasatinib, Nilotinib	62
EGFRvIII mutations	Target sequencing	5	EGFR-TKIs	64
PIK3CA mutations	Target sequencing	3.6	PI3K inhibitors	40
SOX2 amplifications	SNP arrays	23	n.d	65

Abbreviation: n.d, not determined.

V600E is an oncogene driver mutation in lung cancer.[58] Similar to *KRAS* mutation, recent larger analyses suggest that *BRAF* mutations occur most often in former or current smokers compared with patients never smoked.[54,55] In addition, V600E mutations were associated with a more aggressive tumor histotype, and were independently associated with poor prognosis.[54] Whereas oncogenic driver mutations are thought to be mutually exclusive, a recent report has observed concomitant *BRAF* and *EGFR* mutations in 2 of 21 patients harboring V600E mutations.[54]

Oncogene Driver Mutations in Squamous Cell Lung Cancer

Although the genome in the adenocarcinoma of the lung has been extensively characterized, driver mutations in squamous cell lung carcinoma are largely unknown. One plausible reason is that most patients with squamous cancer are smokers. Smoking leads to an acceleration of mutations due to the exposure to tobacco carcinogens.[59] At this time there are no FDA-approved targeted therapies for squamous cell lung cancer; however, several potential therapeutic windows have recently emerged (summarized in Table 5.3).

Fibroblast Growth Factor Receptor Amplification

High-resolution gene copy number analyses of a set of 232 lung cancer specimens, including 155 squamous cell carcinomas, identified frequent and focal fibroblast growth factor receptor 1 (FGFR1) amplification in squamous cell lung cancer, but not in other lung cancer subtypes.[60] FISH confirmed the presence of *FGFR1* amplifications in an independent cohort of squamous cell lung cancer samples (22% of cases). In addition, an FGFR inhibitor suppressed growth and induced apoptosis in vitro and in vivo. Thus, *FGFR1* may be the first driver mutation identified in squamous cell carcinoma.

DDR2

The discoidin domain receptors (DDRs), DDR1 and DDR2, comprise a family of RTKs that function as collagen receptors. Several collagen types, both fibrillar and non-fibrillar types, activate the DDRs, with the two receptors displaying different specificities for certain collagen types. Structurally, the DDRs are characterized by the presence of a collagen-binding discoidin homology domain and a domain unique to the DDRs (stalk region) in their extracellular regions. A transmembrane region is followed by a large cytoplasmic juxtamembrane domain, and, finally a C-terminal tyrosine kinase domain. The DDRs control fundamental cellular processes including cell proliferation, adhesion, and migration. In addition, the DDRs regulate extracellular matrix remodeling by controlling matrix metalloproteinase expression and activity. Both receptors are associated with human diseases, including fibrotic disorders of the lung (DDR1) and several types of malignancies. Although the downstream signaling of DDR2 remains to be elucidated, full activation of DDR2 requires the presence of ShcA and Src-like tyrosine kinases.[61]

DDR2 mutation was found by Sanger re-sequencing of 201 genes including the entire tyrosine kinome. Following validation, cohort analysis identified *DDR2* mutations in 3.2% of tumor samples from 277 lung SCC patients.[62] Mutations were found in both the kinase and in other domains. shRNA knockdown of DDR2 lowered cell proliferation in *DDR2* mutant SCC cell lines and a potent DDR2 inhibitor dasatinib achieved tumor shrinkage in a mouse xenograft model of *DDR2*-mutated lung SCC. Although Src and STAT5 are shown as potential downstream targets, their inhibition might be caused by the off-target effects of dasatinib, a notoriously promiscuous drug.[63] Additionally, it is unclear whether dasatinib can be tolerated by patients at the doses necessary to inhibit DDR2. Nonetheless, this clinically approved drug may be a rational and accessible treatment option for *DDR2*-mutated lung SCC. In addition, more specific DDR2 inhibitors are under development.

EGFR vIII

EGFR variant III (EGFRvIII) is a truncation mutation in the extracellular domain that eliminates exons 2–7 resulting in a distorted ligand-binding region. EGFRvIII does not bind ligand but is constitutively activated in a ligand-independent manner. The presence of EGFRvIII in human tumors has been associated with proliferative advantage, metastasis, and survival in several malignancies. EGFRvIII mutation is most commonly observed in glioblastoma, and also observed in about 5% of human lung squamous cell carcinoma but not in adenocarcinoma.[64] Tissue-specific expression of EGFRvIII in the murine lung led to the development of NSCLC and these tumors are highly sensitive to irreversible EGFR inhibitors.[64] In addition, coexpression of EGFRvIII and PTEN was significantly associated with a clinical response to EGFR-TKI in patients with glioblastoma.

SOX2

SNP arrays of DNA samples derived from lung SCCs identified that the region containing SOX2 on chromosome 3 was amplified in 23% of samples.[65] Interestingly, 8p12, in which FGFR is located, also was shown to be amplified in this study. SOX2 is a well-studied developmental marker of early progenitor cells in various tissues, including tracheal epithelium, and is one of the key components that induce a pluripotency state in differentiated somatic cells. In the bronchoscopic samples, SOX2 amplification effectively segregates high-grade dysplasia from low-grade dysplasia, suggesting that SOX2 gene amplification may be an initial event in the course of SCC development.[66] Furthermore, downregulation of SOX2 expression decreased cell proliferation while exogenous expression of SOX2 led to squamous differentiation, as evidenced by the induced expression of p63 and cytokeratin 6A.[67] In terms of transforming activity of SOX2, somewhat conflicting results were reported. Whereas SOX2 could not transform an immortalized tracheobronchial epithelial cell model in the original report,[65] a second report showed that SOX2 overexpression transformed an immortalized lung epithelial model (BEAS-2B cells).[67] The former result suggests a role for SOX2 as a lineage survival gene in contrast to the latter result that is more consistent with the criteria for a bona-fide oncogene. Despite some conflicting results, SOX2 appears to play a critical role in the survival of a fraction of SCC, thus serving as a therapeutic target.

Other Candidate Genes

In addition to these potential candidates of driver mutations in squamous cell lung cancer, the mutational landscape of head and neck squamous carcinoma (HNSCC) was recently reported.[68,69] Intriguingly, point mutations in NOTCH1 or NOTCH2/3 occurred independently, and both at the same rate of occurrence in HNSCC patients (11%). These mutations are more frequently observed than that of several genes that had previously been implicated in HNSCC—including TP53, CDKN2A, HRAS, PTEN, and PIK3CA. Some similarity between squamous cell lung cancer and HNSCC, especially, chromosomal abnormality, may suggest an abnormality in Notch signaling in lung cancer. Indeed, gain-of-function mutations of NOTCH1 gene were also reported in lung squamous cell carcinoma,[70] a finding worthy of further exploration.

EFFORTS TO DEFINE THE FREQUENCY OF DRIVER MUTATIONS: REPORTS FROM LUNG CANCER MUTATION CONSORTIUM AND OTHER GROUPS

From clinical standpoints, the screening of driver mutations requires a clinically relevant method which is necessary to be cost effective, rapid, reliable, and less labor intensive. Currently, several platforms are used in the clinic for multiplexed analysis of point mutations in DNA from formalin fixed paraffin embedded tissue samples. Among them, Sequenom's MassARRAY system is based on multiplexed PCR, multiplexed single-base primer extension, and analysis of primer extension products using mass spectrometry. The "SNaPshot" system analyzes fluorescently labeled primer-extension products by conventional capillary electrophoresis. The identity of the incorporated nucleotide in these assays indicates the presence or absence of a mutation. In one clinical application, SNaPshot assesses DNA samples simultaneously for 38 somatic recurrent point mutations in eight genes with relevance to targeted therapies specifically in lung cancer.[71] For comparison, while mutant DNA must comprise 25% of the total molecules of DNA for direct sequence analysis to pick up, SNaPshot and sizing assays can detect mutations in samples in which mutant DNA comprises of only 1.56% to 12.5% and 1.56% to 6.25% of the total DNA, respectively. In addition, SNaPshot assays cost 80% less compared to direct sequencing of each mutation. One of the limitations of SNaPshot is that it cannot detect amplifications, insertions, or deletions.

These techniques led 14 leading hospitals in the United States to found the National Cancer Institute's Lung Cancer Mutation Consortium, an initiative created to identify the frequencies and characteristics of

23. Sakamoto H, Tsukaguchi T, Hiroshima S, et al. CH5424802, a selective ALK inhibitor capable of blocking the resistant gatekeeper mutant. Cancer Cell 2011; 19: 679–90.

24. Sasaki T, Koivunen J, Ogino A, et al. A Novel ALK Secondary Mutation and EGFR Signaling Cause Resistance to ALK Kinase Inhibitors. Cancer Res 2011; 71: 6051–60.

25. Pellegrini C, Falleni M, Marchetti A, et al. HER-2/Neu alterations in non-small cell lung cancer: a comprehensive evaluation by real time reverse transcription-PCR, fluorescence in situ hybridization, and immunohistochemistry. Clin Cancer Res 2003; 9(10 Pt 1): 3645–52.

26. Gatzemeier U, Groth G, Butts C, et al. Randomized phase II trial of gemcitabine-cisplatin with or without trastuzumab in HER2-positive non-small-cell lung cancer. Ann Oncol 2004; 15: 19–27.

27. Tomizawa K, Suda K, Onozato R, et al. Prognostic and predictive implications of HER2/ERBB2/neu gene mutations in lung cancers. Lung Cancer 2011; 74: 139–44.

28. Perera SA, Li D, Shimamura T, et al. HER2YVMA drives rapid development of adenosquamous lung tumors in mice that are sensitive to BIBW2992 and rapamycin combination therapy. Proc Natl Acad Sci USA 2009; 106: 474–9.

29. Cappuzzo F, Bemis L, Varella-Garcia M. HER2 mutation and response to trastuzumab therapy in non-small-cell lung cancer. N Engl J Med 2006; 354: 2619–21.

30. Trusolino L, Bertotti A, Comoglio PM. MET signalling: principles and functions in development, organ regeneration and cancer. Nat Rev Mol Cell Biol 2010; 11: 834–48.

31. Onozato R, Kosaka T, Kuwano H, et al. Activation of MET by gene amplification or by splice mutations deleting the juxtamembrane domain in primary resected lung cancers. J Thorac Oncol 2009; 4: 5–11.

32. Bean J, Brennan C, Shih JY, et al. MET amplification occurs with or without T790M mutations in EGFR mutant lung tumors with acquired resistance to gefitinib or erlotinib. Proc Natl Acad Sci USA 2007; 104: 20932–7.

33. Engelman JA, Zejnullahu K, Mitsudomi T, et al. MET amplification leads to gefitinib resistance in lung cancer by activating ERBB3 signaling. Science 2007; 316: 1039–43.

34. Lutterbach B, Zeng Q, Davis LJ, et al. Lung cancer cell lines harboring MET gene amplification are dependent on Met for growth and survival. Cancer Res 2007; 67: 2081–8.

35. Kong-Beltran M, Seshagiri S, Zha J, et al. Somatic mutations lead to an oncogenic deletion of met in lung cancer. Cancer Res 2006; 66: 283–9.

36. Spigel D, Ervin TJ, Ramlau R, et al. Final efficacy results from OAM4558g, a randomized phase II study evaluating MetMAb or placebo in combination with erlotinib in advanced NSCLC. J Clin Oncol 2011; 29: Abst 7505.

37. Schiller JH, Akerley WL, Brugger W, et al. Results from ARQ 197–209: a global randomized placebo-controlled phase II clinical trial of erlotinib plus ARQ 197 versus erlotinib plus placebo in previously treated EGFR inhibitor-naive patients with locally advanced or metastatic non-small cell lung cancer (NSCLC). J Clin Oncol 2010; 28(Suppl 18): LBA7502.

38. Samuels Y, Wang Z, Bardelli A, et al. High frequency of mutations of the PIK3CA gene in human cancers. Science 2004; 304: 554.

39. Endoh H, Yatabe Y, Kosaka T, Kuwano H, Mitsudomi T. PTEN and PIK3CA expression is associated with prolonged survival after gefitinib treatment in EGFR-mutated lung cancer patients. J Thorac Oncol 2006; 1: 629–34.

40. Yamamoto H, Shigematsu H, Nomura M, et al. PIK3CA mutations and copy number gains in human lung cancers. Cancer Res 2008; 68: 6913–21.

41. Engelman JA, Chen L, Tan X, et al. Effective use of PI3K and MEK inhibitors to treat mutant Kras G12D and PIK3CA H1047R murine lung cancers. Nat Med 2008; 14: 1351–6.

42. Yuan TL, Cantley LC. PI3K pathway alterations in cancer: variations on a theme. Oncogene 2008; 27: 5497–510.

43. Malanga D, Scrima M, De Marco C, et al. Activating E17K mutation in the gene encoding the protein kinase AKT1 in a subset of squamous cell carcinoma of the lung. Cell Cycle 2008; 7: 665–9.

44. Bleeker FE, Felicioni L, Buttitta F, et al. AKT1(E17K) in human solid tumours. Oncogene 2008; 27: 5648–50.

45. Do H, Salemi R, Murone C, Mitchell PL, Dobrovic A. Rarity of AKT1 and AKT3 E17K mutations in squamous cell carcinoma of lung. Cell Cycle 2010; 9: 4411–12.

46. Kim MS, Jeong EG, Yoo NJ, Lee SH. Mutational analysis of oncogenic AKT E17K mutation in common solid cancers and acute leukaemias. Br J Cancer 2008; 98: 1533–5.

47. Singh A, Greninger P, Rhodes D, et al. A gene expression signature associated with "K-Ras addiction" reveals regulators of EMT and tumor cell survival. Cancer Cell 2009; 15: 489–500.

48. Sos ML, Fischer S, Ullrich R, et al. Identifying genotype-dependent efficacy of single and combined PI3K- and MAPK-pathway inhibition in cancer. Proc Natl Acad Sci USA 2009; 106: 18351–6.

49. Sos ML, Michel K, Zander T, et al. Predicting drug susceptibility of non-small cell lung cancers based on genetic lesions. J Clin Invest 2009; 119: 1727–40.

50. Luo J, Eumanuele MJ, Li D, et al. A genome-wide RNAi screen identifies multiple synthetic lethal interactions with the Ras oncogene. Cell 2009; 137: 835–48.

51. Barbie DA, Tamayo P, Boehm JS, et al. Systematic RNA interference reveals that oncogenic KRAS-driven cancers require TBK1. Nature 2009; 462: 108–12.

52. Scholl C, Fröhling S, Dunn IF, et al. Synthetic lethal interaction between oncogenic KRAS dependency and STK33 suppression in human cancer cells. Cell 2009; 137: 821–34.

53. Babij C, Zhang Y, Kurzeja RJ, et al. STK33 kinase activity is nonessential in KRAS-dependent cancer cells. Cancer Res 2011; 71: 5818–26.
54. Marchetti A, Felicioni L, Malatesta S, et al. Clinical features and outcome of patients with non-small-cell lung cancer harboring BRAF mutations. J Clin Oncol 2011; 29: 3574–9.
55. Paik PK, Arcila ME, Fara M, et al. Clinical characteristics of patients with lung adenocarcinomas harboring BRAF mutations. J Clin Oncol 2011; 29: 2046–51.
56. Yousem SA, Nikiforova M, Nikiforov Y. The histopathology of BRAF-V600E-mutated lung adenocarcinoma. Am J Surg Pathol 2008; 32: 1317–21.
57. Davies H, Bignell GR, Cox C, et al. Mutations of the BRAF gene in human cancer. Nature 2002; 417: 949–54.
58. Ji H, Wang Z, Perera SA, et al. Mutations in BRAF and KRAS converge on activation of the mitogen-activated protein kinase pathway in lung cancer mouse models. Cancer Res 2007; 67: 4933–9.
59. Pleasance ED, Stephens PJ, O'Meara S, et al. A small-cell lung cancer genome with complex signatures of tobacco exposure. Nature 2010; 463: 184–90.
60. Weiss J, Sos ML, Seidel D, et al. Frequent and focal FGFR1 amplification associates with therapeutically tractable FGFR1 dependency in squamous cell lung cancer. Sci Transl Med 2010; 2: 62ra93.
61. Vogel WF, Abdulhussein R, Ford CE. Sensing extracellular matrix: an update on discoidin domain receptor function. Cell Signal 2006; 18: 1108–16.
62. Hammerman PS, Sos ML, Ramos AH, et al. Mutations in the DDR2 kinase gene identify a novel therapeutic target in squamous cell lung cancer. Cancer Discovery 2011; 1: 78–89.
63. Li J, Rix U, Fang B, et al. A chemical and phosphoproteomic characterization of dasatinib action in lung cancer. Nat Chem Biol 2010; 6: 291–9.
64. Ji H, Zhao X, Yuza Y, et al. Epidermal growth factor receptor variant III mutations in lung tumorigenesis and sensitivity to tyrosine kinase inhibitors. Proc Natl Acad Sci USA 2006; 103: 7817–22.
65. Bass AJ, Watanabe H, Mermel CH, et al. SOX2 is an amplified lineage-survival oncogene in lung and esophageal squamous cell carcinomas. Nat Genet 2009; 41: 1238–42.
66. McCaughan F, Pole JC, Bankier AT, et al. Progressive 3q amplification consistently targets SOX2 in preinvasive squamous lung cancer. Am J Respir Crit Care Med 2010; 182: 83–91.
67. Hussenet T, Dali S, Exinger J, et al. SOX2 is an oncogene activated by recurrent 3q26.3 amplifications in human lung squamous cell carcinomas. PLoS One 2010; 5: e8960.
68. Agrawal N, Frederick MJ, Pickering CR, et al. Exome sequencing of head and neck squamous cell carcinoma reveals inactivating mutations in NOTCH1. Science 2011; 333: 1154–7.
69. Stransky N, Egloff AM, Tward AD, et al. The mutational landscape of head and neck squamous cell carcinoma. Science 2011; 333: 1157–60.
70. Westhoff B, Colaluca IN, D'Ario G, et al. Alterations of the Notch pathway in lung cancer. Proc Natl Acad Sci USA 2009; 106: 22293–8.
71. Su Z, Dias-Santagata D, Duke M, et al. A platform for rapid detection of multiple oncogenic mutations with relevance to targeted therapy in non-small-cell lung cancer. J Mol Diagn 2011; 13: 74–84.
72. Kris MG, Johnson BE, Kwiatkowski DJ, et al. Identification of driver mutations in tumor specimens from 1,000 patients with lung adenocarcinoma: The NCI's Lung Cancer Mutation Consortium (LCMC). J Clin Oncol 2011; 29: CRA7506.
73. Sun Y, Ren Y, Fang Z, et al. Lung adenocarcinoma from East Asian never-smokers is a disease largely defined by targetable oncogenic mutant kinases. J Clin Oncol 2010; 28: 4616–20.
74. Parsons DW, Jones S, Zhang X, et al. An integrated genomic analysis of human glioblastoma multiforme. Science 2008; 321: 1807–12.
75. Weir BA, Woo MS, Getz G, et al. Characterizing the cancer genome in lung adenocarcinoma. Nature 2007; 450: 893–8.
76. Beroukhim R, Mermel CH, Porter D, et al. The landscape of somatic copy-number alteration across human cancers. Nature 2010; 463: 899–905.
77. Starczynowski DT, Lockwood WW, Delehouzee S, et al. TRAF6 is an amplified oncogene bridging the RAS and NF-kappaB pathways in human lung cancer. J Clin Invest 2011; 121: 4095–4105.
78. Paez JG, Janne PA, Lee JC, et al. EGFR mutations in lung cancer: correlation with clinical response to gefitinib therapy. Science 2004; 304: 1497–1500.
79. Ding L, Getz G, Wheeler DA, et al. Somatic mutations affect key pathways in lung adenocarcinoma. Nature 2008; 455: 1069–75.
80. Vicent S, Chen R, Sayles LC, et al. Wilms tumor 1 (WT1) regulates KRAS-driven oncogenesis and senescence in mouse and human models. J Clin Invest 2010; 120: 3940–52.
81. Puyol M, Martin A, Dubus P, et al. A synthetic lethal interaction between K-Ras oncogenes and Cdk4 unveils a therapeutic strategy for non-small cell lung carcinoma. Cancer Cell 2010; 18: 63–73.

6 | First-line therapy of advanced non-small cell lung cancer not harboring an activating EGFR mutation

Cesare Gridelli and Antonio Rossi

INTRODUCTION

Non-small cell lung cancer (NSCLC) represents around 80% of all lung cancers. The three most common histological subtypes of NSCLC are squamous-cell carcinoma, adenocarcinoma, and large cell carcinoma.[1] Unfortunately, a majority of patients have advanced unresectable disease at diagnosis. For advanced disease, systemic therapy is the standard approach with palliation, quality of life (QoL), and prolongation of life being the primary goals of therapy. In this situation, the five-year survival rate measured by the surveillance, epidemiology, and end results (SEER) program in the United States is 16.8%,[2] and Europe's average is 12%.[3]

Recent advances in the knowledge of tumor biology and mechanisms of oncogenesis have led to the identification of specific molecular targets for specific treatment of advanced NSCLC, the first being the epidermal growth factor receptor (EGFR) pathway. Today the identification of activating EGFR mutation is key in the selection of the first-line systemic therapy. This chapter focuses on the first-line treatment of patients with NSCLC with a good performance status (PS 0–1) in the absence of an activating EGFR mutation by elaborating the following aspects of management: chemotherapy, targeted therapy, and maintenance therapy.

CHEMOTHERAPY

During 1970s and 1980s, the role of chemotherapy in the treatment of advanced NSCLC was uncertain. To better understand this issue, an individual patient data (IPD) meta-analysis of 11 randomized trials (1,190 patients and 1,144 deaths) of chemotherapy versus best supportive care (BSC), eight of which used cisplatin-based chemotherapy, was performed. A survival advantage (1.5 months in median overall survival [OS]) for cisplatin-based chemotherapy was reported.[4] All these trials recruited patients during 1980s when old cisplatin-based regimens were used. Starting from these data and with the availability of new generation of chemotherapeutic agents, several additional randomized trials comparing chemotherapy with BSC were performed. These studies were pooled in a new updated IPD meta-analysis to evaluate again the role of chemotherapy in advanced NSCLC.[5] This new meta-analysis, including 16 trials for a total of 2,714 patients (2,533 deaths), confirmed the OS advantage of 1.5 months (from 4.5 to 6 months) for chemotherapy over BSC (hazard ratio [HR] 0.77, 95% confidence interval [CI] 0.71–0.83; $p < 0.0001$) with an absolute survival improvement of 9% at 12 months (from 20% to 29%)[5] (Table 6.1). In both meta-analyses, there was no clear evidence of a difference or trend in the relative effect of chemotherapy in patient subgroups defined by age, sex, stage, histology, or PS.

These data demonstrated conclusively that chemotherapy increases OS for all groups of patients affected by advanced NSCLC and should be always the first choice in the clinical practice.

Third-Generation Chemotherapeutics

During the 1990s, third-generation agents (gemcitabine, docetaxel, paclitaxel, or vinorelbine) were investigated with the following results: (1) single-agent therapy, in most cases, improved survival and QoL versus BSC[6–9]; (2) third-generation cisplatin-based doublets generally improved survival outcomes versus cisplatin alone[10–12]; (3) third-generation cisplatin-based doublets improved the objective response rate (ORR) and QoL, although with no OS benefit, as compared with older combinations such as platinum and etoposide or vindesine.[13–16]

As a result of these observations, the third-generation platinum-based combinations became the first-line therapy for patients with NSCLC. However, no single combination has demonstrated superiority. In fact, at least four large randomized phase III trials failed to demonstrate a clear advantage for any of new regimens. In these studies, an ORR of 17–32%, a median OS ranging from 7.4 to 11.3 months, and one-year survival rates of 31–46% were reported[17–20] (Table 6.2). These results lead to the belief that in clinical practice the different

Table 6.1 Results of Individual Patient Data Meta-Analyses of Randomized Trials Comparing Chemotherapy Versus Best Supportive Care

Author, year	Treatment	No. Trials	No. Pts	HR (95% CI) for OS	*p*-value	% absolute survival benefit
NSCLC Collaborative Group, 1995[4]	Long-term alkylating agents	2	141	1.26 (0.96–1.66)	0.095	– 6
	vs.					
	BSC		85			
	Vinca alkaloids/ etoposide	1	111	0.87 (0.64–1.20)	0.40	4
	vs.					
	BSC		75			
	Cisplatin-based	8	416	0.73 (0.63–0.85)	<0.0001	10
	vs.					
	BSC		362			
NSCLC Collaborative Group, 2008[5]	Anti-metabolic agent only	1	148	0.91 (0.70–1.17)	0.466	
	vs.					
	BSC		152			
	Taxane only	1	79	0.69 (0.49–0.97)	0.032	
	vs.					
	BSC		78			
	Vinca-alkaloid/ Etoposide only	2	191	0.80 (0.64–1.01)	0.057	9[a]
	vs.					
	BSC		156			
	Platinum+vinca- alkaloid/etoposide	9	623	0.77 (0.68–0.86)	<0.0001	
	vs.					
	BSC		578			
	Other platinum regimens	3	358	0.73 (0.63–0.85)	<0.0001	
	vs.					
	BSC		351			

[a]Absolute survival benefit for all chemotherapy treatments versus BSC.
Abbreviations: Pts, patients; HR, hazard ratio; CI, confidence interval; BSC, best supportive care; OS, overall survival.

Table 6.2 Results from Randomized Phase III Trials Investigating the Most Used Third-Generation Platinum-Based Doublets for the Treatment of Advanced Non-Small Cell Lung Cancer

Regimen	ORR (%)	TTP (months)	OS (months)
Cisplatin + Vinorelbine	24–30	4.6–5	9.5–10.1
Cisplatin + Gemcitabine	22–32	4.2–5.3	8.1–9.8
Cisplatin + Docetaxel	17–31	3.7–5	7.4–11.3
Carboplatin + Paclitaxel	17–30	3.1–5.5	8.1–9.9
Cisplatin + Pemetrexed[a]	29	5.5[b]	12.6

[a]Only adenocarcinoma histology.
[b]Progression-free survival.
Abbreviations: ORR, objective response rate; TTP, time-to-progression; OS, overall survival.

regimens were equally effective, albeit having different toxicity profiles. While some differences regarding outcomes were considered to exist, these would have been too small to be detected by insufficiently powered studies.

Some meta-analyses attempted to assess the therapeutic equivalence of available third-generation agents. A meta-analysis including 13 trials (4,556 patients) reported that gemcitabine–platinum regimens produced a statistically significant reduced risk of mortality (HR for survival 0.90, 95% CI 0.84–0.96) with an absolute OS benefit of 3.9% at one year and 2.6% at two years. However, the analysis of all trials with a platinum based third-generation agent comparator showed a trend, favoring gemcitabine–platinum regimens that was not statistically significant (HR 0.93, CI 0.86–1.01).[11] Another meta-analysis of seven trials, including 2,867 patients, comparing docetaxel-containing with vinca alkaloids-containing regimens (vinorelbine in six trials and vindesine in one) showed a significant survival benefit (HR for death 0.89, CI 0.82–0.96; p = 0.004) and more favorable toxicity profile for the former. In fact, grade 3–4 neutropenia and grade 3–4 serious adverse events were less frequent with docetaxel- versus vinca alkaloid-based regimens (odds ratio [OR] 0.59, 95% CI 0.38–0.89; p = 0.013 and OR 0.68, 95% CI 0.55–0.84; p < 0.001, respectively).[22] A further meta-analysis assessed the relative impact of different third-generation drugs on the activity of first-line chemotherapy by considering both ORRs and progressive disease rates as outcome measures. A total of 45 trials, including 11,867 patients, were considered eligible. The odds of obtaining an ORR to treatment were similar across different regimens. Gemcitabine-based chemotherapy was associated with a 14% lower risk for immediate progression, whereas patients receiving paclitaxel showed a 22% higher risk for having progression as the best response. Docetaxel treatment provided a non-significant 9% lower odds for progression.[23]

These data demonstrate that different third-generation agents and regimens have comparable efficacy in chemotherapy-naïve patients with advanced NSCLC. So, the two-drug regimen in which cisplatin or carboplatin is combined with a third-generation agent should be the standard first-line treatment for fit (PS 0–1) patients and the selection of the most appropriate regimen should not be based on efficacy evaluations only but tolerability, convenience, incidence and manageability of adverse side effects, and direct and indirect costs of therapy are all important decision criteria.

Non-Platinum-Based Therapy

The advent of better-tolerated third-generation agents led to the hypothesis that platinum compounds could be excluded from first-line combination therapy to increase patient tolerance in situations of poor PS or comorbidities and to avoid toxicities associated in particular with cisplatin. Several studies investigated the efficacy of platinum-free combination therapies, in particular taxane-based regimens which were the focus of intense research. The combination of docetaxel and gemcitabine reported similar efficacy but better tolerability when compared with cisplatin plus vinorelbine schedule within two randomized phase III trials.[24,25] Also paclitaxel plus gemcitabine combination were equally effective as carboplatin-based regimens, but with different toxicity profiles.[26,27] Our group, in cooperation with the National Cancer Institute of Canada, performed a randomized phase III trial comparing the combination of gemcitabine plus vinorelbine versus a cisplatin-based regimen (cisplatin plus gemcitabine or vinorelbine). The results were similar in terms of ORRs and QoL scores. Hematologic toxicity, renal toxicity, and ototoxicity were seen in the platinum arm to a greater extent, but more hepatic toxicity was seen in the gemcitabine plus vinorelbine arm. The study concluded that the gemcitabine plus vinorelbine regimen is an alternative to platinum-based therapy.[28]

Two main meta-analyses compared platinum-based versus non-platinum-containing regimens.[29,30] The first analyzed 37 randomized trials for a total of 7,633 patients. The one-year survival rate was increased by 5% with platinum-based regimens (34% vs. 29%; OR 1.21, 95% CI 1.09–1.35; p = 0.0003), but there was no statistically significant increase in one-year survival when platinum therapies were compared with third generation-based free-platinum combination regimens (OR 1.11, 95% CI 0.96–1.28; p = 0.17). The toxicity of platinum-based regimens was significantly higher for hematologic toxicity, renal toxicity, and nausea and vomiting, but not for neurotoxicity, febrile neutropenia, or toxic deaths.[29] The second meta-analysis included 11 phase III trials (2,298 and 2,304 patients in platinum-based and non-platinum arms, respectively). Patients treated with a platinum-based regimen reported a 12% reduction in the risk of death at one year (OR 0.88, 95% CI 0.78–0.99; p = 0.044). Forty-four (1.9%) and 29 (1.3%) toxic-related deaths were reported for platinum-based and non-platinum-based regimens, respectively (OR 1.53, 95% CI 0.96–2.49; p = 0.08). A statistically increase in grade 3–4 gastro-intestinal and haematological toxicity for patients receiving platinum-based chemotherapy was demonstrated. No difference in toxic deaths was reported (p = 0.08).[30] For this reason, the most important International guidelines recommend platinum-based regimen for the treatment of fit patients with advanced stage NSCLC; platinum-free combination chemotherapy may represent a feasible alternative, particularly in patients in whom toxicity is a major concern.[31–33]

Cisplatin vs. Carboplatin

The efficacy of cisplatin as compared with carboplatin in the treatment of advanced NSCLC has been addressed by several randomized trials with contrasting results. A meta-analysis based on IPD from nine randomized trials comparing cisplatin- with a carboplatin-based regimen for a total of 2,968 patients was performed.[34] The primary endpoint was median OS which was 9.1 months for cisplatin-based regimens and 8.4 months for carboplatin-based schedules. The risk of death was higher with carboplatin compared with cisplatin, although the difference was not statistically significant (HR 1.07, 95% CI 0.99–1.15; p = 0.10).

The HRs for mortality, in patients treated with carboplatin relative to those treated with cisplatin, were: in non-squamous NSCLC (HR 1.12, 95% CI 1.01–1.23), in squamous histology (HR 0.97, 95% CI 0.85–1.10), treated with second-generation regimens (HR 0.94, 95% CI 0.80–1.11), and third-generation regimens (HR 1.11, 95% CI 1.01–1.21). These subgroup results underlined the different efficacy of the old and new regimens and the importance of histology diagnosis for a more appropriate treatment approach. The ORRs were 24% with carboplatin and 30% with cisplatin with an OR of 1.37 (95% CI 1.16–1.61; p < 0.001). Cisplatin-based doublets were associated with more nausea and vomiting and worse neurotoxicity, while carboplatin induced more thrombocytopenia.[34] Overall, the results of this meta-analysis showed that cisplatin-based chemotherapy provides a higher ORR and a significant OS benefit when the cisplatin is combined with a third-generation agent. Cisplatin should be the first choice in the clinical practice and carboplatin should be employed solely when the use of cisplatin is contraindicated.

Doublets vs. Triplets

The availability of third-generation drugs led several studies evaluating the potential benefit of adding a third drug to standard doublets. A meta-analysis pooled 28 studies including 4,814 patients demonstrated that adding a third agent to a doublet regimen was associated with a significantly increased ORR (OR 0.66, 95% CI 0.58–0.75; p < 0.001). The absolute benefit was 8%, with an increase of ORR from 23% with a doublet regimen to 31% with a triplet regimen. There was no significant difference (p = 0.70) in terms of benefit according to the type of agent added. There was no benefit in one-year survival (OR 1.01, 95% CI 0.85–1.21; p = 0.88) or median survival (median ratio 1.00, 95% CI 0.94–1.06; p = 0.97) by adding a third drug to a doublet regimen. Grade 3–4 toxicities, especially haematological toxicity, occurred more frequently in triplet than in doublet regimens with ORs ranging from 1.4 to 2.9.[35]

Overall, to date, doublets, due to a better safety profile have been considered the standard of care and the platform examining the addition of targeted agents.

Histology-Driven Chemotherapy Choice

In the past the histological subtype of NSCLC has not been taken into account in the choice of the first-line treatment. However, based on the recent evidence of the differential activity of pemetrexed in non-squamous cell carcinoma, the situation has changed.

This has also led to the retrospective re-analyses of trials involving older agents in regard to histology and outcome. A literature review identified 408 publications reporting an association between advanced NSCLC histology, patient prognosis, and/or the efficacy of specific chemotherapeutic agents. Of these, 11 trials reported a prognostic association between histology and clinical outcomes, showing a better survival in patients affected by adenocarcinoma or other type of carcinoma rather than squamous. Seven studies suggested that histological subtype was a predictive factor in patients treated with specific cytotoxic regimens.[36] A retrospective analysis of a randomized phase III trial was performed to assess if histology was predictive of treatment effect or prognostic regardless of treatment. In this trial, patients were randomized to receive carboplatin/paclitaxel, cisplatin/gemcitabine, and cisplatin/vinorelbine. Histology was not predictive of treatment effect for either OS or time-to-progression (TTP). Histology was prognostic for survival with a statistically significant advantage for squamous cell over adenocarcinoma (p = 0.0021).[37] However, none of these data can be considered reliable, since data were derived from the retrospective analysis of studies which were not aimed at assessing the role of histology.

Pemetrexed is a novel multitargeted antifolate which was shown *in vitro* to inhibit at least three different enzymes in the folate pathway: thymidylate synthase (TS), dihydrofolate reductase (DHFR), and glycinamide ribonucleotide formyl transferase (GARFT).[38] Because of its role in the folate pathway, the addition of vitamin B12 and folate to supplement treatment regimens has been investigated as a means of decreasing toxicity. In fact, the toxicity with pemetrexed was higher in patients with elevated pre-therapy homocysteine levels. Based on this information, it was recommended that patients receive vitamin supplementation prior to and during therapy.[39] *In vitro* studies indicated that tumor cell lines expressing high levels of TS or DHFR have a reduced sensitivity to pemetrexed, suggesting that increased expression levels might correlate with reduced clinical efficacy. The baseline TS expression levels are significantly higher in squamous cell carcinoma compared with adenocarcinoma.[40] Moreover, a retrospective analysis of the study comparing pemetrexed with docetaxel in second-line treatment of NSCLC reported a significant treatment-by-histology interactions for both median OS (p = 0.001) and progression-free survival (PFS; p = 0.004) indicating greater efficacy for non-squamous patients treated with pemetrexed.[41] According to all these data a randomized, non-inferiority, phase III trial, enrolled 1,725 chemotherapy-naïve patients with advanced NSCLC to receive either cisplatin 75 mg/m² on day 1 plus gemcitabine 1250 mg/m² on days 1 and 8 or cisplatin at the same dose plus pemetrexed 500 mg/m² on day 1, every three weeks for a maximum of six cycles. All patients received oral folic acid, vitamin B12, and dexamethasone prophylaxis. The primary endpoint was to compare the OS between the two regimens. Median OS was 10.3 months in both arms (HR 0.94, 95% CI 0.84–1.05). Survival rates at one-year were 43.5% and 41.9% for cisplatin/pemetrexed and cisplatin/gemcitabine, respectively. Median PFS was also non-inferior (4.8 vs. 5.1 months, respectively; HR 1.04, 95% CI 0.94–1.15). ORR was 30.6% in the cisplatin/pemetrexed arm and 28.2% in the cisplatin/gemcitabine arm. For cisplatin/pemetrexed, the rates of grade 3–4 neutropenia, anemia, and thrombocytopenia (p ≤ 0.001); febrile neutropenia (p = 0.002); and alopecia (p < 0.001) were significantly lower, whereas grade 3–4 nausea (p = 0.004) was more common for the cisplatin/gemcitabine arm.[42] A pre-planned analysis investigated the treatment outcomes and NSCLC histology subtype relationship. This analysis reported that non-squamous patients had a longer median OS on cisplatin/pemetrexed (11 months) than on cisplatin/gemcitabine (10.1 months; HR 0.84, 95% CI 0.74–0.96; p = 0.011) particularly evident for the adenocarcinoma histology (12.6 vs. 10.9 months, respectively; HR 0.84, 95% CI 0.71–0.99; p = 0.03) (Table 6.2) whereas squamous patients had a shorter median OS on cisplatin/pemetrexed than on cisplatin/gemcitabine (9.4 vs. 10.8 months, respectively; HR 1.23, 95% CI 1.00–1.51; p = 0.05). Non-squamous patients reported a better PFS on cisplatin/pemetrexed than on cisplatin/gemcitabine (5.26 vs. 4.96 months, respectively; HR 0.95, 95% CI 0.84–1.06; p = 0.349). Squamous patients had a shorter PFS on cisplatin/pemetrexed than on cisplatin/gemcitabine (4.4 vs. 5.5 months, respectively; HR 1.36, 95% CI 1.12–1.65; p = 0.002). ORR was higher in the cisplatin/pemetrexed arm than in the cisplatin/gemcitabine arm in patients with adenocarcinoma (28.9% vs. 21.7%); higher ORR occurred in patients with squamous cell carcinoma (23.4% vs. 31.4%) on cisplatin/gemcitabine.[43] Conversely, a phase III trial, comparing carboplatin (area under the curve [AUC] 6, day 1) with pemetrexed (500 mg/m², day 1) or with gemcitabine (1000 mg/m², day 1 and 8), recycled every three weeks, reported no significant differences for the primary health-related QoL endpoint or in OS between the two treatment arms (n = 446; pemetrexed/carboplatin, 7.3 months; gemcitabine/carboplatin, 7.0 months; p = 0.63). Multivariate analyses and interaction tests did not reveal any significant associations between histology and survival.[44] However, this trial was not designed to assess a survival difference; it used carboplatin which scored lower than cisplatin in OS,[34] and it was not designed for subgroup analyses, so the results should be interpreted with caution.

According to these results, pemetrexed in combination with platinum has been granted as first-line treatment of patients with advanced NSCLC other than predominantly squamous cell histology.

TARGETED THERAPY

Chemotherapeutic agents seem to have reached a plateau of effectiveness in the treatment of advanced NSCLC[31–33] leading to an increase in research to better understand the cancer biology. The major progresses made in recent years toward the mechanisms of oncogenesis allowed the development of novel therapeutic agents that specifically target growth factor pathways dysregulated in tumor cells. Targeting the vascular endothelial growth factor (VEGF) and the EGFR pathways has played a central role in advancing NSCLC research, treatment, and patients' outcome over the last years. Two monoclonal antibodies were developed for the treatment of advanced NSCLC: bevacizumab against the VEGF pathway and cetuximab against the EGFR pathway.

Bevacizumab

The anti-VEGF humanized monoclonal antibody bevacizumab is directed against the VEGF. Bevacizumab consists of 93% human and 7% murine components and it recognizes all isoforms of VEGF ligands. Bevacizumab exerts its antiangiogenic effects by binding to free circulating VEGF, thereby inhibiting the binding of VEGF to its receptors, preventing VEGF ligand receptor downstream signaling.[45]

A randomized phase II study enrolled 99 patients to carboplatin (AUC 6) plus paclitaxel (200 mg/m²) on day 1 alone or with bevacizumab 7.5 mg/kg or 15 mg/kg on day 1, every three weeks. ORRs were 31.5%, 28.1%, and 18.8% in the high-dose bevacizumab group, low-dose bevacizumab group, and chemotherapy alone group, respectively. Median TTP was 7.4, 4.3, and 4.2 months, and median OS 17.7, 11.6, and 14.9 months, respectively. Bevacizumab therapy appeared to be associated with an increased risk of major haemoptysis with four fatal episodes.[46] Bleeding arose in centrally located tumors close to major blood vessels, and the cavitation or necrosis frequently occurred, typically on location of squamous histological subtype. As a consequence, all the following trials excluded to enroll squamous histology. The phase III trial, the Eastern Cooperative Oncology Group (ECOG-E4599), randomized 878 patients with recurrent or advanced non-squamous NSCLC to carboplatin plus paclitaxel alone or in combination with bevacizumab 15 mg/kg for a maximum of six cycles and then, in non-progressed patients, bevacizumab until progression or unacceptable toxicity.[47] Patients with squamous-cell tumors, brain metastases, and clinically significant haemoptysis were excluded. The median OS, the primary endpoint, was 12.3 months in the group assigned to chemotherapy plus bevacizumab, as compared with 10.3 months in the chemotherapy-alone group (HR for death 0.80, 95% CI 0.69–0.93; p = 0.003). The median PFS in the two groups was 6.2 and 4.5 months, respectively (HR for disease progression 0.66, 95% CI 0.57–0.77; p < 0.001), with ORRs of 35% and 15% (p < 0.001). Rates of clinically significant bleeding were 4.4% and 0.7%, respectively (p < 0.001). There were 15 treatment-related deaths in the chemotherapy plus bevacizumab group, including five from pulmonary hemorrhage.[47] This study represents a clear superior efficacy of a targeted therapy combined with chemotherapy over chemotherapy alone in the treatment of advanced NSCLC. A retrospective analysis of the E4599 trial reported very interesting data concerning the adenocarcinoma patients (n = 602), with a median OS of 14.2 months for the bevacizumab arm versus 10.3 months for the control arm (HR 0.69, 95% CI 0.58–0.83). For large cell carcinoma patients (n = 48), median OS was 10 months for bevacizumab and 8.7 months for placebo while for NSCLC not otherwise specified (NOS; n = 165) it was 9.5 and 10 months, respectively.[48] Of interest was the survival difference reported according to gender. In fact, median OS in the chemotherapy and bevacizumab group was 8.7 and 11.7 months for males, 13.1 and 13.3 months for females, respectively.[49] Possible explanations include imbalances between the two groups with respect to baseline prognostic factors, in the use of further lines of therapy or statistical chance. A further retrospective analysis of the E4599 trial explored the impact of hypertension (a bevacizumab side effect) on NSCLC outcomes. Administration of bevacizumab is postulated to decrease nitric oxide synthesis and lead to hypertension, which may be a physiological sign that the VEGF pathway is being blocked. Comparing patients on bevacizumab group who experienced a high blood pressure with those on chemotherapy arm reported a HR for OS of 0.60 (95% CI 0.43–0.81; p = 0.001) while HR for OS was 0.86 (95% CI 0.74–1.00; p = 0.05) in patients who did not experience hypertension. It means that the onset of hypertension during treatment with bevacizumab may be associated with improved outcomes.[50] However, we do not advise a side effect be used as a potential marker of outcome.

A further, placebo-controlled, phase III study, the AVAiL (AVAstin in Lung) trial, used the combination of cisplatin 80 mg/m² on day 1 plus gemcitabine 1250 mg/m² on days 1 and 8, recycled every three weeks.[51,52] In this trial, chemotherapy plus placebo was compared with chemotherapy plus two different doses of bevacizumab, 7.5 and 15 mg/kg. Also in this trial after a maximum of six cycles, in non-progressed patients, bevacizumab was administered until progression or unacceptable toxicity. A total of 1,043 patients with non-squamous NSCLC were randomized to the three arms. Median PFS, the main endpoint of the trial, was significantly prolonged with the bevacizumab administration, 6.7 versus 6.1 months for placebo (HR 0.75, 95% CI 0.62–0.91; p = 0.003) in the low-dose group, and 6.5 versus 6.1 months for placebo (HR 0.82, 95% CI 0.68–0.98; p = 0.03) in the high-dose group compared with placebo. ORRs were 20.1%, 34.1%, and 30.4% for placebo, low-dose bevacizumab, and high-dose bevacizumab plus chemotherapy, with a response duration of 4.7, 6.1, and 6.1 months, respectively. Median OS was 13.1 months for chemotherapy alone, 13.6 months for bevacizumab at 7.5 mg/kg plus chemotherapy (HR vs. placebo 0.93, 95% CI 0.78–1.11; p = 0.42), and 13.4 months for bevacizumab at 15 mg/kg plus chemotherapy (HR vs. placebo 1.03, 95% CI 0.86–1.23; p = 0.76). Incidence of grade > 3 adverse events was similar across arms occurring in 75%, 76%, and 81% in chemotherapy alone, low dose bevacizumab, and high dose bevacizumab, respectively. Grade > 3 pulmonary hemorrhage rates were ≤ 1.5% for all arms despite the fact that 9% of patients received therapeutic anticoagulation. No difference according to the gender was observed minimizing the gender issue of the E4599 trial (Table 6.3).

The safety and efficacy of adding bevacizumab to first-line chemotherapy in a daily oncology practice population has been assessed in two multicenter, open-label and single-arm studies. Both trials further documented, in a real-world population, the safety and efficacy outcomes seen in phase III clinical trials of bevacizumab administered in combination with any chemotherapeutics, as first-line therapy.[53,54]

Bevacizumab in non-squamous cell carcinoma has also been evaluated in phase II studies with other chemotherapy doublets (oxaliplatin plus gemcitabine, oxaliplatin plus pemetrexed, carboplatin plus docetaxel). However, the results are still preliminary and no firm conclusions should be drawn.[55]

There is interest in determining if patients with brain metastases and with squamous histology can still be candidates for therapy with bevacizumab. The PASSPORT trial was a phase II single-arm study of bevacizumab in combination with first- or second-line therapy in non-squamous NSCLC patients with treated central nervous system (CNS) metastases. Patients received bevacizumab (15 mg/kg) every three weeks with platinum-based doublets or erlotinib as first-line therapy, or with single-agent chemotherapy or erlotinib as second-line treatment, according to institutional standards. Patients with brain metastases were allowed to

Table 6.3 Phase III Trials with Bevacizumab or Cetuximab Plus Chemotherapy in the First-Line Treatment of Advanced Non-Small-Cell Lung Cancer

Author, year	Regimen	No. pts	ORR (%)	PFS (months)	OS (months)
Sandler, 2006[47]	CbP + BEV	434	35	6.2	12.3
	vs.				
	CbP	444	15	4.5	10.3
Reck, 2010[51,52]	CG + BEV 7.5 mg/kg	345	34.1	6.7[o]	13.6
	vs.				
	CG + BEV 15 mg/kg	351	30.4	6.5[a]	13.4
	vs.				
	CG + Placebo	347	20.1	6.1[oa]	13.1
Pirker, 2009[60]	CV + CET	557	36	4.8	11.3
	vs.				
	CV	568	29	4.8	10.1
Lynch, 2010[62]	CbTAX + CET	338	25.7[b]	4.4[b]	9.69
	vs.				
	CbTAX	338	17.2[b]	4.24[b]	8.38

[a]Statistically significant.
[b]Assessed by independent radiologic review committee.
Abbreviations: No. pts, number of patients; ORR, objective response rate; PFS, progression-free survival; OS, overall survival; BEV, bevacizumab; CET, cetuximab; Cb, carboplatin; P, paclitaxel; C, cisplatin: G, gemcitabine; V, vinorelbine; TAX, taxanes.

enter the trial after completion of whole brain radiotherapy and/or neurosurgery. The primary endpoint was to assess the rate of grade ≥ 2 symptomatic brain hemorrhage during bevacizumab therapy. Among the 106 evaluable patients, no grade 1–5 brain hemorrhages were reported; however, two grade 5 pulmonary hemorrhages occurred thus suggesting that bevacizumab treatment can be administered with acceptable condition of the patient.[56] The phase II BRIDGE trial investigated the use of bevacizumab in 31 squamous advanced NSCLC patients treated with two cycles of carboplatin and paclitaxel followed by the addition of bevacizumab in the following four cycles. Grade > 3 pulmonary hemorrhage, the primary endpoint, occurred in one patient (3.2%). However, despite the low incidence of grade > 3 pulmonary hemorrhage, the treatment of squamous NSCLC patients with bevacizumab must be considered experimental.[57]

The search for predictive biomarkers for the use of bevacizumab in NSCLC has not been successful so far. VEGF, basic fibroblast growth factor (bFGF), soluble intercellular adhesion molecule-1 (ICAM), and E-selectin, were evaluated in the pretreatment plasma of patients enrolled in the E4599 trial. Baseline ICAM levels were prognostic for survival and predicted response to chemotherapy with or without bevacizumab. VEGF levels were predictive of response to bevacizumab but not survival.[58]

To date, bevacizumab is licensed in combination with platinum-based chemotherapy as first-line therapy of advanced non-squamous NSCLC patients, including pretreated brain metastases; however, according to the reported results, carboplatin/paclitaxel combination should be considered as the chemotherapy backbone.

Cetuximab

Cetuximab is a chimeric (human-murine) mAb directed against the extracellular domain of the EGFR that blocks ligand (TGF-α, EGF) access to the receptor.[59]

In the large phase III trial FLEX (First-Line ErbituX in lung cancer), 1,125 advanced NSCLC patients, with EGFR-detectable by immunohistochemistry (IHC), were randomized to cisplatin (80 mg/m² day 1) plus vinorelbine (25 mg/m² day 1 and 8), every three weeks for a maximum of six cycles with or without cetuximab (400 mg/m² initial dose, then 250 mg/m²/week) as first-line treatment. Cetuximab was administered until progression or unacceptable toxicity also after completing the six cycles of chemotherapy in patients without progression of disease. The median PFS was 4.8 months in both groups (HR 0.943, 95% CI 0.825–1.077; p = 0.39). The median OS, the main endpoint, was 11.3 months in the cetuximab arm and 10.1 months in the control arm (HR 0.871; 95% CI 0.762–0.996; p = 0.044). A survival benefit was seen in all histological subgroups of NSCLC, with median OS of 12 versus 10.3 months, respectively for patients with adenocarcinomas (n = 413), 10.2 versus 8.9 months, respectively for those with squamous cell carcinomas (n = 347), and 9 versus 8.2 months, respectively for patients with other histological subtypes (n = 185; large-cell, adenosquamous carcinoma and NSCLC NOS).[60] The FLEX study is the first to demonstrate a survival benefit from the use of a targeted agent in combination with platinum-based chemotherapy across all histological subtypes in first-line treatment of advanced NSCLC. The main cetuximab-related adverse event was grade 3 acne-like rash in 57 (10%) patients. This side effect has been considered as a potential predictive factor in selecting patients who much benefit from cetuximab-based therapy. In fact, in the FLEX trial, 290 patients who had been randomized to chemotherapy plus cetuximab arm and who developed an acne-like rash of any grade within the first three weeks of treatment (and were still alive after the first cycle) had a longer OS than the 228 patients without acne-like rash (14.3 vs. 8.1 months).[61] However, in this case too we do not advise a side effect be used as a potential marker of outcome in such a poor prognosis population.

A multicenter, open-label, phase III study (BMS099), enrolled 676 chemotherapy-naïve patients with advanced NSCLC, without restrictions based on histology or EGFR expression. Patients were randomly assigned to carboplatin (AUC 6) plus paclitaxel (225 mg/m²) or docetaxel (75 mg/m²), all drugs given on day 1 and recycled every three weeks, with or without cetuximab at 400 mg/m² as loading dose and then 250 mg/m²/week. Also in this trial the administration of cetuximab continued until progression or unacceptable toxicity. The primary endpoint was PFS, assessed by independent radiologic review committee (IRRC). Median PFS-IRRC was 4.4 months with cetuximab plus chemotherapy versus 4.24 months with chemotherapy alone (HR 0.902, 95% CI 0.761–1.069; p = 0.236). Median OS was 9.69 versus 8.38 months, respectively (HR 0.890, 95% CI 0.754–1.051; p = 0.169). ORR-IRRC was 25.7% with cetuximab plus chemotherapy versus 17.2% with chemotherapy (p = 0.007). The safety profile of this combination was manageable and consistent with its individual components: QoL did not differ across treatment arms. This trial failed to reach its main endpoint; however, there was a significant improvement in ORR-IRRC and the difference in OS favored cetuximab but did not reach statistical significance (Table 6.3).[62]

The different results reported by these two trials were explained with the insufficient number of patients enrolled in the BMS099 trial, making impossible to detect an outcome difference between the two arms. Other hypotheses were the type of chemotherapy used, and the possible influence of any molecular selection.

A meta-analysis based on IPD of four randomized phase II/III studies investigating cetuximab in advanced NSCLC patients involving 2,018 patients demonstrated a significant benefit for the cetuximab combination over chemotherapy alone across all investigated efficacy endpoints, irrespective of the type of platinum doublet and the histological subtype used. The HRs were for OS 0.878 (95% CI 0.795–0.969; p = 0.010), and for PFS 0.899 (95% CI 0.814–0.993, p = 0.036). The OR for ORR was 1.463 (95% CI 1.201–1.783, p < 0.001).[63]

Despite these positive results cetuximab is not registered for the treatment of advanced NSCLC. However, interesting results have emerged from examining the degree of EGFR expression in sections submitted at the beginning of the FLEX trial taking into account the degree and the proportion of cells measured by the expression of EGFR by IHC. The EGFR expression levels were determined via a continuous EGFR-IHC scoring system (H-score) ranging from 0–300 based on a composite score consisting of proportion of positive cells and membrane staining intensity. Above a cut-off of 200, a clear benefit of the addition of cetuximab to chemotherapy compared with chemotherapy alone was seen. In fact, patients with high EGFR-IHC score reported a higher ORR (44.4%) in the cetuximab arm than those receiving chemotherapy only (ORR 28.1%; p = 0.002) or also cetuximab but with a low EGFR-IHC score (ORR 32.6%). Median OS of patients with high EGFR-IHC score and treated with cetuximab was 12.0 versus 9.6 months of those receiving chemotherapy only (HR 0.73, 95% CI 0.58–0.93; p = 0.011).[64]

Based on these results, a new request for its registration in patients selected for EGFR-IHC high score has been submitted to the regulatory agencies.

MAINTENANCE THERAPY
The rationale for this approach is based on the Goldie and Coldman hypothesis, which states that the proportion of chemotherapy-resistant cells in a tumor increases over time[65] and so, the early administration of non-cross-resistant agents might increase the probability of killing more cancer cells before they become resistant. The potential role of the prolonged treatment has been addressed by a systematic review and meta-analysis of 13 randomized controlled trials, including 3,027 patients, addressing this issue. The primary endpoint was OS which was improved by extending therapy (HR 0.92, 95% CI 0.86–0.99; p = 0.03) and PFS, too (HR 0.75, 95% CI 0.69–0.81; p < 0.00001). Subgroup analysis revealed that improvement of PFS was greater in trials using chemotherapy with third-generation regimens rather than older regimens (HR 0.70 interaction vs. 0.92 interaction; p = 0.003). Extending chemotherapy was associated with more frequent side effects in all trials where it was reported, and impaired QoL in two of seven trials.[66] While this meta-analysis suggests that prolonged chemotherapy might improve the outcomes in advanced NSCLC, it suffers from the flaw concerning different methodological designs used in individual trials. It is of particular

importance to define the prolonged duration of therapy as either the continued administration of therapy in patients who did not report a progression of disease after a defined number of induction cycles of therapy (continuation maintenance) or the introduction of new agents (switch maintenance) at this point.[67] A sort of continuing maintenance was already performed by the trials in which targeted agents, such as bevacizumab and cetuximab, were administered behind the six cycles of chemotherapy. However, these studies were not designed to evaluate the maintenance step of the trial. In the last few years, several randomized trials addressed the issue of switch and continuing maintenance investigating both chemotherapeutics and targeted agents.

Switch Maintenance

A randomized, double-blind, phase III trial compared the efficacy and safety of pemetrexed (500 mg/m^2 on day 1), every three weeks plus BSC versus placebo plus BSC in patients who had not progressed on four cycles of platinum-based induction chemotherapy not containing pemetrexed. The primary endpoint was PFS which was 4.3 versus 2.6 months, in the 663 randomized patients (441 in the pemetrexed arm and 222 in the placebo group), in the pemetrexed and the placebo arms, respectively (HR 0.50, 95% CI 0.42–0.61; p < 0.0001). Median OS was 13.4 months with pemetrexed and 10.6 months with placebo (HR 0.79, 95% CI 0.65–0.95; p = 0.012), respectively. Treatment with pemetrexed reported 5% serious adverse events versus 1% for placebo and 16% grade 3–4 adverse events versus 4% for placebo (p < 0.0001).[68] A prespecified analysis for efficacy by NSCLC histology reported that in squamous NSCLC patients the PFS was 2.4 months in the pemetrexed arm and 2.5 months in the placebo group (HR 1.03, 95% CI 0.71–1.49; p = 0.896) with an OS of 9.9 and 10.8 months (HR 1.07, 95% CI 0.77–1.50; p = 0.678), respectively. On the contrary, in patients with non-squamous NSCLC the median PFS was 4.4 months with pemetrexed versus 1.8 months for placebo (HR 0.47, 95% CI 0.37–0.60; p < 0.0001) with a median OS of 15.5 versus 10.3 months, respectively (HR 0.70, 95% CI 0.56–0.88; p = 0.002).[68] This trial suffered from a main flaw. In fact, among patients who were randomized to the pemetrexed group, 98% received the treatment (pemetrexed) effectively, and 51% received post-study therapy. By contrast, among patients randomized to placebo, only 67% received, at progression, a post-study therapy, which was pemetrexed in only 18%. This means that not all patients enrolled in this trial had the same possibility of treatment, and this discrepancy might affect the final results.

However, according to these results, pemetrexed is the first agent to be licensed for maintenance therapy of patients affected by advanced NSCLC and non-progressed after induction of platinum-based doublets therapy not containing pemetrexed.

The randomized phase III SATURN (Sequential Tarceva in Unresectable Lung Cancer) trial enrolled 889 patients with no evidence of disease progression after four cycles of platinum-based chemotherapy to receive either oral erlotinib 150 mg/day or placebo until progression or unacceptable toxicity. The primary endpoint was PFS in all patients, and the co-primary endpoint was PFS in EGFR IHC-positive patients. Median PFS in all patients was 12.3 weeks with erlotinib and 11.1 weeks for placebo (HR 0.71, 95% CI 0.62–0.82; p < 0.0001) and the same results were reported also in EGFR IHC-positive patients (HR 0.69, 95% CI 0.58–0.82; p < 0.0001). All biomarker subgroups showed a PFS benefit with erlotinib, including patients whose tumors had wild-type EGFR (HR 0.78, 95% CI 0.63–0.96; p = 0.0185), or those with EGFR mutations (HR 0.10, 95% CI 0.04–0.25; p < 0.0001). Median OS, for all the population, was, in the erlotinib arm, 12 months and 11 months in the placebo group (HR 0.81, 95% CI 0.70–0.95; p = 0.0088). The ORRs were 11.9% with erlotinib versus 5.4% with placebo. QoL was similar in both arms. Erlotinib significantly extended time to pain (HR 0.61; p = 0.008) and time to analgesic use (HR 0.66; p = 0.02). The main treatment-related adverse events were grade 1–2. Surprisingly, in patients achieving a stable disease after induction therapy, median OS was 11.9 months with maintenance erlotinib versus 9.6 months with placebo (HR 0.72, 95% CI 0.59–0.89; p = 0.0019).[69] Unfortunately, also in this trial the same flaw reported in the maintenance pemetrexed study should be pointed out. Among the patients randomized in the placebo arm, 72% were able, at the time of disease progression, to receive a second-line therapy and only 21% received an EGFR-tyrosine kinase inhibitors (TKIs). These data could influence the final results of this trial underlining the need of studies whose design should also define the further therapies.

Overall, the results coming from this trial led to the registration of erlotinib as monotherapy for maintenance treatment in patients whose disease has not progressed after four cycles of standard platinum-based chemotherapy by Food and Drug Administration (FDA) while European Medicines Agency (EMA) restricted this registration only to patients who achieved a stable disease.

The main goal of the switch maintenance approach is to deliver second-line treatment to all possible patients not progressing during induction therapy. This could be of particular importance because over one-third of patients generally do not receive a second-line therapy at progression mainly due to worsening of their general condition. These data were confirmed by the drop-out rates of the control arm of the previous reported maintenance trials.[68,69] As stated before, a possible flaw of these studies was the fact that not all patients enrolled had the same possibility of receiving the same treatment, i.e., pemetrexed or erlotinib. A randomized phase III trial enrolled 398 patients who did not progress to four cycles of induction carboplatin plus gemcitabine to receive immediate six cycles or delayed, at progression, docetaxel 75 mg/m² on day 1 every three weeks. The primary endpoint was OS, which was not reached, with 12.3 and 9.7 months, in the immediate and delayed arms, respectively (p = 0.0853). But, an improved PFS was reported with immediate docetaxel (5.7 and 2.7 months, respectively; p ≤ 0.0001). Also in this trial, only the 63% of patients enrolled in the delayed docetaxel arm received the drug effectively while the same therapeutic approach was used in all patients. In fact, looking to the median OS of the patients who effectively received docetaxel in the delayed arm, it was similar to that reported in the immediate group (12.5 vs. 12.3 months, respectively).[70] Recently, the ASCO guidelines reported that for patients with stable disease or response after four cycles, immediate treatment with an alternative, single-agent chemotherapy such as pemetrexed in patients with non-squamous histology, docetaxel, or erlotinib in unselected patients may be considered. However, these data are limited by the fact that a break from cytotoxic chemotherapy after a fixed course starting a second-line chemotherapy at disease progression is also acceptable.[71] In fact, deriving the drop-outs of patients from the survival curves of the experimental arm of these three trials,[68–70] it was approximately one-third like the percentage of patients unable to receive therapy at progression in the control arm. This means that there is a portion of patients who do not benefit in any manner from further therapy and so, for them, a possible further toxicity should be avoided. Therefore, there is the need of investigating the real role of switch maintenance versus second-line treatment at progression using the same drug in the experimental and control arm. This kind of trial has been requested by regulatory agencies for erlotinib. This is the only way of confirming if the switch maintenance is able to rescue the percentage of patients otherwise lost to second-line therapy and also getting information in order to select patients who could really benefit from a further therapy.[72]

Erlotinib was investigated as switch maintenance also in the randomized phase III ATLAS study. A total of 743 patients who did not progress after four cycles of platinum-based regimens plus bevacizumab received erlotinib 150 mg/day plus bevacizumab or placebo plus bevacizumab. The Data Monitoring Committee recommended stopping the trial at the second planned interim efficacy analysis, because it had met the primary endpoint of improved PFS with the addition of erlotinib to bevacizumab. Median PFS was 4.76 months for bevacizumab plus erlotinib and 3.71 months for bevacizumab plus placebo (HR 0.71, 95% CI 0.58–0.86; p = 0.0006). Median OS was 15.9 versus 13.9 months, respectively (HR 0.90, 95% CI 0.74–1.09; p = 0.2686). Moreover, in both arms, the same percentage (39.7%) of patients received further therapy with EGFR-TKIs. Grade 3–4 adverse events were observed in 44.1% of patients enrolled in the bevacizumab plus erlotinib arm and 30.4% of patients in the bevacizumab arm only.[73]

Gefitinib was investigated as maintenance therapy, too. A randomized phase III trial enrolled 173 non-progressing patients after 2–6 cycles of any platinum-based induction chemotherapy to receive gefitinib 250 mg daily (n = 86) or placebo (n = 87). Median OS, the primary endpoint, was 10.9 months for gefitinib and 9.4 months for placebo (HR 0.81, 95% CI 0.59–1.12; p = 0.204), while median PFS was 4.1 versus 2.9 months, respectively (HR 0.61, 95% CI 0.45–0.83; p = 0.002). Treatment was very well tolerated. Unfortunately this trial closed early due to a slow accrual; however, the advantage in PFS reported by gefitinib was very promising while survival endpoint was biased by the low number of enrolled patients.[74] In the randomized phase III INFORM study, performed in Asian population, 296 patients who had not progressed after four cycles of platinum-based chemotherapy were assigned to gefitinib (250 mg daily) or placebo until progression or unacceptable toxicity. Median PFS, the primary endpoint, was 4.8 months for gefitinib group and 2.6 months for placebo arm (HR 0.42, 95% CI 0.33–0.55; p < 0.0001). Median PFS was particularly high in the 30 EGFR-mutated patients (15 assigned per each arm) with 16.6 months for gefitinib and 2.8 months for placebo (HR 0.17, 95% CI 0.07–0.42). The ORRs were 23.6% and 0.7% (OR 54.1, 95% CI 7.17–408; p = 0.0001). Median OS was 18.7 and 16.9 months, respectively (HR 0.84, 95% CI 0.62–1.14; p = 0.26). About 50% of patients enrolled in the gefitinib arm received a further therapy, and about 65% of patients randomized in the placebo arm received second-line therapy which was mainly chemotherapy in both groups. Gefitinib was well tolerated (Table 6.4).[75]

The results of these last two trials confirmed that both erlotinib and gefitinib, when investigated as switch maintenance in the general population, improved the outcomes of advanced NSCLC patients with good toxicity profiles. These results are a lot better in EGFR-mutated patients. However, what is the impact on the results of the EGFR mutations not detectable in the most of randomized population due to the unavailability of enough tissue is still unknown.

Table 6.4 Results of Randomized Phase III Trials Investigating the Switch Maintenance in Advanced Non-Small Cell Lung Cancer Patients

Author, year	Induction therapy	Randomization	No. pts	ORR (%)	PFS (months)	OS (months)
Ciuleanu, 2009[68]	Platinum-based doublets (excluding pemetrexed) for four cycles	Placebo vs. PEM	222	1.8	2.6	10.6
			441	6.8	4.3	13.4
Cappuzzo, 2010[69]	Platinum-based doublets for four cycles	Placebo vs. ERL	447	5.4	11.1[a]	11.0
			437	11.9	12.3[a]	12.0
Kabbinavar, 2010[73]	Platinum-based doublets + bevacizumab for four cycles	BEV+Placebo vs. BEV+ERL	373	NR	3.71	13.9
			370		4.76	15.9
Gaafar, 2011[74]	Platinum-based regimens for 2–6 cycles	Placebo vs. GEF	87	NR	2.9	9.4
			86		4.1	10.9
Zhang, 2012[75]	Platinum-based doublets for four cycles	Placebo vs. GEF	148	0.7	2.6	16.9
			148	23.6	4.8	18.7

[a]Weeks.

Abbreviations: No. pts, number of patients; ORR, objective response rate; PFS, progression-free survival; OS, overall survival; NR, not reported; PEM, pemetrexed; ERL, erlotinib; BEV, bevacizumab; GEF, gefitinib.

Continuing Maintenance

A phase III randomized trial, enrolled 255 patients who had not progressed after 4 cycles of carboplatin plus gemcitabine chemotherapy to receive maintenance gemcitabine (1000 mg/m² on day 1 and 8, every three weeks; n = 128) with BSC or BSC alone (n = 127). The primary endpoint was median OS which was 8.0 months for gemcitabine and 9.3 months for BSC (HR 0.97, 95% CI 0.72–1.30; p = 0.84) with a median PFS of 7.4 and 7.7 months, respectively (HR 1.09, 95% CI 0.81–1.45; p = 0.575).[76] However, this trial suffered from a bias due to its early closure because of the slow accrual and the high rate (64%) of PS 2 patients included.

Given the efficacy of pemetrexed as a maintenance agent, when not used in the induction regimen, the PARAMOUNT randomized phase III study investigated its role in this setting in patients with advanced non-squamous NSCLC who did not progress after four cycles of induction chemotherapy with cisplatin plus pemetrexed. A total of 539 patients were randomized with a ratio 2:1 to receive pemetrexed 500 mg/m² on day 1 every three weeks (n = 359) or placebo (n = 180) until progression or unacceptable toxicity. Median independently reviewed PFS was the primary endpoint and it was 3.9 months for pemetrexed therapy and 2.6 months for placebo treatment (HR 0.64, 95% CI 0.51–0.81; p = 0.0002). The ORRs were 2.8% versus 0.6%, respectively. The final median OS, from randomization, was 13.9 and 11 months (HR 0.78, 95% CI 0.64–0.96; p = 0.0195), respectively with benefit seen across all subgroups. Drug-related serious adverse events were 8.9% and 2.8%, respectively.[77,78] Moreover, long-term maintenance pemetrexed did not affect QoL.[79]

A mixed approach was investigated in the randomized phase III IFCT-GFPC 0502 trial in which 464 non-progressing patients to four cycles of cisplatin and gemcitabine induction treatment received observation (n = 152) or gemcitabine (1.250 mg/m² on day 1 and 8, every three weeks; n = 149) or erlotinib (n = 153). Median PFS, primary endpoint, was 3.8 months for gemcitabine group versus 1.9 months for control arm (HR 0.55, 95% CI 0.43–0.70; p < 0.0001), whereas it was 2.9 months for erlotinib arm (HR 0.82, 95% CI 0.73–0.93; p = 0.002). Preliminary OS of gemcitabine versus observation reported a HR of 0.86, while for erlotinib versus observation the HR was 0.91. Grade 3–4 adverse events were 2.6% for observation arm, 27.9% for gemcitabine arm, and 15.5% for erlotinib group (Table 6.5).[80] This is the only trial in which the two maintenance approach, switch and continuing, were compared contemporarily with the standard arm of observation. However, the results are still preliminary and, unfortunately, the trial was not designed to compare the two approaches.

CONCLUSION

The choice of first-line therapy for fit patients affected by advanced NSCLC with EGFR wild-type is driven by histotype (Fig. 6.1). For non-squamous histology, the best choice might be a platinum-based doublet including pemetrexed, although other third-generation doublets are also acceptable. In this histology,

Table 6.5 Results of Randomized Phase III Trials Investigating the Continuing Maintenance in Advanced Non-Small Cell Lung Cancer Patients

Author, year	Induction therapy	Randomization	No. pts	ORR (%)	PFS (months)	OS (months)
Belani, 2010[76]	CBDCA+GEM for four cycles	BSC vs.	127	6	7.7	9.3
		GEM+BSC	128	28	7.4	8.0
Paz-Ares, 2012[77,78]	CDDP+PEM for four cycles	Placebo vs.	180	0.6	2.6	11.0
		PEM	359	2.8	3.9	13.9
Perol, 2010[80]	CDDP+GEM for four cycles	Observation vs.	155		1.9	
		GEM vs.	154	NR	3.8	HR 0.86[a]
		ERL	155		2.9	HR 0.91[a]

[a]Versus observation.

Abbreviations: No. pts, number of patients; ORR, objective response rate; PFS, progression-free survival; OS, overall survival; NR, not reported; NA, not applicable; CBDCA, carboplatin; CDDP, cisplatin; GEM, gemcitabine; PEM, pemetrexed; BSC, best supportive care; ERL, erlotinib.

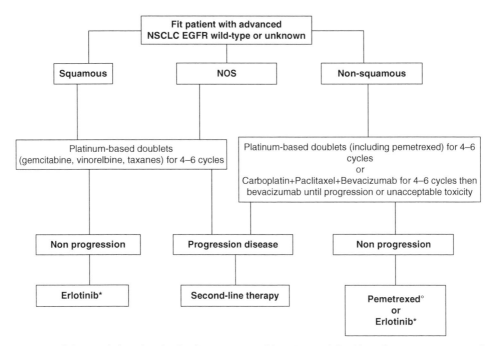

Figure 6.1 Suggested decisional algorithm for first-line treatment of fit patients, adult with performance status 0–1, affected by advanced NSCLC with EGFR wild-type or unknown. (°Not allowed by regulatory agencies in patients receiving first-line pemetrexed-based regimens; *Approved, in this setting, by European Medicines Agency only for patients achieving a stable disease). *Abbreviations*: NSCLC: non-small cell lung cancer; EGFR: epidermal growth factor receptor; NOS: not otherwise specified.

bevacizumab-based chemotherapy is a valid option for patients considered eligible to this therapy; however, carboplatin plus paclitaxel should be considered the chemotherapy backbone. For squamous cell histology any third-generation platinum-based doublet, with the exception of pemetrexed, is the treatment of choice, and the potential side effects will influence the individual decision. For the occasional patient whose tumor was or could not be otherwise specified, the use of immunohistochemical panel including markers of squamous and glandular cell differentiation is recommended.

Maintenance pemetrexed can be considered for patients with advanced non-squamous NSCLC who did not progress after four cycles of platinum-based chemotherapy. While maintenance erlotinib can be considered for patients with all histotypes advanced NSCLC who have stable disease, for EMA, or not progressed for FDA, after completing first-line chemotherapy consisting of 4 cycles of platinum-based chemotherapy.

REFERENCES

1. Govindan R, Page N, Morgensztern D, et al. Changing epidemiology of small-cell lung cancer in the United States over the last 30 years: analysis of the Surveillance, Epidemiologic, and End Results database. J Clin Oncol 2006; 24: 4539–44.

2. Altekruse SF, Kosary CL, Krapcho N, et al. SEER Cancer Statistics Review 1975–2007, National Cancer Institute. Bethesda, MD. [Available from: http://seer.cancer.gov/csr/1975_2007/based on November 2009 SEER data submission, posted to the SEER web site, 2010] [Accessed on 15th September 2011].

3. EUROCARE-4: Survival of cancer patients in Europe diagnosed 2000–2002. [[Available from: http://www.eurocare.it/Results/tabid/79/Default.aspx#longsurv0002] [Accessed on 15th September 2011].

4. Non-small Cell Lung Cancer Collaborative Group. Chemotherapy in non small cell lung cancer: a meta-analysis using updated data on individual patients from 52 randomised clinical trials. Br Med J 1995; 311: 899–909.

5. Non-small Cell Lung Cancer Collaborative Group. Chemotherapy in addition to supportive care improves survival in advanced non-small-cell lung cancer: a systematic review and meta-analysis of individual patient data from 16 randomized controlled trials. J Clin Oncol 2008; 26: 4617–25.

6. Ranson M, Davidson N, Nicolson M, et al. Randomized trial of paclitaxel plus supportive care versus supportive care for patients with advanced non–small-cell lung cancer. J Natl Cancer Inst 2000; 92: 1074–80.

7. Roszkowski K, Pluzanska A, Krzakowski M, et al. A multicenter, randomized, phase III study of docetaxel plus best supportive care versus best supportive care in chemotherapy-naïve patients with metastatic or non-resectable localized non–small cell lung cancer (NSCLC). Lung Cancer 2000; 27: 145–57.

8. The Elderly Lung Cancer Vinorelbine Italian Study Group. Effects of vinorelbine on quality of life and survival of elderly patients with advanced non small cell lung cancer. J Natl Cancer Inst 1999; 91: 66–72.

9. Anderson H, Hopwood P, Stephens RJ, et al. Gemcitabine plus best supportive care (BSC) vs BSC in inoperable non–small cell lung cancer—a randomized trial with quality of life as the primary outcome. UK NSCLC Gemcitabine Group. Non–small Cell Lung Cancer. Br J Cancer 2000; 83: 447–53.

10. Sandler AB, Nemunaitis J, Denham C, et al. Phase III trial of gemcitabine plus cisplatin versus cisplatin alone in patients with locally advanced or metastatic non–small-cell lung cancer. J Clin Oncol 2000; 18: 122–30.

11. Wozniak AJ, Crowley JJ, Balcerzak SP, et al. Randomized trial comparing cisplatin with cisplatin plus vinorelbine in the treatment of advanced non–small-cell lung cancer: a Southwest Oncology Group study. J Clin Oncol 1998; 16: 2459–65.

12. Gatzemeier U, von Pawel J, Gottfried M, et al. Phase III comparative study of high-dose cisplatin versus a combination of paclitaxel and cisplatin in patients with advanced non–small-cell lung cancer. J Clin Oncol 2000; 18: 3390–9.

13. Le Chevalier T, Pujol JL, Douillard JY, et al. A three-arm trial of vinorelbine (Navelbine) plus cisplatin, vindesine plus cisplatin, and single-agent vinorelbine in the treatment of non–small cell lung cancer: an expanded analysis. Semin Oncol 1994; 21: 28–33.

14. Bonomi P, Kim K, Fairclough D, et al. Comparison of survival and quality of life in advanced non–small-cell lung cancer patients treated with two dose levels of paclitaxel combined with cisplatin versus etoposide with cisplatin: results of an Eastern Cooperative Oncology Group trial. J Clin Oncol 2000; 18: 623–31.

15. Cardenal F, Lopez-Cabrerizo MP, Anton A, et al. Randomized phase III study of gemcitabine-cisplatin versus etoposide-cisplatin in the treatment of locally advanced or metastatic non–small-cell lung cancer. J Clin Oncol 1999; 17: 12–18.

16. Kubota K, Watanabe K, Kunitoh H, et al. Phase III randomized trial of docetaxel plus cisplatin versus vindesine plus cisplatin in patients with stage IV non–small-cell lung cancer: the Japanese Taxotere Lung Cancer Study Group. J Clin Oncol 2004; 22: 254–61.

17. Kelly K, Crowley J, Bunn PA Jr, et al. Randomized phase III trial of paclitaxel plus carboplatin versus vinorelbine plus cisplatin in the treatment of patients with advanced non–small-cell lung cancer: a Southwest Oncology Group trial. J Clin Oncol 2001; 19: 3210–18.

18. Schiller JH, Harrington D, Belani CP, et al. Comparison of four chemotherapy regimens for advanced non–small-cell lung cancer. N Engl J Med 2002; 346: 92–8.

19. Scagliotti GV, De Marinis F, Rinaldi M, et al. Phase III randomized trial comparing three platinum-based doublets in advanced non–small-cell lung cancer. J Clin Oncol 2002; 20: 4285–91.

20. Fossella F, Pereira JR, von Pawel J, et al. Randomized, multinational, phase III study of docetaxel plus platinum combinations versus vinorelbine plus cisplatin for advanced non–small-cell lung cancer: the TAX 326 study group. J Clin Oncol 2003; 21: 3016–24.

21. Le Chevalier T, Scagliotti G, Natale R, et al. Efficacy of gemcitabine plus platinum chemotherapy compared with other platinum containing regimens in advanced non-small-cell lung cancer: a meta-analysis of survival outcomes. Lung Cancer 2005; 47: 69–80.

22. Douillard JY, Laporte S, Fossella F, et al. Comparison of docetaxel- and vinca alkaloid-based chemotherapy in the first-line treatment of advanced non small cell lung cancer: a meta-analysis of seven randomized clinical trials. J Thorac Oncol 2007; 2: 939–46.

23. Grossi F, Aita M, Defferrari C, et al. Impact of third-generation drugs on the activity of first-line chemotherapy in advanced non-small cell lung cancer: a meta-analytical approach. Oncologist 2009; 14: 497–510.

24. Georgoulias V, Ardavanis A, Tsiafaki X, et al. Vinorelbine plus cisplatin versus docetaxel plus gemcitabine in advanced nonsmall-cell lung cancer: a phase III randomized trial. J Clin Oncol 2005; 23: 2937–45.

25. Pujol JL, Breton JL, Gervais R, et al. Gemcitabine-docetaxel versus cisplatin-vinorelbine in advanced or metastatic nonsmall-cell lung cancer: a phase III study addressing the case for cisplatin. Ann Oncol 2005; 16: 602–10.
26. Kosmidis PA, Kalofonos C, Christodoulou C, et al. Paclitaxel and gemcitabine versus carboplatin and gemcitabine in patients with advanced non-small-cell lung cancer. A phase III study of the Hellenic Cooperative Oncology Group. Ann Oncol 2008; 19: 115–22.
27. Treat J, Gonin R, Socinski MA, et al. A randomized, phase III multicenter trial of gemcitabine in combination with carboplatin or paclitaxel versus paclitaxel plus carboplatin in patients with advanced or metastatic non-small cell lung cancer. Ann Oncol 2010; 21: 540–7.
28. Gridelli C, Gallo C, Shepherd FA, et al. Gemcitabine plus vinorelbine compared with cisplatin plus vinorelbine or cisplatin plus gemcitabine for advanced non-small-cell lung cancer: a phase III trial of the Italian GEM-VIN investigators and the National Cancer Institute of Canada Clinical Trials Group. J Clin Oncol 2003; 21: 3025–34.
29. D'Addario G, Pintilie M, Leighl NB, et al. Platinum-based versus non-platinum-based chemotherapy in advanced non-small-cell lung cancer: a meta-analysis of the published literature. J Clin Oncol 2005; 23: 2926–36.
30. Pujol JL, Barlesi F, Daures JP. Should chemotherapy combinations for advanced non-small cell lung cancer be platinum-based? A meta-analysis of phase III randomized trials. Lung Cancer 2006; 51: 335–45.
31. Azzoli CG, Baker S Jr, Temin S, et al. American Society of Clinical Oncology clinical practice guideline update on chemotherapy for stage IV non-small-cell lung cancer. J Clin Oncol 2009; 27: 6251–66.
32. Felip E, Gridelli C, Baas P, et al. Metastatic non-small-cell lung cancer: consensus on pathology and molecular tests, first-line, second-line, and third-line therapy: 1st ESMO Consensus Conference in Lung Cancer; Lugano 2010. Ann Oncol 2011; 221: 507–19.
33. NCCN clinical practice guidelines in oncology: non-small cell lung cancer. Version 3.2011. [Available from: www.nccn.com] [Accessed on 15th September 2011].
34. Ardizzoni A, Boni L, Tiseo M, et al. Cisplatin-versus carboplatin-based chemotherapy in first-line treatment of advanced non-small-cell lung cancer: an individual patient data meta-analysis. J Natl Cancer Inst 2007; 99: 847–57.
35. Delbaldo C, Michiels S, Syz N, et al. Benefits of adding a drug to a single-agent or a 2-agent chemotherapy regimen in advanced non-small-cell lung cancer: a meta-analysis. JAMA 2004; 292: 470–84.
36. Hirsch FR, Spreafico A, Novello S, et al. The prognostic and predictive role of histology in advanced non-small cell lung cancer: a literature review. J Thorac Oncol 2008; 3: 1468–81.
37. Scagliotti GV, de Marinis F, Rinaldi M, et al. The role of histology with common first-line regimens for advanced non-small cell lung cancer: a brief report of the retrospective analysis of a three-arm randomized trial. J Thorac Oncol 2009; 4: 1568–71.
38. Shih C, Chen VJ, Gossetti LS, et al. LY231514, a pyrrolo [2,3-d] pyrimidine-based antifolate that inhibits multiple folate-requiring enzymes. Cancer Res 1997; 57: 1116–23.
39. Hazarika M, White RM, Johnson JR, et al. FDA drug approval summaries: pemetrexed (Alimta). Oncologist 2004; 9: 482–8.
40. Schultz RM, Chen VJ, Bewley JR, et al. Biological activity of the multitargeted antifolate, MTA (LY231514), in human cell lines with different resistance mechanisms to antifolate drugs. Sem Oncol 1999; 26(Suppl 6): 68–73.
41. Peterson P, Park K, Fossella F, et al. Is pemetrexed more effective in adenocarcinoma and large cell lung cancer than in squamous cell carcinoma? A retrospective analysis of a phase III trial of pemetrexed vs docetaxel in previously treated patients with advanced non-small cell lung cancer (NSCLC). J Thorac Oncol 2007; 2(Suppl 4): S851 (abstr P2–328).
42. Scagliotti GV, Parikh P, von Pawel J, et al. Phase III study comparing cisplatin plus gemcitabine with cisplatin plus pemetrexed in chemotherapy-naive patients with advanced-stage non-small-cell lung cancer. J Clin Oncol 2008; 26: 3543–51.
43. Scagliotti G, Hanna N, Fossella F, et al. The differential efficacy of pemetrexed according to NSCLC histology: a review of two Phase III studies. Oncologist 2009; 14: 253–63.
44. Gronberg BH, Bremnes RM, Flotten O, et al. Phase III study by the Norwegian lung cancer study group: pemetrexed plus carboplatin compared with gemcitabine plus carboplatin as first-line chemotherapy in advanced non-small-cell lung cancer. J Clin Oncol 2009; 27: 3217–24.
45. Ferrara N, Hillan KJ, Gerber HP, et al. Discovery and development of bevacizumab, an anti-VEGF antibody for treating cancer. Nat Rev Drug Discov 2004; 3: 391–400.
46. Johnson DH, Fehrenbacher L, Novotny WF, et al. Randomized phase II trial comparing bevacizumab plus carboplatin and paclitaxel with carboplatin and paclitaxel alone in previously untreated locally advanced or metastatic non-small-cell lung cancer. J Clin Oncol 2004; 22: 2184–91.
47. Sandler A, Gray R, Perry MC, et al. Paclitaxel-carboplatin alone or with bevacizumab for non-small-cell lung cancer. New Engl J Med 2006; 355: 2542–50.
48. Sandler A, Yi J, Dahlberg S, et al. Treatment outcomes by tumor histology in Eastern Cooperative Group Study 4599 of bevacizumab with paclitaxel/carboplatin for advanced non-small cell lung cancer. J Thorac Oncol 2010; 5: 1416–23.
49. Brahmer JR, Dahlberg SE, Gray RJ, et al. Sex differences in outcome with bevacizumab therapy: analysis of patients with advanced-stage non-small cell lung cancer treated with or without bevacizumab in combination with paclitaxel and carboplatin in the Eastern Cooperative Oncology Group Trial 4599. J Thorac Oncol 2011; 6: 103–8.

50. Dahlberg SE, Sandler AB, Brahmer JR, et al. Clinical course of advanced non-small-cell lung cancer patients experiencing hypertension during treatment with bevacizumab in combination with carboplatin and paclitaxel on ECOG 4599. J Clin Oncol 2010; 28: 949–54.

51. Reck M, von Pawel J, Zatloukal P, et al. Phase III trial of cisplatin plus gemcitabine with either placebo or bevacizumab as first-line therapy for nonsquamous non-small-cell lung cancer: AVAiL. J Clin Oncol 2009; 27: 1227–34.

52. Reck M, von Pawel J, Zatloukal P, et al. Overall survival with cisplatin-gemcitabine and bevacizumab or placebo as first-line therapy for nonsquamous non-small-cell lung cancer: results from a randomised phase III trial (AVAiL). Ann Oncol 2010; 21: 1804–9.

53. Crinò L, Dansin E, Garrido P, et al. Safety and efficacy of first-line bevacizumab-based therapy in advanced non-squamous non-small-cell lung cancer (SAiL, MO19390): a phase 4 study. Lancet Oncol 2010; 11: 733–40.

54. Wozniak AJ, Garst J, Jahanzeb M, et al. Clinical outcomes (CO) for special populations of patients (pts) with advanced non-small cell lung cancer (NSCLC): Results from ARIES, a bevacizumab (BV) observational cohort study (OCS). J Clin Oncol 2010; 28: 567s.

55. Rossi A, Maione P, Ferrara C, et al. New angiogenic agents and non-small cell lung cancer: current results and future development. Targ Oncol 2007; 2: 211–23.

56. Socinski MA, Langer CJ, Huang JE, et al. Safety of bevacizumab in patients with non-small-cell lung cancer and brain metastases. J Clin Oncol 2009; 27: 5255–61.

57. Hainsworth JD, Fang L, Huang J, et al. BRIDGE: An open-label phase II trial evaluating the safety of bevacizumab + carboplatin/paclitaxel as first-line treatment for patients with advanced, previously untreated, squamous non-small cell lung cancer. J Thorac Oncol 2011; 6: 109–14.

58. Dowlati A, Gray R, Sandler AB, et al. Cell adhesion molecules, vascular endothelial growth factor, and basic fibroblast growth factor in patients with non-small cell lung cancer treated with chemotherapy with or without bevacizumab - an Eastern Cooperative Oncology Group Study. Clin Cancer Res 2008; 14: 1407–12.

59. Humblet Y. Cetuximab: an IgG(1) monoclonal antibody for the treatment of epidermal growth factor receptor-expressing tumours. Expert Opin Pharmacother 2004; 5: 1621–33.

60. Pirker R, Pereira JR, Szczesna A, et al. Cetuximab plus chemotherapy in patients with advanced non-small-cell lung cancer (FLEX): an open-label randomised phase III trial. Lancet 2009; 373: 1525–31.

61. Gatzemeier U, von Pawel J, Vynnychenko I, et al. First-cycle rash and survival in patients with advanced non-small-cell lung cancer receiving cetuximab in combination with first-line chemotherapy: a subgroup analysis of data from the FLEX phase 3 study. Lancet Oncol 2011; 12: 30–7.

62. Lynch TJ, Patel T, Dreisbach L, et al. Cetuximab and first-line taxane/carboplatin chemotherapy in advanced non-small-cell lung cancer: results of the randomized multicenter phase III trial BMS099. J Clin Oncol 2010; 28: 911–17.

63. Thatcher N, Lynch TJ, Butts C, et al. Cetuximab plus platinum-based chemotherapy as 1stline treatment in patients with non-small cell lung cancer (NSCLC): a meta-analysis of randomized phase II/III trials (Abstract A3.7). J Thorac Oncol 2009; 4(Suppl 1): S297 (abstr A37).

64. Pirker R, Pereira JR, von Pawel J, et al. EGFR expression as a predictor of survival for first-line chemotherapy plus cetuximab in patients with advanced non-small-cell lung cancer: analysis of data from the phase 3 FLEX study. Lancet Oncol 2012; 13: 33–42.

65. Goldie JH, Coldman AJ. A mathematic model for relating the drug sensitivity of tumors to their spontaneous mutation rate. Cancer Treat Rep 1979; 63: 1727–33.

66. Soon YY, Stockler MR, Askie LM, et al. Duration of chemotherapy for advanced non-small-cell lung cancer: a systematic review and meta-analysis of randomized trials. J Clin Oncol 2009; 27: 3277–83.

67. Gridelli C, Rossi A, Maione P, et al. The role of maintenance treatment in advanced non-small-cell lung cancer: reality or early second line? Clin Lung Cancer 2010; 6: 374–82.

68. Ciuleanu T, Brodowicz T, Zielinski C, et al. Maintenance pemetrexed plus best supportive care versus placebo plus best supportive care for non-small-cell lung cancer: a randomised, double-blind, phase 3 study. Lancet 2009; 374: 1432–40.

69. Cappuzzo F, Ciuleanu T, Stelmakh L, et al. Erlotinib as maintenance treatment in advanced non-small-cell lung cancer: a multicentre, randomised, placebo-controlled phase 3 study. Lancet Oncol 2010; 11: 521–9.

70. Fidias P, Dakhil S, Lyss AP, et al. Phase III study of immediate compared with delayed docetaxel after front-line therapy with gemcitabine plus carboplatin in advanced non-small-cell lung cancer. J Clin Oncol 2008; 27: 591–8.

71. Azzoli CG, Temin S, Aliff T, et al. 2011 focused update of 2009 American Society of Clinical Oncology clinical practice guideline update on chemotherapy for stage IV non-small-cell lung cancer 2011. J Clin Oncol 2011; 29: 3825–31.

72. Rossi A, Torri V, Gridelli C. Switch maintenance versus second-line treatment in non-small cell lung cancer. J Thorac Oncol 2011; 6: 1298–9.

73. Kabbinavar FF, Miller VA, Johnson BE, et al. Overall survival (OS) in ATLAS, a phase IIIb trial comparing bevacizumab (B) therapy with or without erlotinib (E) after completion of chemotherapy (chemo) with B for first-line treatment of locally advanced, recurrent, or metastatic non-small cell lung cancer (NSCLC). J Clin Oncol 2010; 28: 544s (abstr 7526).

74. Gaafar RM, Surmont VF, Scagliotti GV, et al. A double-blind, randomised, placebo-controlled phase III intergroup study of gefitinib in patients with advanced NSCLC, non-progressing after first line platinum-based chemotherapy (EORTC 08021/ILCP 01/03). Eur J Cancer 2011; 47: 2331–40.

75. Zhang L, Ma S, Song X, et al. Gefitinib versus placebo as maintenance therapy in patients with locally-advanced or metastatic non-small-cell lung cancer (INFORM; C-TONG 0804): a multicentre, double-blind randomised phase 3 trial. Lancet Oncol 2012; 13: 466–75.
76. Belani CP, Waterhouse DM, Ghazal H, et al. Phase III study of maintenance gemcitabine (G) and best supportive care (BSC) versus BSC, following standard combination therapy with gemcitabine-carboplatin (G-Cb) for patients with advanced non-small cell lung cancer (NSCLC). J Clin Oncol 2010; 28: 540s (abstr 7506).
77. Paz-Ares L, de Marinis F, Dediu M, et al. Maintenance therapy with pemetrexed plus best supportive care verus placebo versus best supportive care after induction therapy with pemetrexed plus cisplatin for advanced non-squamous non-small-cell lung cancer (PARAMOUNT): a double-blind, phase 3, randomised controlled trial. Lancet Oncol 2012; 13: 247–55.
78. Paz-Ares L, de Marinis F, Dediu M, et al. PARAMOUNT: Final overall survival (OS) results of the phase III study of maintenance pemetrexed (pem) plus best supportive care (BSC) versus placebo (plb) plus BSC immediately following induction treatment with pem plus cisplatin (cis) for advanced nonsquamous (NS) non-small cell lung cancer (NSCLC). J Clin Oncol 2012; 30: 481s (abstr LBA7507).
79. Gridelli C, de Marinis F, Pujol JL, et al. Safety, resource use, and quality of life (QOL) from PARAMOUNT: A phase III study of maintenance pemetrexed plus best supportive care (BSC) versus placebo plus BSC immediately following induction treatment with pemetrexed-cisplatin for advanced nonsquamous non-small cell lung cancer (NSCLC). J Thorac Oncol 2011; 6(Suppl 2): S323–4 (abstr O11.06).
80. Perol M, Chouaid C, Milleron BJ, et al. Maintenance with either gemcitabine or erlotinib versus observation with predefined second-line treatment after cisplatin-gemcitabine induction chemotherapy in advanced NSCLC: IFCT-GFPC 0502 phase III study. J Clin Oncol 2010; 28: 540s (abstr 7507).

Table 7.1 EGFR TKIs as First-Line Treatment for Patients with Advanced NSCLC

Authors	Study phase	Agent	Case number	ORR (%)	Median PFS/ TTP (mo)	Median OS (mo)
Giaccone et al. 2006[22]	Phase II	Erlotinib	53	22.7	84 (days)	391 (days)
Lee et al. 2009[28]	Phase II (ineligible for chemotherapy)	Erlotinib	24	21	1.5	3.2
Niho et al. 2006[24]	Phase II	Gefitinib	40	30	N/A	13.9
Yang et al. 2008[25]	Phase II	Gefitinib	106	50.9	5.5	22.4
Janne, et al. 2010[26]	Phase II (adeno, ever smokers)	Erlotinib	81	35	6.7	24.3
		Erlotinib+Carbo+Pac	100	48	6.6	19.6
Mok et al. 2009[27]	Phase III (adeno, ever smokers)	Gefitinib	609	43.0	5.7	18.6
		Carbo+Pac	608	32.2	5.8	17.3
Lee et al. 2009[28]	Phase III (adeno, never smokers)	Gefitinib	159	53.5	6.1	21.3
		Gem+cis	150	45.3	6.6	23.3

Abbreviations: EGFR, epidermal growth factor receptor; PFS, progression free survival; TTP, time to progression; ORR, objective response rate; OS, overall survival; Cis, cisplatin; Carbo, carboplatin; Pac, paclitaxel; Doc, docetaxcel; Gem, gemicitabine.

erlotinib alone with erlotinib intercalated with chemotherapy in chemotherapy-naïve patients with advanced NSCLC who were positive for EGFR protein expression and/or with high *EGFR* gene copy number. The six-month PFS was 26% and 31% for the combined and erlotinib alone arms, the median were 4.57 and 2.69 months, respectively. Patients with tumors harboring *EGFR* activating mutations did better on erlotinib alone (median PFS, 18.2 vs. 4.9 months). This study did not support erlotinib intercalated with chemotherapy in advanced NSCLC selected by EGFR expression.[34]

There is increasing recognition that patients with certain clinicopathological characteristics appear to derive more benefit from EGFR TKIs. These patients tend to be female gender, of Asian ethnicity, never-smokers, and adenocarcinoma histology, all known to be associated with a higher prevalence of *EGFR* mutations. On the basis of these observations, three randomized trials have compared first-line EGFR TKI to platinum-based chemotherapy in the patients selected by these clinical characteristics (adenocarcinoma histology, never or light smokers). CALGB 30406[26] is a Caucasian study and IPASS[27] and First-Signal[28] East Asian studies. These studies showed that first-line EGFR TKI was not inferior to standard chemotherapy in terms of ORR, PFS, and OS, but superior in terms of toxicity profile and quality of life.

Further exploratory biomarker analysis of IPASS suggested that *EGFR* mutation was a major predictive factor for clinical benefit from first-line EGFR TKI. Improvement in PFS with gefitinib was confined to those with *EGFR* mutations. In fact, first-line EGFR TKI seems to have a detrimental effect in those without an *EGFR* mutation. These results were confirmed by the FIRST-SIGNAL and CALGB 30406 trials. Thus, clinical characteristics alone are not sufficient to correctly predict benefit from EGFR TKIs because they allow to identify the presence of an *EGFR* mutation only in up to 60% of patients. In addition, it is not always possible to rule out the possibility of an *EGFR* mutation solely on the basis of clinical characteristics. About 10% of patients with non-adenocarcinoma harbor *EGFR* mutations.[14,15] Thus the molecular diagnosis of *EGFR* mutation is considered the "gold standard" for patient selection for first-line EGFR TKI therapy. Taken together, these trials suggest that EGFR TKIs are not appropriate for front-line therapy in unselected populations, in those with negative *EGFR* mutation, or with unknown *EGFR* genotyping.

EGFR TKIs AS FIRST-LINE TREATMENT FOR ADVANCED NSCLC PATIENTS WITH *EGFR* MUTATIONS

The presence of *EGFR* mutations has proven to be the most reliable predictor of clinical benefit associated with EGFR TKIs. Several phase II clinical trials have screened *EGFR*-mutant patients for first-line therapy. iTARGET[35] was a prospective phase II study of first-line gefitinib in advanced NSCLC patients harboring *EGFR* mutations. Efficacy was encouraging, with an ORR of 55% (95% confidence interval [CI] 33–70), PFS of 9.2 months (95% CI 6.2–11.8), and OS of 17.5 months (95% CI 13.5–21.3). Another study screened 2105 advanced NSCLC patients for *EGFR* mutations. Of them, 350 patients were found to harbor the mutation (16.6%).[36] There were 217 patients who were given erlotinib, including

Table 7.2 EGFR TKIs as First-Line Treatment for EGFR-Mutant Patients

Authors	Study phase	Treatment	Case number	ORR (%)	Median PFS/ TTP (mo)	Median OS(mo)
Inoue et al. 2009[42]	Phase II (unfit)	Gefitinib	30	66	6.5	17.8
Sequist et al. 2008[35]	Phase II	Gefitinib	34	55	9.2	17.5
Rosell et al. 2009[36]	Phase II	Erlotinib	113	52.1	14	28
Yang et al. 2008[25]	Phase II	Gefitinib	55	69	8	24
De Greve et al. 2011	Phase II	Erlotinib	30	56.5	13	NA
Janne et al. 2010[26]	Phase II	Erlotinib	33	67	14.1	31.3
		Erlotinib+ Carbo+Pac	33	73	17.2	39.0
Mok et al. 2009[27]	Phase III	Gefitinib	132	71.2	9.5	21.6
		Carbo+Pac	129	47.3	6.3	21.9
Lee et al. 2009[28]	Phase III	Gefitinib	26	84.6	8.4	30.6
		Gem+Cis	16	37.5	6.7	26.5
Maemondo et al. 2010[37]	Phase III	Gefitinib	115	73.7	10.8	30.5
		Carbo+Pac	115	30.7	5.4	23.6
Mitsudomi et al. 2010[38]	Phase III	Gefitinib	88	62.1	9.2	NA
		Cis+Doc	89	32.2	6.3	NA
OPTIMAL (Zhou et al. 2011[41])	Phase III	Erlotinib	82	83	13.1	NA
		Carbo+Gem	72	36	4.6	NA
EURTAC (Rosell et al. 2011[40])	Phase III	Erlotinib	86	58	9.7	NA
		Carbo/Cis+Doc/ Gem	87	15	5.2	NA

113 patients receiving erlotinib as the first-line therapy. Median PFS and OS was 14 months (95% CI 9.7–18.3) and 28.0 months (95% CI 22.7–33) in first-line treatment, respectively. The study showed that large-scale screening for *EGFR* mutations was feasible and that EGFR TKI as first-line therapy seemed more effective (Table 7.2).

Recently, there have been four randomized phase III studies comparing first-line EGFR TKI to standard chemotherapy in the patients with advanced NSCLC harboring *EGFR* mutations. Two studies were with gefitinib[37,38] in Japanese patients and two with erlotinib,[39,40] one from China and the other from Europe. In NEJ002, 230 *EGFR*-mutant patients were randomly assigned to receive gefitinib or carboplatin/paclitaxel. Median PFS (10.8 months vs. 5.4 months, hazard ratio [HR] = 0.30, p < 0.001) and ORR (73.7% vs. 30.7%, p < 0.001) were significantly improved by gefitinib. However, OS was comparable between the two arms. In WJTOG 30405, 177 chemotherapy-naïve patients were enrolled and randomized to receive either gefitinib (n = 88) or cisplatin/ docetaxel (n = 89) for 3–6 cycles. ORR and PFS were also much better in the gefitinib arm compared with the chemotherapy arms.

OPTIMAL was a randomized phase III trial conducted in China, comparing erlotinib to carboplatin/ gemcitabine for four cycles in advanced NSCLC patients harboring *EGFR* mutations. The primary endpoint was PFS. Erlotinib was significantly superior to chemotherapy in terms of PFS (13.1 vs. 4.6 months, HR 0.16, 95% CI 0.10–0.26, p < 0.0001), and ORR (83% vs. 36%, p < 0.001). Subgroup analysis showed that most subgroups (including male gender, smokers, non-adenocarcinoma histology) had a better clinical benefit from erlotinib, suggesting tumor biology is more important than clinical characteristics in prediction of efficacy to EGFR TKIs. The EURTAC trial, the only available study conducted in Caucasian patients with *EGFR* mutations, is an ongoing multicenter, randomized phase III study, comparing erlotinib to platinum-based doublet chemotherapy (cisplatin or carboplatin plus gemcitabine or docetaxel). The planned interim analysis showed that, compared to doublet chemotherapy, erlotinib significantly extended PFS (9.7 vs. 5.2 months, HR = 0.37, p < 0.001) and improved ORR (58% vs. 15%).

Treatment with EGFR TKIs has also been found to be associated with improvement of quality of life. We found improvement rates for FACT-L, the trial outcome index and lung cancer subscale was 72–76% in the erlotinib arm versus 24 –32% in the chemotherapy arm (p < 0.001). When adjusted by PS, smoking history, and gender, or by *EGFR* mutation type, smoking history, and histology, OR ranged from 6.63 to 8.63, substantially favoring the erlotinib arm.[41] These results are consistent with those of the IPASS and first-SIGNAL trials.

Molecular selection is also of particular importance in unfit patients. Disappointing results have been obtained in clinical trials testing EGFR TKIs in unselected patients, as mentioned above; EGFR TKIs did not improve OS in those unfit for chemotherapy, compared with placebo. On the other hand, when gefitinib was administered to chemo-naïve patients with poor PS, selected by the presence of *EGFR* mutations, very encouraging results in terms of ORR, PFS, and OS were obtained. One study[25] retrospectively investigated the role of gefitinib in advanced NSCLC with poor PS (ECOG PS 3 or 4). They found that clinical features associated with *EGFR* mutations such as female gender, adenocarcinoma histology, and never-smoking history predicted longer survival time. Another group[42] reported the results of phase II study on first-line gefitinib in advanced NSCLC patients with *EGFR* mutations who could not tolerate chemotherapy. Thirty patients were enrolled and 22 had ECOG PS 3 or 4. After gefitinib, 68% patients had significant improvement in PS (from ECOG PS 3 or 4 to PS 0 or 1). Median PFS was 6.5 months and OS was 17.8 months.

The question of whether there is any difference in efficacy of EGFR TKIs between *EGFR* exon 19 deletions and exon 21 L858R mutation has not been answered. Clinical data seem to indicate that exon 19 deletions are more susceptible to the EGFR TKI activity compared with L858 mutation. One group[43] found that exon 19 deletions were associated with longer TTP and OS compared with L858R. Another observed a trend toward more durable responses in those with exon 19 deletions. We found PFS for erlotinib tended to be longer in those with exon 19 deletions than with L858R mutation (15.3 vs. 12.5 months, HR = 0.58, p = 0.057). However, in the IPASS study (two Japanese phase III trials and the iTARGET trial) there was no significant difference in PFS between exon 19 deletions and L858R. Both patients with exon 19 deletions and L858R got substantial clinical benefit from EGFR TKIs compared with chemotherapy. Based on these limited data, it is not possible to conclude if a specific *EGFR* mutation affects EGFR TKI response.

A recently pooled analysis further supports first-line EGFR TKI use over standard chemotherapy in advanced NSCLC patients with *EGFR* mutations.[44] About 60 prospective or retrospective studies were included in the analysis, of which 12 evaluated erlotinib (365 patients), 39 gefitinib (1069 patients), and 9 chemotherapy (375 patients). Median PFS was 13.2 months with erlotinib, 9.8 months with gefitinib, and 5.9 months with chemotherapy. Erlotinib and gefitinib achieved a longer median PFS versus chemotherapy, both individually (P = 0.000 and P = 0.002, respectively) and as a combined group (EGFR TKI vs. chemotherapy, P = 0.000). EGFR TKIs appear to be the most effective agents for patients with advanced NSCLC harboring *EGFR* mutations.

EGFR TKIs are well tolerated. According to several phase III studies of *EGFR*-mutant patients, TKIs are seldom associated with hematological toxicity. Treatment-related toxicity, in general, is comparatively lower for EGFR TKIs than standard chemotherapy. Significantly fewer cases need dose reductions or discontinuation due to adverse events. Among typical side effects, dermatologic toxicity (including rash, acne, dry skin, and pruritus) and diarrhea are the most common. Rash is of mild to moderate intensity and, in most cases, easily manageable. Liver toxicity and interstitial lung disease should also be mentioned, especially in the Japanese. Elevation of alanine and/or aspartate aminotransferase and bilirubin are relatively common, although these laboratory abnormalities are usually asymptomatic and reversible upon drug cessation. Occurrence of interstitial lung disease is potentially lethal, but the incidence is ~1–3%. EGFR TKI therapy also appears feasible in unfit NSCLC patients. No treatment-related death was reported with the EGFR TKI in the TOPICAL study.

EGFR TKIS IN PATIENTS WITH RARE *EGFR* MUTATIONS

Rare *EGFR* mutations are defined as mutations in exon 18 and 20, uncommon mutations in exon 19 and 21, and/or complex mutations. Little is known about efficacy of first-line EGFR TKIs in this population. *EGFR* T790M mutation is believed to be responsible for acquired resistance to EGFR TKIs and was believed not to exist in EGFR TKI-naïve tumors. However, a recent study demonstrated it could be found in the tumors before TKI treatment and usually co-existed with the other *EGFR* activation mutations. Its existence in pre-treatment tumors might not affect tumor response to EGFR TKIs but shorten PFS.[45,46]

One group[43] found 12 patients with rare *EGFR* mutations. Four patients developed progressive disease, two partial responses (one with exon 19 duplication, and another with G719A+G779C) and two with durable stable disease (20.5 months with exon 19 del+L861Q, 25.8 months with exon 19 deletion + KRAS mutation). In a series of 10 patients with rare *EGFR* mutations,[47] 3 achieved partial responses to erlotinib and six developed progressive disease. The three with partial responses harbored *EGFR* E709A+ G719C, G719S, and del I744_K745insKIP-VAI, respectively. Thus, most rare *EGFR* mutations seem to be associated with primary EGFR TKI resistance.

SECOND-GENERATION EGFR TKIs

Erlotinib and gefitinib act as ATP-mimetic and reversible inhibitors of EGFR. In contrast, second-generation, irreversible EGFR TKIs not only act as ATP mimetic but also covalently bind to EGFR, thereby inhibiting EGFR phosphorylation, even in the presence of a T790M secondary mutation.[48]

Compounds as second generation EGFR TKIs under clinical development include Afatinib and PF299804. Afatinib is a highly selective and irreversible ErbB-family blocker and found to be effective in inhibiting growth of NSCLC cell with the *EGFR* T790M mutation, both *in vitro* and *in vivo*. On the basis of these pre-clinical studies, clinical trials are under way to determine its efficacy in NSCLC patients. Lux-lung 2 was a multicenter phase II open-label trial in which staged IIIB-IV NSCLC patients harboring *EGFR* mutations were enrolled and given afatinib, 50 mg/day, until disease progression or intolerable toxicity. Median PFS and OS were 14 and 24 months, respectively. The ORR was quite similar between the subgroups with exon 19 deletions or L858R mutation, 67% and 69%, respectively.[49]

PF 299804 is a pan-HER inhibitor. A phase II trial showed its efficacy in those with *EGFR* mutations. Tumor response rate was 59% and PFS at the ninth months was 90%.[50]

There are 20–30% of *EGFR*-mutated patients who do not respond to a first-generation of EGFR TKIs. Moreover, virtually all patients with *EGFR* mutations who initially respond to EGFR TKIs eventually develop progressive disease. Thus, irreversible EGFR TKIs may be more or as effective as reversible EGFR TKIs in patients with the common *EGFR* or even T790M mutations. Certainly, further randomized phase III studies are required to demonstrate their efficacy.

FIRST-LINE VS. SECOND-LINE EGFR TKIs

No studies comparing first-line EGFR TKI with chemotherapy in advanced NSCLC patients with *EGFR* mutation showed a difference in OS, as discussed above. The possible explanation is that a relevant number of patients in the chemotherapy arm received EGFR TKIs after failure to chemotherapy. EGFR TKIs as first- or second-line therapy have proven to be effective. One group found that PFS and OS were comparable between those receiving first-line and second-line erlotinib. However, it should be kept in mind that the use of an EGFR TKI makes the biggest contribution to outcomes of NSCLC patients with EGFR mutations. OS was not different between the patients with and without *EGFR* mutations before gefitinib was approved in Japan (13.2 vs. 10.4 months, HR = 0.79, p = 0.13). However, OS was significantly improved in those with *EGFR* mutations (27.2 vs. 13.6 months, HR = 0.48, p < 0.001) after its approval.[51] Therefore, patients with *EGFR* mutations should be given the opportunity to use EGFR TKIs during the course of their disease; however, it is not clear when they should receive it. In our practice, not all patients have the chance to receive second-line therapy. Many patients' conditions and PS deteriorate rapidly after failure of first-line chemotherapy, preventing use of second-line EGFR TKIs.[52] In the TORCH trial, a significant proportion of patients assigned to first-line chemotherapy did not receive second-line TKIs.[32] These results emphasize the risk of never receiving an EGFR TKI, if not administered as first-line.[52]

EGFR TKIs have demonstrated to result in a significantly prolonged PFS, superior quality of life, and better toxicity profile in the several randomized clinical trials. Thus, first-line EGFR TKIs seem the best option for the patients with *EGFR* mutations and are so recommended by the recent NSCLC guidelines.

TREATMENT OF PATIENTS WITH ACQUIRED RESISTANCE TO EGFR TKIs

Although patients with *EGFR* mutations benefit more from EGFR TKIs, almost all patients will finally develop disease progression or acquired resistance. The definition of "acquired resistance" to EGFR TKIs has now been published.[53] Several mechanisms have been proposed to be strongly associated with acquired resistance, including the *EGFR* T790M mutation, c-MET amplification, and others. T790M mutation and *c-MET* amplification account for acquired resistance in approximately 50% and 20% of patients, respectively. Occasionally, resistant tumors with *MET* amplification have a concurrent *EGFR* T790M mutation.[54,55] A D761Y secondary mutation is also associated with acquired resistance, but occurs in <1% of patients.[56] T790M mutation detected in pretreatment tumors may not be associated with EGFR TKI resistance or prevent tumor response to retreatment of EGFR TKIs if co-existing with activating *EGFR* mutations.[45] One group suggested that the balance of single activating mutations and activating mutations plus T790M mutations will influence the probability of a response to EGFR TKIs and also its clinical benefit.[57]

There are several treatment options after failure of first-line EGFR TKIs. Switching to standard chemotherapy is recommended by NCCN guidelines and the ESMO consensus statement.[3] According to PS and histology, chemotherapy regimen can be determined. One group[37] found that 67.5% of patients assigned to the gefitinib arm received post-study carboplatin/paclitaxel and achieved a tumor response similar (28.5%) to its use as first-line chemotherapy (30.7%), suggesting that first-line EGFR TKIs do not change the sensitivity of NSCLC to standard chemotherapy.

Continuation of an EGFR TKI beyond disease progression may be effective. In patients with acquired resistance to EGFR TKIs, discontinuation of therapy may be associated with a clinical significant risk of accelerated disease progression or even a disease "flare." Acquired resistant tumors may contain both TKI-resistant and -sensitive cancer cells. Because of more indolent courses seen in tumors with the T790M mutation, TKI-sensitive cancer cells may quickly repopulate after TKI discontinuation. One study found that 23% of patients experienced a disease flare. Median time to disease flare was only eight days. They found factors related to flare were shorter TTP on initial EGFR TKIs and the presence of pleural or brain disease.[58]

Some patients develop disease progression only in central nervous system during EGFR TKI therapy. The blood–brain barrier may prevent penetration of EGFR TKIs into brain. Indeed, metastatic tumors to the brain may still be sensitive to higher doses of EGFR TKIs since an increased TKI dose has been shown to be effective in some cases.[59]

Some studies have tried re-administration of EGFR TKIs after failure of an EGFR TKI.[60–62] One group[63] performed serial CT and PET imaging of patients with acquired resistance at three time points: before stopping EGFR TKI, three weeks after TKI discontinuation, and three weeks after its re-administration. Tumor volume and FDG avidity increased significantly after stopping TKI but decreased in many cases when TKIs were restarted.

Because of different dosing schedules, erlotinib at its clinically recommended dose produces greater drug exposure than gefitinib. Several studies have investigated the role of erlotinib in those with prior failure to gefitinib. One study[64] retrospectively analyzed 11 patients who had obtained a partial response or stable disease with gefitinib and were then treated with erlotinib after disease progression. Among them, one patient (9%) achieved a response and seven patients (64%) had stable disease, giving a disease control rate of 73% (95% CI 43–91), median PFS of 3.4 months (95% CI 2–5.2), and OS of 7.3 months (95% CI 2.7–13). Another group[65] made a pooled analysis of reports of erlotinib after gefitinib failure. A total of 106 patients were pooled. This group found that erlotinib could produce clinical benefit in patients who had shown a long duration of stable disease (>6 months) with prior gefitinib therapy, but not in those with partial response. However, these studies were either of empiric observations or were retrospective analyses. Thus, such results should be interpreted with caution.

Irreversible EGFR TKIs are another possible option for overcoming acquired TKI resistance. Many compounds are under study and have proved effective in preclinical studies. Lux-lung 1 compared afatinib to placebo in patients previously treated with chemotherapy and an EGFR TKI. Tumor response and PFS was improved but the primary endpoint of OS was not met.[66]

Mouse studies have examined what combination of EGFR-targeted therapies had maximal efficacy against T790M-harboring transgenic tumors and found that the combination of an irreversible EGFR TKI plus cetuximab effectively reduced tumor burden, while neither agent was effective alone.[67] However, a phase II study did not find any patient achieving a response to combination of cetuximab and erlotinib. A recent phase II study[68] investigated the combination of afatinib and cetuximab in those previously treated with chemotherapy and an EGFR TKI. Forty-five patients were enrolled and a 40% partial response and 90% disease control rate were achieved. Tumor responses were observed in those with and without an *EGFR* T790M mutation. These results need to be confirmed in a randomized phase III study.

CONCLUSION

Lung cancer is the leading cause of cancer-related deaths, world-wide, and remains to be for some time. Evidence shows that lung cancer is heterogeneous and that *EGFR*-mutant lung cancer is a distinct subgroup. EGFR TKIs, namely gefitinib and erlotinib, have obtained marked progress in treating this group. Compared with standard chemotherapy, EGFR TKIs obtain much longer PFS, a favorable toxicity profile, and an improved quality of life in the first-line setting for *EGFR*-mutant cancer patients. Thus, EGFR TKIs are now considered to be appropriate first-line treatment for this group. Second generation of EGFR TKIs have been developed and are in clinical trials, hopefully giving oncologists more options for targeting NSCLC.

REFERENCES

1. Jemal A, Siegel R, Xu J, et al. Cancer statistics. CA Cancer J Clin 2010; 60: 277–300.
2. Rinaldi M, Cauchi C, Gridelli C. First line chemotherapy in advanced or metastatic NSCLC. Ann Oncol 2006; 5(Suppl): v64–7.
3. Felip Em, Gridelli C, Baas P, et al. Metastatic non-small-cell lung cancer: consensus on pathology and molecular tests, first-line, second-line, and third-line therapy. 1st ESMO Consensus Conference in Lung Cancer; Lugano 2010. Ann Oncol 2011; 22: 1507–19.

4. Non-small Cell Lung Cancer Collaborative Group. Chemotherapy in non-small cell lung cancer: a meta-analysis using updated data on individual patients from 52 randomised clinical trials. BMJ 1995; 311: 899–909.

5. Schiller JH, Harrington D, Belani CP, et al. Comparison of four chemotherapy regimens for advanced non-small-cell lung cancer. N Engl J Med 2002; 346: 92–8.

6. Mendelsohn J, Baselga J. The EGF receptor family as targets for cancer therapy. Oncogene 2000; 19: 6550–65.

7. Riely GJ, Politi KA, Miller VA. Update on epidermal growth factor receptor mutations in non-small cell lung cancer. Clin Cancer Res 2006; 12: 7232–41.

8. Grunwald V, Hidalgo M. Developing inhibitors of the epidermal growth factor receptor for cancer treatment. J Natl Cancer Inst 2003; 95: 851–67.

9. Jorissen RN, Walker F, Pouliot N, et al. Epidermal growth factor receptor: mechanisms of activation and signalling. Exp Cell Res 2003; 284: 31–53.

10. Normanno N, Bianco C, De Luca A, et al. Target-based agents against ErbB receptors and their ligands: a novel approach to cancer treatment. Endocr Relat Cancer 2003; 10: 1–21.

11. Bronte G, Rizzo S, Paglia LL, et al. Driver mutations and differential sensitivity to targeted therapies: a new approach to the treatment of lung adenocarcinoma. Lung Cancer 2010; 36: S21–9.

12. Lynch T, Bell DW, Sordella R, et al. Activating mutations in the epidermal growth factor receptor underlying responsiveness of non-small-cell lung cancer to gefitinib. N Eng J Med 2004; 304: 2129–39.

13. Paez JG, Janne PA, Lee JC, et al. EGFR mutations in lung cancer: correlation with clinical response to gefitinib therapy. Science 2004; 304: 1497–500.

14. Mitsudomi T, Kosaka T, Yatabe Y. Biological and clinical implications of EGFR mutations in lung cancer. Int J Clin Oncol 2006; 113: 190–8.

15. Wu YL, Zhong WZ, Li LY, et al. Epidermal growth factor receptor mutations and their correlation with gefitinib therapy in patients with non-small cell lung cancer: a meta-analysis based on updated individual patient data from six medical centers in mainland China. JTO 2007; 25: 430–9.

16. Zhang X, Gureasko J, Shen K, et al. An allosteric mechanism for activation of the kinase domain of epidermal growth factor receptor. Cell 2006; 125: 1137–49.

17. Politi K, Zakowski MF, Fan PD, et al. Lung adenocarcinomas induced in mice by mutant EGF receptors found in human lung cancers respond to a tyrosine kinase inhibitor or to down-regulation of the receptors. Genes Dev 2006; 20: 1496–510.

18. Carey KD, Garton AJ, Romero MS, et al. Kinetic analysis of epidermal growth factor receptor somatic mutant proteins shows increased sensitivity to the epidermal growth factor receptor tyrosine kinase inhibitor, erlonib. Cancer Res 2006; 66: 8163–71.

19. Zhu CQ, da Cunha Santos G, Ding K, et al. Role of KRAS and EGFR as biomarkers of response to erlotinib in National Cancer Institute of Canada Clinical Trials Group Study BR.21. J Clin Oncol 2008; 26: 4268–75.

20. Clark GM, Zborowski DM, Culbertson JL, et al. Clinical utility of epidermal growth factor receptor expression for selecting patients with advanced non-small cell lung cancer for treatment with erlotinib. J Thorac Oncol 2006; 1: 837–46.

21. Wu YL, Zhou C, Chen G, et al. Efficacy results from the randomized phase III OPTIMAL(CTONG 0802) study comparing first-line erlotinib versus carboplatin plus gemcitabine in Chinese advanced non-small cell lung cancer patients with EGFR activating mutations. Ann of Oncol 2010; 21: viii6.

22. Giaccone G, Ruiz MG, Le Chevalier T, et al. Erlotinib for frontline treatment of advanced non-small cell lung cancer: a phase II study. Clin Cancer Res 2006; 12: 6049–55.

23. Lee DH, Kim HT, Lee JS. Phase II study of erlotinib for chemotherapy-naive patients with advanced or metastatic non-small cell lung cancer who are ineligible for platinum doublets. Clin Lung Cancer 2009; 105: E14.

24. Niho N, Kubota K, Goto K, et al. First-line single agent treatment with gefitinib in patients with advanced non-small-cell lung cancer: a phase II study. J Clin Oncol 2006; 24: 64–9.

25. Yang CH, Yu CJ, Shih JY, et al. Specific EGFR mutations predict treatment outcome of stage IIIB/IV patients with chemotherapy-naive non-small-cell lung cancer receiving first-line gefitinib monotherapy. J Clin Oncol 2008; 26: 2745–53.

26. Janne PA, Wang XF, Socinski MA, et al. Randomized phase II trial of erlotinib (E) alone or in combination with carboplatin/paclitaxel (CP) in never or light former smokers with advanced lung adenocarcinoma: CALGB 30406. J Clin Oncol 2010; 28: 7503a.

27. Mok TS, Wu YL, Thongprasert S, et al. Gefitinib or carboplatin-paclitaxel in pulmonary adenocarcinoma. N Engl J Med 2009; 361: 947–57.

28. Lee JS, Park K, Kim SW, et al. A randomized phase III study of gefitinib (IRESSATM) versus standard chemotherapy (gemcitabine plus cisplatin) as a first-line treatment for never-smokers with advanced or metastatic adenocarcinoma of the lung. JTO 2009; 4: s283–4.

29. Crino L, Cappuzzo F, Zatloukal P, et al. Gefitinib versus vinorelbine in chemotherapy-naive elderly patients with advanced non-small-cell lung cancer (INVITE). a randomized, phase II study. J Clin Oncol 2008; 26: 4253–60.

30. Lee S, Rudd R, khan I, et al. TOPICAL: randomized phase III trial of erlotinib compared with placebo in chemotherapy-naïve patients with advanced non-small cell lung cancer (NSCLC) and unsuitable for first-line chemotherapy. J Clin Oncol 2010; 28: 7504a.

31. Goss G, Ferry D, Wierzbicki R, et al. Randomized phase II study of gefitinib compared with placebo in chemotherapy-naïve patients with advanced non-small-cell lung cancer and poor performance status. J Clin Oncol 2009; 27: 2253–60.

32. Gridelli C, Ciardiello F, Feld R, et al. International multicenter randomized phase III study of first-line erlotinib (E) followed by second-line cisplatin plus gemcitabine (CG) versus first-line CG followed by second-line E in advanced non-small cell lung cancer (aNSCLC): The TORCH trial. J Clin Oncol 2010; 28–7508a.

33. Stinchcombe TE, Peterman AH, Lee CB, et al. A randomized phase II trial of first-line treatment with gemcitabine, erlotinib, or gemcitabine and erlotinib in elderly patients (Age ≥70 Years) with stage IIIB/IV non-small cell lung cancer. J Thorac Oncol 2011; 6: 1569–77.

34. Hirsch R, Kabbinavar F, Eisen T, et al. Phase II, biomarker-selected study comparing erlotinib to erlotinib intercalated with chemotherapy in first-line therapy for advanced non-small-cell lung cancer. J Clin Oncol 2011; 29: 3567–73.

35. Sequist LV, Martins RG, Spigel D, et al. First-line gefitinib in patients with advanced non-small-cell lung cancer harboring somatic EGFR mutations. J Clin Oncol 2008; 26: 2442–9.

36. Rosell R, Moran T, Queralt C, et al. Screening for epidermal growth factor receptor mutations in lung cancer. N Engl J Med 2009; 361: 958–67.

37. Maemondo M, Inoue A, Kobayashi K, et al. Gefitinib or chemotherapy for non-small-cell lung cancer with mutated EGFR. N Engl J Med 2010; 362: 2380–8.

38. Mitsudomi T, Morita S, Yatabe Y, et al. Gefitinib versus cisplatin plus docetaxel in patients with non-small-cell lung cancer harbouring mutations of the epidermal growth factor receptor (WJTOG3405): an open label, randomised phase 3 trial. Lancet Oncol 2010; 11: 121–8.

39. Zhou C, Wu Y, Chen G, et al. Erlotinib versus chemotherapy as first-line treatment for patients with advanced EGFR mutation-positive non-small-cell lung cancer (OPTIMAL, CTONG-0802): a multicentre, open-label, randomised, phase 3 study. Lancet Oncol 2011; 128: 735–42.

40. Rosell R, Gervais R, Vergnenegre A, et al. Erlotinib versus chemotherapy (CT) in advanced non-small cell lung cancer (NSCLC) patients (p) with epidermal growth factor receptor (EGFR) mutations: Interim results of the European Erlotinib Versus Chemotherapy (EURTAC) phase III randomized trial. J Clin Oncol 2011; 29: 7503a.

41. Zhou C, Wu Y, Chen G, et al. Updated median PFS and analysis of quality of life (QOL) in OPTIMAL, a phase III, randomized , open-label, first line study of erlotinib vs. carboplatin/gemcitabine in patients with advanced non-small cell lung cancer (NSCLC) with EGFR activating mutations. JTO 2011; 6: s315–16.

42. Inoue A, Kobayashi K, Usui K, et al. First-line gefitinib for patients with advanced non-small-cell lung cancer harboring epidermal growth factor receptor mutations without indication for chemotherapy. J Clin Oncol 2009; 27: 1394–400.

43. De Greve, J. P. Van Meerbeeck, J. F. Vansteenkiste, et al. First-line erlotinib in advanced non-small cell lung cancer (NSCLC) carrying an activating EGFR mutation: A multicenter academic phase II study in Caucasian patients (pts) (NCT00339586)-FIELT study group. J Clin Oncol 29: 2011

44. Jackman DM, Yeap BY, Sequist LV, et al. Exon 19 deletion mutations of epidermal growth factor receptor are associated with prolonged survival in non-small cell lung cancer patients treated with gefitinib or erlotinib. Clin Cancer Res 2006; 12: 3908–14.

45. Paz-Ares L, Soulieres D, Melezinek I, et al. Clinical outcomes in non-small-cell lung cancer patients with EGFR mutations: pooled analysis. J Cell Mol Med 2010; 14: 51–69.

46. Fukuoka M, Wu YL, Thongprasert S, et al. Biomarker analysis and final overall survival results from a phase III, randomized, open-label, first-line study of gefitinib versus carboplatin/paclitaxel in clinical selected patients with advanced non-small-cell lung cancer in Asia (IPASS). JCO 2010; 29: 2866–74.

47. Rosell R, Molina MA, Costa C, et al. Outcome to erlotinib in non-small cell lung cancer (NSCLC) patients (p) according to the presence of the EGFR T790M mutation and BRCA1 mRNA expression levels in pretreatment biopsies. J Clin Oncol 2010; 28(Suppl 15): 7514.

48. De Pas T, Toffalorio F, Manzotti M, et al. Activity of epidermal growth factor receptor-tyrosine kinase inhibitors in patients with non-small cell lung cancer harboring rare epidermal growth factor receptor mutations. J Thorac Oncol 2011; 6: 1895–901.

49. Takezawa K, Okamoto I, Tanizaki J, et al. Enhanced anticancer effect of the combination of BIBW 2992 and thymidylate synthase-targeted agents in non-small cell lung cancer with the T790M mutation of epidermal growth factor receptor. Molecular Cancer Therapeutics 2010; 96: 1647–56.

50. Yang C, Shih J, Su W, et al. A Phase II study of BIBW 2992 in patients with adenocarcinoma of the lung and activating EGFR mutations (LUX-Lung 2). J Clin Oncol 2010; 28: 7521a.

51. Mok T, Spigel DR, Park K, et al. Efficacy and safety of PF-00299804 (PF299), an oral irreversible, pan-human epidermal growth factor receptor (pan-HER) tyrosine kinase inhibitor (TKI), as first-line treatment (tx) of selected patients (pts) with advanced (adv) non-small cell lung cancer (NSCLC). J Clin Oncol 2010; 28: 7537a.

52. Takano T, Fukui T, Ohe Y, et al. EGFR mutations predict survival benefit from gefitinib in patients with advanced lung adenocarcinoma: a historical comparison of patients treated before and after gefitinib approval in Japan. J Clin Oncol 2008; 2634: 5589–95.

53. Gridelli C, De Marinis F, Di Maio M. Gefitinib as first-line treatment for patients with advanced non-small-cell lung cancer with activating Epidermal Growth Factor Receptor mutation: implications for clinical practice and open issues. Lung Cancer 2011; 721: 3–8.

54. Jackman D, Pao W, Riely GJ, et al. Clinical definition of acquired resistance to epidermal growth factor receptor tyrosine kinase inhibitors in non-small-cell lung cancer. J Clin Oncol 2010; 28: 357–60.
55. Engelman JA, Zejnnullahu K, Mitsudomi T, et al. MET amplification leads to gefitinib resistance in lung cancer by activating ERBB3 signaling. Science 2007; 316: 1039–43.
56. Bean J, Brennan C, Shih JY, et al. MET amplification occurs with or without T790M mutations in EGFR mutant lung tumors with acquired resistance to gefitinib or erlotinib. Proc Natl Acad Sci USA 2007; 10452: 20932–7.
57. Balak MN, Gong Y, Riely GJ, et al. Novel D761Y and common secondary T790M mutations in epidermal growth factor receptor-mutant lung adenocarcinomas with acquired resistance to kinase inhibitors. Clin Cancer Res 2006; 12: 6494–501.
58. Becker A, Crombag L, Heideman DAM, et al. Retreatment with erlotinib: regain of TKI sensitivity following a drug holiday for patients with NSCLC who initially responded to EGFR-TKI treatment. Eur J Cancer 2011; 47: 2603–6.
59. Chaft JE, Oxnard GR, Sima CS, et al. Disease flare after tyrosine kinase inhibitor discontinuation in patients with EGFR-mutant lung cancer and acquired resistance to erlotinib or gefitinib. Clin Cancer Res 2011; 17: 6298–303.
60. Jackman DM, Holmes AJ, Lindeman N, et al. Response and resistance in a non-small-cell lung cancer patient with an epidermal growth factor receptor mutation and leptomeningeal metastases treated with high-dose gefitinib. J Clin Oncol 2006; 24: 4517–20.
61. Chang JW, Chou CL, Huang SF, et al. Erlotinib response of EGFR-mutant gefitinib-resistant non-small-cell lung cancer. Lung Cancer 2007; 58: 414–17.
62. Gridelli C, Maione P, Galetta D, et al. Three cases of long-lasting tumor control with erlotinib after progression with gefitinib in advanced non-small cell lung cancer. J Thorac Oncol 2007; 2: 758–61.
63. Costa DB, Nguyen KS, Cho BC, et al. Effects of erlotinib in EGFR mutated non-small cell lung cancers with resistance to gefitinib. Clin Cancer Res 2008; 14: 7060–7.
64. Riely GJ, Politi PA, Miller VA, et al. Update on epidermal growth factor receptor mutations in non-small cell lung cancer. Clin Cancer Res 2006; 12: 7232–41.
65. Watanabe S, Tanaka J, Ota T, et al. Clinical responses to EGFR-tyrosine kinase inhibitor retreatment in non-small cell lung cancer patients who benefited from prior effective gefitinib therapy: a retrospective analysis. BMC Cancer 2011; 11: 1.
66. Kaira K, Naito T, Takahashi T, et al. Pooled analysis of the reports of erlotinib after failure of gefitinib for non-small cell lung cancer. Lung Cancer 2010; 68: 99–104.
67. Metro G, Crino L. The LUX-Lung clinical trial program of afatinib for non-small-cell lung cancer. Expert Rev Anticancer Ther 2011; 115: 673–82.
68. Janjigian YY, Azzoli CG, Krug LM, et al. Phase I/II trial of cetuximab and erlotinib in patients with lung adenocarcinoma and acquired resistance to erlotinib. Clin Cancer Res 2011; 178: 2521–7.
69. Janjigian YY, Groen HJ, Horn L, et al. Activity and tolerability of afatinib (BIBW 2992) and cetuximab in NSCLC patients with acquired resistance to erlotinib or gefitinib. J Clin Oncol 2011; 29(Suppl): 7525a.

8 | Second-line therapy of non-small cell lung cancer

David F. Heigener, Sabine Bohnet, and Martin Reck

INTRODUCTION

In this chapter we describe the current standard of second-line chemotherapy of non-small cell lung cancer (NSCLC) as well as future directions. Second line is here defined as therapy after disease progression. Maintenance—defined as continued treatment after first-line therapy without tumor progression—will be discussed in a different chapter.

CURRENT STANDARDS

For many years, chemotherapy in NSCLC was restricted to one regimen. No second-line therapy proved to be effective. One year survival was well below 20%. This changed after the introduction of docetaxel monotherapy in a three weekly regimen achieving a one-year survival rate of 37% compared to 11% with best supportive care alone. In this three-arm trial, docetaxel was tested in two doses (100 mg/m² and 75 mg/m² every three weeks, respectively) against best supportive care. Time to progression was longer for docetaxel patients than for best supportive care patients (10.6 vs. 6.7 weeks, respectively; $p < 0.001$), as was median survival (7.0 vs. 4.6 months; log-rank test, $p = 0.047$). The difference between docetaxel 100 mg and best supportive care regarding overall survival was not significant, probably due to the higher toxicity and the resulting lower dose delivery. There was a higher rate of febrile neutropenia resulting in one and two deaths in the 75 and 100 mg/m² dose group, respectively.[1] Because of superior efficacy, 75 mg/m² became standard in second-line therapy.

The next agent that was introduced into second-line therapy was the multi-targeted antifolate pemetrexed. In a head-to-head trial with docetaxel, non-inferiority was proven with both agents achieving a one-year survival rate of 29.7%. Progression-free survival (PFS) was also similar with 2.9 months in each arm. Overall survival (OS) was 8.3 and 7.9 months for pemetrexed and docetaxel, respectively. This difference was not statistically significant ($p = 0.105$). Off note, the hematologic toxicity of pemetrexed was significantly lower than that of docetaxel.[2] In a retrospective analysis which was performed following the growing body of evidence, that the efficacy of the agent was restricted to non-squamous histology,[3] it was indeed shown that patients with squamous histology did not benefit from pemetrexed (hazard ratio [HR] compared to docetaxel 1.56) but had superior efficacy in patients harboring tumors with non-squamous histology (HR compared to docetaxel 0.78).[4] The label of pemetrexed has thus been restricted to non-squamous histology.

Erlotinib is a small molecule inhibiting the intracellular domain of the epidermal-growth factor receptor (EGFR), which is commonly overexpressed in NSCLC. This compound was tested in a second- and third-line setting in NSCLC patients. The study was not stratified for any molecular marker, especially not EGFR mutation. The recognition, that EGFR tyrosine kinase inhibitors (TKIs) like erlotinib or its sister agent gefitinib are particularly effective in patients harboring EGFR-activating mutations, came up later[5] when recruitment of the study was finished. So this study was done in an "all comer" (i.e., unselected) population of NSCLC patients receiving either erlotinib 150 mg plus best supportive care or placebo plus best supportive care. Of 731 patients randomized, 49% received two prior regimens of chemotherapy and 93% received a platinum-based chemotherapy. PFS was 2.2 versus 1.8 months for erlotinib and placebo, respectively (HR 0.61; $p < 0.001$), OS was 6.7 versus 4.7 months, respectively (HR 0.70; $p < 0.001$), in favor of erlotinib.[6] These results were reproduced in a recent phase IV trial showing 8.6 months of OS with a one-year survival rate of 39.4%.[7]

The efficacy of erlotinib and gefitinib in unselected patients is doubted by many colleagues. Indeed gefitinib failed to show a significant effect on OS versus best supportive care alone in a phase III trial in pretreated patients (5.6 months for gefitinib and 5.1 months for placebo; HR 0.89 [95% confidence interval (CI) 0.77–1.02], $p = 0.087$).[8] However, this trial had methodical flaws: the study population consisted of "refractory" patients, that is, patients which progressed within three months after first-line therapy. These patients are hard to treat anyway. Often it is postulated that the positive observed effect of erlotinib in "all comers" is driven by the fraction of patients harboring an activating EGFR mutation (~10%) who usually achieve long survival times. However, in a phase III trial comparing the sister agent gefitinib with docetaxel in second- or third-line treatment, there was no difference in terms of OS (7.6 vs. 8.0 months with gefitinib and docetaxel, respectively, HR 1.02). In a pre-specified analysis of patients with a high copy number of EGFR genes (measured by fluorescence in-situ hybridization (FISH), which is a weak surrogate of an activating EGFR mutation) there too was no difference (8.4 vs. 7.5 for gefitinib and docetaxel, respectively, HR 1.09). Even the EGFR mutation itself had no predictive role regarding OS.[9] Only PFS was prolonged in patients receiving gefitinib.[10] This argues strongly against the hypothesis that the clinical efficacy of EGFR tyrosine inhibitors like gefitinib or erlotinib is restricted to patients with an activating EGFR mutation. However, a prospective trial of these agents in patients with proven "EGFR wild-type" has never been performed and presumably will never be done.

EXPERIMENTAL CHEMOTHERAPEUTIC APPROACHES

Recent trails have evaluated the use of new cytotoxic agents, which are not yet approved in second-line treatment of advanced NSCLC. Oral topotecan, vinflunine, and poly-glutamated paclitaxel were studied in phase III trials.

Topotecan

Topotecan is an orally available topoisomerase I inhibitor, which is widely used in second-line therapy of small cell lung cancer (SCLC). A randomized phase III trial in 829 patients compared oral topotecan (2.3 mg/m^2 orally, days 1–5) to standard intravenous docetaxel (75 mg/m^2) in second-line treatment of advanced NSCLC. One-year survival rates were 25.1% with topotecan and 28.7% with docetaxel. This difference met the pre-specified 10% non-inferiority margin. Although not statistically significant, OS (27.9 vs. 30.7 weeks, p = 0.057) was slightly in favor for docetaxel and time to disease progression was longer in the docetaxel group (11.3 vs. 13.1 weeks, p = 0.02). The risk for hematologic and non-hematologic side effects was similar in both treatment arms; however, the toxicity profile of the two substances was different. Grade 3 or 4 neutropenia occurred more frequently with docetaxel (60% vs. 50%), grade 3 or 4 anemia and thrombopenia occurred more frequently with topotecan (26% vs. 10%, and 26% vs. 7%, respectively). Nausea, vomiting and diarrhea were more frequent in the topotecan group, whereas neuropathy and fever were more frequent in the docetaxel group. Both treatments showed a progressive worsening of the quality of life symptom scores, which were probably not only related to therapy side effects but also to disease progression.[11] This study demonstrated that topotecan provides activity in the second-line treatment of advanced NSCLC—albeit slightly inferior to docetaxel—and may thus become an option for patients who desire orally available treatment and who are not eligible for targeted protocols.

Vinflunine

Vinflunine is a novel tubulin-targeted agent affecting the mitotic spindle function consecutively leading to modification of cell cycle progression and cell killing.[12] It has a lesser affinity to axonal tubulin than older vinca alkaloids and thus a favorable neurotoxic profile.[13] In a multicenter phase II trial, 63 previously treated patients with advanced NSCLC received vinflunine (320 mg/m^2 every three weeks). Response rate was 7.9%, median PFS 2.6 months and OS 7.0 months. Non-hematologic toxicities included myalgia (15.9%) and constipation (9.5%), and were manageable.[14] These encouraging results lead to a phase III study comparing vinflunine to standard docetaxel treatment. Five hundred and fifty-one patients with disease progression after first-line platinum-based chemotherapy were randomized to receive either vinflunine 320 mg/m^2 or docetaxel 75 mg/m^2 every three weeks. The primary endpoint was PFS and the non-inferiority analysis was based on a 10% difference. Secondary endpoints included response rate, overall survival, safety and quality of life assessment. The study met the primary endpoint since PFS was 2.3 months for both treatment groups. Response rate and overall survival were 4.4% versus 5.5% [not significant (ns)] and 6.7 versus 7.2 months (ns), respectively. No significant difference was observed in patient benefit and quality of life. Higher rates of adverse events occurred in the vinflunine group (higher than grade 0: abdominal pain 20.1% vs. 3.6%, constipation 39.2% vs. 11.7%, injection site reaction 31.9% vs. 0.7%).[15] In summary, vinflunine proved to be effective in this setting. However, due to the modestly disfavorable toxicity profile it cannot be recommended to be used in the second-line setting instead of the already approved agents.

Paclitaxel Poliglumex

Paclitaxel poliglumex (PPX) is a macro-molecule agent conjugate that reduces systemic exposure to peak concentrations of free paclitaxel. Macromolecules such as PPX passively accumulate in tumor tissues due to the hyperpermeable tumor vascularization and the reduced lymphatic clearance, which results in a 10- to 100-fold increase in intra-tumoral agent concentrations when compared with an equivalent dose of the agent given conventionally.[16,17] Paz-Ares and colleagues conducted a randomized phase III study comparing 175 mg/m^2 (in patients with performance status [PS] 2) or 210 mg/m^2 (PS 0–1) PPX to the standard docetaxel regimen in previously treated patients with NSCLC. Total 849 patients were enrolled. The primary end point of this study was OS. Secondary objectives included response rate, time to disease progression (TTP), safety, and quality of life. Median survival was 6.9 months in both arms (p = 0.257). One-year and two-year survival were 25% and 8%, respectively, for PPX, and 29% and 12%, respectively, for docetaxel, which was not statistically significant. The overall response rate for the PPX arm was 8%, with no complete responses (CRs). The overall response rate for the docetaxel arm was 12%, with two CRs. Disease control was achieved 40% in the PPX arm compared with 45% in the docetaxel arm. Time to disease progression were 2.0 and 2.6 months, respectively (p = 0.075). In the docetaxel arm, significantly more grade 3 and 4 neutropenia (37% vs. 14%, p < 0.001) and febrile neutropenia (6% vs. 2%, p = 0.006) occurred. Patients enrolled in the PPX arm were significantly more likely to experience grade 3 or 4 hypersensitivity reaction (3% vs. <1%, p = 0.007) and neuropathy (19% vs. 3%, p < 0.001). Severe neuropathy was observed in 19% of patients in the PPX arm and 3% of patients in the docetaxel arm, respectively.[18] In this study PPX produced similar survival to docetaxel as second-line treatment in NSCLC with less febrile neutropenia and greater ease of administration. The higher incidence of neuropathy, however, was clinically significant and required dose reduction. Considering these results, PPX—probably at a slightly modified dosage—might become an interesting second-line alternative for patients with limited bone marrow reserve in the future.

Combination Chemotherapy

Several randomized trials have been conducted to compare single agent with doublet chemotherapy in second-line treatment of NSCLC. In one recently published meta-analysis, data from six trials and 847 patients were analyzed. Response rate and median PFS was higher in the doublet arms compared to single agent arms (15.1% vs. 7.3%, p = 0.0004; 14 weeks vs. 11.7 weeks, p = 0.0009). However, OS was not different (37.7 weeks vs. 34.7 weeks, p = 0.32) and patients receiving doublet chemotherapy experienced significantly more grade 3 and 4 toxicities (hematologic: 41% vs. 25%, p < 0.0001, non-hematologic: 28% vs. 22%, p = 0.034).[19]

Two newer phase II second-line trails investigated pemetrexed in combination with platin derivates. Smit and colleges performed a randomized phase II trial comparing pemetrexed monotherapy to pemetrexed plus carboplatin. A total of 240 patients were randomized in this quite large phase II trial. As expected, overall response rate (4% vs. 9%) and median time to disease progression were better in the combination arm (2.8 months vs. 4.2 months, p = 0.005). However, there was no difference in overall survival (7.6 months vs. 8.0 months).[20] In another phase II trial, pemetrexed combination with either carboplatin or cisplatin was investigated. In this trial 53 patients were enrolled. Median PFS and OS were quite high (6 and 10 months, respectively[21]) compared to other published second-line trials. Both trials included patients with squamous histology, since the trials started recruitment before the use of pemetrexed was restricted to non-squamous tumor types.

To date, combination chemotherapy has been restricted to clinical trials and cannot be recommended for general use in a second-line setting.

EXPERIMENTAL THERAPEUTIC CONCEPTS: TARGETED THERAPY
EGFR Resistance

EGFR resistance has been defined as a state of disease progression after treatment with gefitinib or erlotinib in patients who have a known activating mutation or had an unknown mutation status coupled with a durable response to these agents.[22]

Second-line therapy in patients with an activating EGFR mutation, who received gefitinib or erlotinib as first-line treatment is particularly challenging. A switch to platinum-based chemotherapy is—albeit feasible— often jeopardized by a poor performance status of second-line patients. A more elegant approach, however, is to continue to target the pathway the tumor cell is addicted to. The key problem is to identify the cause of acquired resistance. At least two mechanisms have been proposed: First, a secondary mutation in exon 20 (T790M) resulting in a conformational change in the intracellular domain of the receptor leading to blockage of the binding cleft for erlotinib or gefitinib. Second, an amplification of a parallel pathway, the cMET (mesothelial to epithelial transformation)-receptor pathway, with its ligand hepatocyte growth factor (HGF).This pathway triggers the same downstream effectors as EGFR and thereby renders EGFR-inhibition useless.

Irreversible Tyrosine Kinase Inhibitors

In case of a T790M mutation, second generation "irreversible" TKIs seem to be a reasonable treatment option. Afatinib (BIBW 2992) is an orally available irreversible inhibitor of EGFR and human epidermal receptor (HER) 2. In the LUX-LUNG 1 trial, patients with one or two prior lines of therapy who must have been at least three months under gefitinib or erlotinib were randomized to afatinib 50 mg plus best supportive care or placebo plus best supportive care. The primary endpoint, OS, was not met: Survival was 10.78 months with BSC and afatinib versus 11.96 months with BSC and placebo. PFS, however, was three-fold higher in the afatinib arm from 1.1 to 3.3 months (HR = 0.38; p < 0.0001).[23] One reason for the failure of this trial might be the high number of subsequent therapies favouring the placebo-arm.

The question whether afatinib is superior to a conventional therapy remains unanswered as well, because this trial had no active control arm.

There are several other trials running with afatinib. Sequist and colleagues are running a single arm phase II trial recruiting patients with an activating EGFR mutation who have not been treated with a first-generation EGFR-TKI yet. They will be treated with afatinib instead. At the time of progression, another biopsy will be taken to search for a T790M mutation. The purpose is to assess for the presence or absence of a T790M mutation compared to historical controls after therapy with gefitinib or erlotinib (Clinical Trials. gov number NCT01074177).

Another irreversible pan HER-inhibitor (PF 00299804) inhibits the tyrosine kinases of HER1, −2, and −4. In a single-arm phase I dose escalation study, patients who had at least two lines of prior therapy containing gefitinib or erlotinib and had an adenocarcinoma with KRAS wild-type received 30 mg (first 12 patients) or 45 mg of PF 00299804 daily. The primary endpoint was PFS at four months (which was 48%) and OS at six months (which was 87%). Of these patients, 16.7% had an activating EGFR mutation, 7.1% had the EGFR wild-type, but only 4.8% had the T790M mutation. In 71.4%, the mutational status was unknown.[24] There is now a phase III trial running. Eligible are patients who had one or two prior regimens of chemotherapy. Patients receive either erlotinib 150 mg or PF00299804 in a double-blind randomized fashion. Primary endpoint is PFS. There is no biomarker-driven patient selection; however, tissue sampling for biomarker analysis is implemented (Clinical Trials.gov number NCT01360554). A phase I protocol will combine PF00299804 with the cMET inhibitor crizotinib in a dose-escalation design. Primary endpoint of this study is the safety profile. Rationale of this trial is to combine inhibition of EGFR (and HER2) with cMET inhibition and therefore blocking two major pathways responsible for acquired resistance to first-generation TKIs. A drawback is, again the lack of biomarker-driven enrolment. This study is open to patients regardless of their pre-therapeutic EGFR mutational status (Clinical Trials.gov number NCT001121575).

cMET

As mentioned above, the activation of the cMET pathway can lead to acquired resistance. Three agents are in advanced clinical development: The dual EML4-ALK and cMET inhibitor crizotinib has already been discussed regarding cMET inhibition and will be discussed with regard to EML4-ALK inhibition in the next section. The monoclonal antibody MetMAb binds to the cMET receptor and prevents binding by HGF, its activating ligand. In a phase-II protocol, MetMAb was given in combination with erlotinib compared to erlotinib alone. Patients were stratified according to cMET protein expression in the tumor as "Met high" (staining intensity of 2 or 3) compared to "Met low" (staining intensity 0 or 1). There was no difference in PFS or OS regarding the entire cohort (PFS 9.6 vs. 11.1 weeks for MetMAb plus erlotinib and erlotinib alone, respectively; p = 0.069; OS 8.2 vs. 7.1 months, respectively; p = 0.76). In the "Met high" group (n = 65), PFS was significantly longer in the patients receiving MetMAb (3.0 vs. 1.5 months; HR 0.47; p = 0.01), as was OS (12.6 vs. 4.6 months, HR = 0.37; p = 0.002), in the "Met low" group, the results were vice versa with a significantly lower PFS and OS for MetMAb and erlotinib compared to erlotinib alone (PFS 6.0 vs. 11.4 weeks, p = 0.035; OS 5.5 vs. 9.2 months, p = 0.021).[25,26] Why there is a detrimental effect of MetMAb in patients with no or low expression of cMET remains elusive.

ARQ197 (tivantinib) is the third agent in advanced clinical development that targets cMET. It is a non-ATP dependent competitive inhibitor of cMET ought to stabilize the molecule in its inactive form. In a randomized, placebo-controlled phase II study, ARQ197 was given together with erlotinib compared with erlotinib plus placebo in pretreated patients who must not have had prior anti-FGFR therapy. PFS was similar in both arms in a univariate analysis (3.8 months for ARQ197 plus erlotinib and 2.3 months for erlotinib + placebo, HR 0.81; p = 0.24). In a pre-specified multivariate analysis (including male sex, one prior regimen, PD as best response to prior therapy, longer than six months since diagnosis, and EGFR wt-status), the hazard ratio became significant toward a benefit of the combination regimen (HR 0.68, p = 0.04). OS was not significantly different in uni- or multivariate analysis. Interestingly, patients with a kRAS mutation (although small in number, n = 15) seem to benefit most from the combination regimen (HR 0.18, CI 0.05 to 0.7; p < 0.01). In 84% of patients Met-FISH analysis could be done. There was a trend for better PFS with rising gene copy numbers, not reaching statistical significance. The hazard ratios for gene copy numbers of >2, 3, 4, and 5 were 0.92, 0.75, 0.71, and 0.42, respectively.[27]

A phase III trial is now running with a similar design and OS as the primary endpoint. Again, no biomarker-driven selection of patients is undertaken (Clinical Trials.gov number NCT01244191).

EML4-ALK

Approximately 4–6% of patients with NSCLC harbor a genetic translocation of two genes: echinoderm microtubule-associated protein-like 4 (EML4) and the anaplastic lymphoma kinase (ALK). The resulting protein is a constitutively activated tyrosine kinase resulting in malignant growth and inhibition of apoptosis. See more details about the molecular biology of this target in the chapter "oncogenic drivers." Crizotinib (Crizotinib®) is a small molecule blocking this fusion protein as well as cMET (see above).

Kwak et al. screened 1500 patients for the presence of an EML4-ALK translocation and found 82 harboring this driver mutation. In a phase I-part of the study, 2 × 250 mg was found to be the optimal dose. Patients entering phase II were heavily pre-treated with 57% having had three or more prior therapies. At the time of publication, 77% of patients were still on therapy and PFS-probability at six months was 72%. One complete and 46 partial remissions could be confirmed.[28] Results like this have—to our knowledge—never been achieved before in a NSCLC-subpopulation. Indeed, crizotinib recently was approved by the Food and Drug Administration (FDA) for patients harboring an EML4-ALK translocation relying on these phase I/II trial results. In Europe, a phase III trial is still recruiting (profile 1007). In this trial, patients with an EML4-ALK translocation who had one prior line of therapy will be randomized to crizotinib or mono-chemotherapy with pemetrexed or docetaxel as chosen by the investigator. In the light of the approval of crizotinib in the United States, recruitment will be more and more difficult because of the excellent results with the study agent. However, it is not proven yet that crizotinib is superior to chemotherapy, although retrospective evidence suggests that survival has not improved in patients with an EML4-ALK translocation versus wild-type receiving conventional chemotherapy.[29] The multi-targeted antifolate pemetrexed might be an exception, because it showed superior PFS rates in patients harboring an EML4-ALK translocation compared to patients with an EGFR- or no mutation.[30] These somewhat controversial results definitely justify the completion of phase III trials before approval in Europe. It is, however, mandatory to offer cross-over to patients allocated to the chemotherapy arm.

Antiangiogenesis

Angiogenesis is a necessary factor for malignant growth. The monoclonal antibody to vascular endothelial growth factor (VEGF), bevacizumab, is effective in combination with standard chemotherapy in the first-line setting. Other "pure" anti-angiogenic agents include the recombinant fusion-protein aflibercept, which binds VEGF, so it cannot interact with its receptor ("VEGF-trap"). In a phase III randomized trial, 913 patients after failure of a platinum-based first-line therapy were randomized to docetaxel plus placebo or docetaxel plus aflibercept. The primary endpoint was OS, which was 10.05 months for aflibercept compared to 10.41 months for placebo (HR 1.01, CI 0.87–1.17; p = 0.898). There was a small benefit in PFS for aflibercept (HR 0.882, CI 0.72–0.94, p = 0.0035).[31]

Another mechanism is vascular disruption as provided by ASA 404 (vadimezan). In a phase III trial, vadimezan aflibercept plus docetaxel was tested against aflibercept plus placebo (ATTRACT-2, Clinical Trials.gov number NCT00738387). However, this trial was terminated after the results of ATTRACT-1 became available, showing no benefit of aflibercept in combination with carboplatin and paclitaxel in the first-line setting.[32] The exact results are not yet available, but it seems unlikely to detect any positive signal from this substance in the second-line setting.

Multi-Targeted Small Molecules

There is a large amount of so-called multi-kinase inhibitors, which are orally available agents targeting different oncogenic drivers besides vascular endothelial growth factor receptor (VEGFR). To date, no such agent has been approved for the treatment of NSCLC; however, many of them are in advanced clinical testing.

Vandetanib is a dual inhibitor of EGFR and VEGFR. The agent was tested in different second-line settings: in addition to docetaxel (the ZODIAC trial), in addition to pemetrexed (the ZEAL-trial), and against erlotinib (the ZEST-trial). Only the ZODIAC-trial reached its primary endpoint of a significant PFS-advantage

(HR 0.79, CI 0.70–0.90; p < 0.0001).[33] However, this difference was not deemed clinically relevant. The other trials failed to show superiority over their competitors.[34,35] As long as we lack clinical or biological predictors of response, the fate of this agent in second-line treatment of NSCLC remains uncertain.

Sorafenib is a multi-kinase inhibitor with activity against VEGFR, RAF, and others. In a randomized phase II trial, sorafenib was tested against placebo in addition to erlotinib in patients who had received one or two prior lines of chemotherapy. The PFS was 3.38 months for sorafenib plus erlotinib compared to 1.94 months for erlotinib plus placebo. The difference was not statistically significant (HR 0.86, CI 0.60–1.22; p = 0.196). In a retrospective analysis, patients with EGFR wild-type had a significant advantage of the combination of sorafenib and erlotinib (3.38 vs. 1.77 months for erlotinib plus placebo, p = 0.018) which translated into an OS benefit (8 months vs. 4.5 months, p = 0.019). However, these data have to be validated prospectively. The benefit in EGFR wild-type tumors might be related to the RAS-downstream effector RAF, which is inhibited by sorafenib. In many EGFR wild-type patients a kRAS mutation is evident. There are hints, that sorafenib is beneficial in patients with a kRAS mutation: In the BATTLE-trial retrospective analyses showed, that disease control rate in patients with a kRAS mutation in the tumor was 61% with sorafenib compared to 31% with erlotinib.[36] Sorafenib monotherapy was tested in a phase II discontinuation trial in an enriched, heavily pre-treated NSCLC population: All patients received the agent for two months as a run-in phase. Then only patients with stable disease continued in the study. Those with progression dropped out, those with remission continued with sorafenib outside the study. Patients with stable disease were randomized to sorafenib or placebo. In this group, PFS was significantly better for the sorafenib-treated patients (3.6 vs. 1.9 months, p = 0.01).[37] However, prospective data in selected patients are lacking.

Another multi-kinase inhibitor is BIBF 1120; this agent is, in particular, interesting because it targets the fibroblast growth factor receptor and platelet-derived growth factor-receptor (PDGFR) besides VEGFR. In a phase II study comparing two doses of BIBF 1120 (i.e., 150 mg and 250 mg bid), median PFS was 6.9 weeks with no difference between the arms. Disease stabilization was achieved in all histologic subgroups in a similar manner (46% of patients, 59% in patients with good performance status)[38] suggesting efficacy in squamous-cell carcinoma as well. Results of a phase III study in combination with docetaxel in the second-line setting are expected soon.

CONCLUSION

To date, three agents are approved for the second- and third-line treatment of NSCLC as monotherapy, namely docetaxel, pemetrexed and erlotinib. It seems, that conventional chemotherapy has reached a plateau of efficacy in this setting and combination therapy is too toxic in these pretreated patients. Future attempts should focus on the combination of targeted agents or the identification of other "drugable" (i.e. a target-inhibiting drug exists) driver mutations to improve outcomes.

The authors are aware of the fact, that numerous other drugs are in clinical development and evidence changes fast especially in the targeted treatment approaches, but due to space restrictions we focused on the most relevant drugs in the recent situation.

REFERENCES

1. Shepherd FA, Dancey J, Ramlau R, et al. Prospective randomized trial of docetaxel versus best supportive care in patients with non-small-cell lung cancer previously treated with platinum-based chemotherapy. J Clin Oncol 2000; 1810: 2095–103.
2. Hanna N, Shepherd FA, Fossella FV, et al. Randomized phase III trial of pemetrexed versus docetaxel in patients with non-small-cell lung cancer previously treated with chemotherapy. J Clin Oncol 2004; 22: 1589–97.
3. Scagliotti GV, Parikh P, von PJ, et al. Phase III study comparing cisplatin plus gemcitabine with cisplatin plus pemetrexed in chemotherapy-naive patients with advanced-stage non-small-cell lung cancer. J Clin Oncol 2008; 26: 3543–51.
4. Scagliotti G, Hanna N, Fossella F, et al. The differential efficacy of pemetrexed according to NSCLC histology: a review of two Phase III studies. Oncologist 2009; 14: 253–63.
5. Lynch TJ, Bell DW, Sordella R, et al. Activating mutations in the epidermal growth factor receptor underlying responsiveness of non-small-cell lung cancer to gefitinib. N Engl J Med 2004; 350: 2129–39.
6. Shepherd FA, Rodrigues PJ, Ciuleanu T, et al. erlotinib in previously treated non-small-cell lung cancer. N Engl J Med 2005; 353: 123–32.
7. Heigener DF, Wu YL, van ZN, et al. Second-line erlotinib in patients with advanced non-small-cell lung cancer: Subgroup analyses from the TRUST study. Lung Cancer 2011; 74: 274–9.

8. Thatcher N, Chang A, Parikh P, et al. Gefitinib plus best supportive care in previously treated patients with refractory advanced non-small-cell lung cancer: results from a randomised, placebo-controlled, multicentre study (Iressa Survival Evaluation in Lung Cancer). Lancet 2005; 366: 1527–37.

9. Kim ES, Hirsh V, Mok T, et al. Gefitinib versus docetaxel in previously treated non-small-cell lung cancer (INTEREST): a randomised phase III trial. Lancet 2008; 372: 1809–18.

10. Douillard JY, Shepherd FA, Hirsh V, et al. Molecular predictors of outcome with gefitinib and docetaxel in previously treated non-small-cell lung cancer: data from the randomized phase III INTEREST trial. J Clin Oncol 2010; 28: 744–52.

11. Ramlau R, Gervais R, Krzakowski M, et al. Phase III study comparing oral topotecan to intravenous docetaxel in patients with pretreated advanced non-small-cell lung cancer. J Clin Oncol 2006; 24: 2800–7.

12. Ngan VK, Bellmann K, Panda D, et al. Novel actions of the antitumor agents vinflunine and vinorelbine on microtubuluses. Cancer Res 2000; 60: 5045–51.

13. Lobert S, Ingram JW, Hill BT, Correia JJ. A comparison of thermodynamic parameters for vinorelbine- and vinflunine-induced tubulin self-association by sedimentation velocity. Mol Pharmacol 1998; 53: 908–15.

14. Bennouna J, Breton JL, Tourani JM, et al. Vinflunine – an active chemotherapy for treatment of advanced non-small-cell lung cancer previously treated with a platinum-based regimen: results of a phase II study. Br J Cancer 2006; 94: 1383–8.

15. Krzakowski M, Ramlau R, Jassem J, et al. Phase III trial comparing vinflunine with docetaxel in second-line advanced non-small-cell lung cancer previously treated with platinum-containing chemotherapy. J Clin Oncol 2010; 28: 2167–73.

16. Matsumura Y, Maeda H. A new concept for macromolecular therapeutics in cancer chemotherapy: mechanism of tumoritropic accumulation of proteins and the antitumor agent smancs. Cancer Res 1986; 46(12 Pt 1): 6387–92.

17. Greish K, Fang J, Inutsuka T, Nagamitsu A, Maeda H. Macromolecular therapeutics: advantages and prospects with special emphasis on solid tumour targeting. Clin Pharmacokinet 2003; 42: 1089–105.

18. Paz-Ares L, Ross H, O'Brien M, et al. Phase III trial comparing paclitaxel poliglumex vs docetaxel in the second-line treatment of non-small-cell lung cancer. Br J Cancer 2008; 98: 1608–13.

19. Di MM, Chiodini P, Georgoulias V, et al. Meta-analysis of single-agent chemotherapy compared with combination chemotherapy as second-line treatment of advanced non-small-cell lung cancer. J Clin Oncol 2009; 27: 1836–43.

20. Smit EF, Burgers SA, Biesma B, et al. Randomized phase II and pharmacogenetic study of pemetrexed compared with pemetrexed plus carboplatin in pretreated patients with advanced non-small-cell lung cancer. J Clin Oncol 2009; 27: 2038–45.

21. Guan-Zhong Z, Jiao SC, Zhao-Ting M. Pemetrexed plus cisplatin/carboplatin in previously treated locally advanced or metastatic non-small cell lung cancer patients. J Exp.Clin Cancer Res 2010; 29: 38–44.

22. Jackman D, Pao W, Riely GJ, et al. Clinical definition of acquired resistance to epidermal growth factor receptor tyrosine kinase inhibitors in non-small-cell lung cancer. J Clin Oncol 2010; 28: 357–60.

23. Miller VA, Hirsh V, Cadranel J, Chen YM. Phase IIB/III double-blind randomized trial of Afatinib (BIBW2992, irreversible inhibitor of EGFR/HER1 and HER2) + Best supportive care versus placebo and BSC in patients failing 1–2 lines of chemotherapy and erlotinib or gefitinib (LUX-Lung 1). Ann Oncol 2010; 21: Suppl 8.

24. Park K, Heo DS, Cho D, Kim M. PF-00299804 (PF299) in Asian patients (pts) with non-small cell lung cancer(NSCLC) refractory to chemotherapy (CT) and erlotinib(E) or gefitinib (G): A phase (P) I/II study. J Clin Oncol 2010; 28: Suppl 15s.

25. Spigel D, Ervin T, Ramlau R, Daniel D. Randomised multicenter double-blind placebo controlled phase II study evaluating METMAB, an antibody to MET-Receptor in combination with erlotinib in patients with advanced non-small cell lung cancer. Ann Oncol 2010; 21: Suppl 18.

26. Spigel D, Ervin T, Ramlau R, Daniel DB. Final efficacy results from OAM4558g, a randomized phase II study evaluating MetMAb or placebo in combination with erlotinib in advanced NSCLC. J Clin Oncol 2011; 29(Suppl): Abstr 7505.

27. Sequist LV, von PJ, Garmey EG, et al. Randomized phase ii study of erlotinib plus tivantinib versus erlotinib plus placebo in previously treated non-small-cell lung cancer. J Clin Oncol 2011; 29: 3307–15.

28. Kwak EL, Bang YJ, Camidge DR, et al. Anaplastic lymphoma kinase inhibition in non-small-cell lung cancer. N Engl J Med 2010; 363: 1693–703.

29. Shaw AT, Yeap BY, Mino-Kenudson M, et al. Clinical features and outcome of patients with non-small-cell lung cancer who harbor EML4-ALK. J Clin Oncol 2009; 27: 4247–53.

30. Camidge DR, Kono SA, Lu X, et al. Anaplastic lymphoma kinase gene rearrangements in non-small cell lung cancer are associated with prolonged progression-free survival on pemetrexed. J Thorac Oncol 2011; 6: 774–80.

31. Novello S, Ramlau R, Corbunova VA, Ciuleanu T. Aflibercept in combination with docetaxel for second-line treatment of locally advanced or metastatic non-small-cell lung cancer (NSCLC): Final results of a multinational placebo-controlled phase III trial (EFC10261-VITAL). J Thorac Oncol 2011. Abstract No. O43.06.

32. Lara PN Jr, Douillard JY, Nakagawa K, et al. Randomized phase III placebo-controlled trial of carboplatin and paclitaxel with or without the vascular disrupting agent vadimezan (ASA404) in advanced non-small-cell lung cancer. J Clin Oncol 2011; 29: 2965–71.

33. Herbst RS, Sun Y, Eberhardt WE, et al. Vandetanib plus docetaxel versus docetaxel as second-line treatment for patients with advanced non-small-cell lung cancer (ZODIAC): a double-blind, randomised, phase 3 trial. Lancet Oncol 2010; 11: 619–26.
34. de Boer RH, Arrieta O, Yang CH, et al. Vandetanib plus pemetrexed for the second-line treatment of advanced non-small-cell lung cancer: a randomized, double-blind phase III trial. J Clin Oncol 2011; 29: 1067–74.
35. Natale RB, Thongprasert S, Greco FA, et al. Phase III trial of vandetanib compared with erlotinib in patients with previously treated advanced non-small-cell lung cancer. J Clin Oncol 2011; 29: 1059–66.
36. Herbst R, Blumenschein G, Kim ES, Lee J, Tsao M. Sorafenib treatment efficacy and KRAS biomarker status in the Biomarker-Integrated Approaches of Targeted Therapy for Lung Cancer Elimination (BATTLE) trial. J Clin Oncol 2010; 28: 15s.
37. Schiller J, Lee JW, Hanna N, Traynor A, Carbone D. A randomized discontinuation phase II study of sorafenib versus placebo in patients with non-small cell lung cancer who have failed at least two prior chemotherapy regimens: E2501. J Clin Oncol 2008; 26(Suppl 15): Abstr 8014.
38. Reck M, Kaiser R, Eschbach C, et al. A phase II double-blind study to investigate efficacy and safety of two doses of the triple angiokinase inhibitor BIBF 1120 in patients with relapsed advanced non-small-cell lung cancer. Ann Oncol 2011; 22: 1374–81.

9 | Adjuvant and neoadjuvant therapy of non-small cell lung cancer

Alejandro Navarro Mendivil and Enriqueta Felip

INTRODUCTION

Lung cancer remains the leading cause of cancer-related mortality worldwide, responsible for 1.18 million deaths in 2002.[1,2] More than 80% of all newly diagnosed cases of lung cancer are non-small cell lung cancer (NSCLC). For patients with early stage disease, from clinical stage IA through IIB, surgical resection represents the standard of care.[3] However, those patients represent only one-third of all newly diagnosed cases, and even if they undergo complete resection, approximately 50% of patients will relapse and die of recurrent disease within 5 years.[4] Most of these relapses are distant metastases to central nervous system, bone, contra-lateral lung, liver, and adrenals, whereas loco-regional relapse is less common (Table 9.1).[5-8] Relapse at distant organs is thought to be a result of occult micrometastatic disease, undetectable at preoperative staging.[9]

In order to improve survival in patients with early stage NSCLC, efforts have been focused on the use of chemotherapy and radiotherapy before or after surgery with the aim of reducing the risk of relapse. At present, the benefit of adjuvant chemotherapy is widely accepted and it should be offered to patients with resected stage II–IIIA NSCLC. However, some areas such as the treatment of patients with IB stage tumors, the role of postoperative radiotherapy (PORT) in stage IIIAN2 and the neoadjuvant approach still require elucidation.[10]

New approaches are now under investigation in early stage NSCLC. Increasing knowledge of molecular biology has led to the development of novel targeted agents and immunotherapies that are also being investigated in this setting.[11] Ongoing randomized trials are also examining the relevance of pharmacogenomic approaches which may enable the choice of adjuvant chemotherapy to be more tailor-made.

ADJUVANT SETTING
Adjuvant Chemotherapy

Adjuvant chemotherapy treatment has long been used in dealing with certain types of tumors and seems to be a reasonable option in order to improve the outcome of NSCLC patients who have undergone surgical resection.

The history of adjuvant chemotherapy in completely resected NSCLC started in the 1960s with the use of alkylating agents and nonspecific immunotherapies that failed to demonstrate any survival benefit. Cisplatin-based chemotherapy also was tested in randomized trials in resectable NSCLC patients prompted by the activity observed in the metastatic setting. However, these studies had considerable design limitations and yielded inconclusive findings.[12-17]

In 1995, a meta-analysis of 52 studies conducted between 1965 and 1991 including data from 9387 patients was published.[18] Performed on the basis of individual data, it overviewed eight cisplatin-based studies (n = 1394) and showed an absolute survival benefit of 5% at 5 years with the use of adjuvant chemotherapy, which was not statistically significant (HR = 0.87, p = 0.08). Conversely, adjuvant chemotherapy with older alkylating agents had a detrimental impact on survival. Analyses of individual data from five studies (n = 2145) using alkylating agents showed an absolute decrease in survival of 5% at 5 years (HR = 1.15, p = 0.005). Results from this meta-analysis generated optimism and prompted additional evaluation of platinum-based regimens in resectable NSCLC resulting in further prospective randomized phase III trials.

The North American Intergroup trial ECOG 3590 evaluated the efficacy of four cycles of postoperative cisplatin-etoposide plus concomitant radiotherapy *versus* PORT alone in resected stage II and IIIA NSCLC.[19] A total of 463 patients were included and no significant differences in survival between the study arms were found. Radiation toxicity caused by the concomitant administration of chemotherapy could explain the lack of efficacy. This is the only study in which adjuvant concurrent chemoradiation is compared to PORT alone.

The ALPI-EORTC trial evaluated the efficacy of three cycles of mitomycin, vindesine, and cisplatin (MVP) *versus* observation in resected stage I, II, and IIIA NSCLC.[20] The decision to give PORT after surgery in the observation group or after chemotherapy in the adjuvant treatment group was made by each of the centers

Table 9.1 Patterns of Relapse after Surgery in Early Stage NSCLC

Study	Stage and histology	Number of patients	Pattern of relapse (%)	
			Loco-regional only	Distant only
Martini et al.[6]	T1-2 N1 squamous	93	16	31
	T1-2 N1 adenocarcinoma	114	8	54
	T2-3 N2 squamous	46	13	52
	T2-3 N2 adenocarcinoma	103	17	61
Pairolero et al.[7]	T1N0	170	6	15
	T2N0	158	6	23
	T1N1	18	28	39
Thomas and Rubenstein[8]	T1N0 squamous	226	5	7
	T1N0 adenocarcinoma	346	9	17

and, overall, 43% of patients were treated with radiotherapy. A total of 1209 patients were included and randomly assigned to the two arms with no significant difference in survival being observed. Subgroup analysis showed a 10% survival advantage at 5 years for chemotherapy-treated stage II patients, although without statistical significance. It is worth mentioning that only 69% of patients completed three cycles of MVP and that a considerable proportion of patients required dose reductions.

The Big Lung trial (BLT) also evaluated the efficacy of three cycles of cisplatin-based chemotherapy (a doublet with vindesine or vinblastine or a triplet with mitomycin and ifosfamide or MVP) *versus* observation in resected stage I, II, and III NSCLC.[21] PORT was also given in 14% of the cases. A total of 381 patients were enrolled with no survival differences between arms, although this study may well have been underpowered to detect any survival benefit.

The International Adjuvant Lung Cancer trial (IALT) was published in 2004 and was the first relevant study to show statistically significant benefit from the use of adjuvant chemotherapy in both disease-free survival (DFS) and overall survival (OS).[22] A total of 1867 completely resected stage I, II, and III NSCLC patients were randomized to receive chemotherapy with cisplatin in combination with vinblastine or vinorelbine or etoposide *versus* observation. PORT was also given in 27% of the cases. All stages were represented in this trial: 10% stage IA, 27 % stage IB, 24 % stage II, and 39 % stage III. Overall survival was longer for patients in the chemotherapy group (HR = 0.86, CI 0.76–0.98, p < 0.03). Median DFS was 40.2 *versus* 30.5 months and median OS was 50.8 *versus* 44.4 months for the chemotherapy arm and the control arm, respectively. Stage III patients obtained the greatest benefit from adjuvant chemotherapy. Results of IALT were updated with long-term follow-up in 2008, reporting that the survival benefit from adjuvant chemotherapy was non-significant after a median follow-up of 7.5 years. One possible explanation for the loss of survival benefit with long-term follow-up could be a higher mortality rate because of potential late chemotherapy effects.[23]

The Adjuvant Navelbine International Trial Association (ANITA) evaluated the efficacy of cisplatin and vinorelbine *versus* observation in resected stage IB, II, and III NSCLC patients.[24] A total of 840 patients were included: 36% stage IB, 25% stage II, and 39% stage III. PORT was given to 232 patients (22% in the chemotherapy arm and 33% in the observation arm). After a median follow-up of 76 months, median survival was significantly longer in the chemotherapy arm (65.7 months) in comparison with the observation arm (43.7 months). When subgroup analysis was performed, the benefit appeared to be limited to stage II and III patients. A descriptive analysis suggested that radiotherapy could play a positive role in stage III.[25]

The National Cancer Institute of Canada Clinical Trials Group designed a similar trial, known as NCIC-BR10, but limited it to stage IB and II (excluding T3N0) NSCLC.[26] A total of 482 patients were enrolled and randomized to cisplatin and vinorelbine *versus* observation. PORT was not given in this study. OS was significantly longer (HR = 0.69, p = 0.04) in the chemotherapy group (94 months) in comparison with the observation group (73 months). There was an absolute gain of 15% in 5-year survival rate, from 54% to 69%. Subgroup analyses showed that benefit was limited to stage II patients. In this study, the chemotherapy schedule was four cycles of cisplatin 50 mg/m^2 days 1 and 8 every 4 weeks and vinorelbine 25 mg/m^2 weekly for 16 weeks. Grade 3–4 neutropenia was documented in 73% of patients, febrile neutropenia in 7%, and there were two treatment-related deaths (0.8%). The results of this study were updated with long-term follow-up (median follow-up 9.3 years) and the improvement in survival obtained with adjuvant chemotherapy was maintained.[27]

In the NCIC-BR10 study a retrospective analysis was made to evaluate the impact of age on survival, chemotherapy compliance, and toxicity.[28] Data from 327 young and 155 elderly patients (65 years or older)

Table 9.2 Summary of Adjuvant Platinum-Based Chemotherapy Trials

Study	Number of patients	Stage	Treatment	OS (HR, 95% CI) p value	Port use per arm Experimental/ control (%)	Absolute improvement in 5-year survival (%)
ECOG 3590 (1991–1997)	488	II–IIIA	Cisplatin plus etoposide and concurrent radiotherapy	0.93 (0.74–1.18) p = 0.56	YES	
ALPI-EORTC (1994–1999)	1209	I–IIIA	Mitomycin C, vindesine and cisplatin	0.96 (0.81–1.13) p = 0.589	64/70	1.0
ANITA (1994–2000)	840	IB–IIIA	Cisplatin plus vinorelbine	0.80 (0.66–0.96) P = 0.017	21/33	8.6
JBR.10 (1994–2001)	482	IB–II	Cisplatin and vinorelbine	0.69 (0.52–0.91) P = 0.04	0/0	15.0
BLT (1995–2001)	381	I–IV	Cisplatin doublet with vindesine, vinorelbine or mitomycin or triplet vinblastine and mitomycin	1.02 (0.77–1.35) P = 0.9	NS	−2
IALT (1995–2000)	1867	IA–IIIB	Cisplatin doublet with vindesine, vinorelbine, vinblastine or etoposide	0.86 (0.76–0.98) P < 0.03	64/70	4.1
CALGB 9633 (1996–2003)	344	IB	Carboplatin and paclitaxel	0.83 (0.64–1.08) P = 0.12	0/0	3

were analyzed. Younger patients had a major prevalence of adenocarcinoma and had better performance status. Elderly patients received significant fewer doses of chemotherapy with no significant differences in toxicities when compared with the younger study population. It is important to mention that OS in elderly patients was significantly better in those treated with chemotherapy than in the observation group (HR = 0.61, p = 0.04), but in the few patients older than 75 years (n = 23) survival was shorter than in those aged 65 to 75.

The Cancer and Leukemia Group B (CALGB) designed a randomized trial known as CALGB 9633, including only resected stage IB NSCLC patients.[29] It was the first study to use the carboplatin-paclitaxel regimen. This study was closed early based on a positive interim analysis with a total of 344 patients randomized. Although a significant survival benefit was shown at 4 years, it was not confirmed at 6-year follow-up. In an unplanned analysis, patients with tumors of at least 4 cm in size obtained a survival benefit from chemotherapy (HR = 0.66, p < 0.04) in contrast with patients with smaller tumors (HR = 1.02, p = 0.51). In this study, the chemotherapy schedule followed was carboplatin AUC = 6 and paclitaxel 200 mg/m^2 every 3 weeks for four cycles. In contrast with other schedules, tolerability of this combination was excellent, with nearly 85% of patients receiving all four planned cycles. In 36% of patients, grade 3–4 toxicity was registered but there were no treatment-related deaths. Table 9.2 summarizes a number a randomized trials addressing the role of adjuvant platinum-based chemotherapy in resected NSCLC patients.

The lung adjuvant cisplatin evaluation (LACE) pooled individual data of 4854 patients from five randomized adjuvant trials using adjuvant cisplatin combinations, ALPI, ANITA, BLT, IALT, and NCIC-BR10.[30] Adjuvant chemotherapy was associated with an improvement in OS with an 11% relative reduction in the risk of death (HR = 0.89, CI 0.82–0.96, p = 0.04). However, the degree of benefit varied depending on stage. In stages II and III, OS benefit was 5.3 % at 5 years (HR = 0.83, CI 0.73–0.95 and HR = 0.83, CI 0.72–0.94, respectively), whereas a small but not statistically significant benefit was observed in stage IB (HR = 0.93, CI 0.78–1.10), and a detrimental effect in stage IA (HR = 1.40, CI 0.95–2.06).

The NSCLC Meta-analyses Collaborative Group recently undertook two systematic reviews and meta-analyses to establish the effect of adding chemotherapy to surgery, or to surgery plus radiotherapy.[31] The first meta-analysis of surgery plus chemotherapy *versus* surgery alone was based on 34 trials and 8447 patients (3323 deaths). They reported a benefit of adding chemotherapy after surgery (HR = 0.86, CI 0.81–0.92, p < 0.0001), with an absolute increase in survival of 4% at 5 years. The second meta-analysis of surgery plus radiotherapy and chemotherapy *versus* surgery plus radiotherapy was based on 13 trials and 2660 patients (1909 deaths). They reported a benefit of adding chemotherapy to surgery plus radiotherapy (HR = 0.88, CI 0.81–0.97, p = 0.009), representing an absolute improvement in survival of 4% at 5 years.

A number of studies addressed the role of uracil-tegafur (UFT) in the adjuvant setting. UFT is an oral fluoropyrimide extensively used in Japan in different tumors, even in adjuvant or metastatic setting. A large trial evaluated the efficacy of adjuvant UFT in NSCLC.[32] A total of 979 patients with completely resected stage I adenocarcinoma were randomized to UFT $250\,mg/m^2$ or observation. There was an increase in OS in the UFT arm (HR = 0.71, CI 0.52–0.98), limited to T2N0 subgroup. UFT is thought to have a particular sensitivity in Japanese populations. No study addressing the role of adjuvant UFT has been performed outside Japan, which is a clear limitation for its use in the clinical practice.

Adjuvant Radiotherapy

Loco-regional recurrence after resection in patients with NSCLC occurs in up to 50% of patients with stage III disease. Based on these facts, multiple studies examining the potential role of PORT were conducted during the 1970s and 1980s.

A meta-analysis was published in 1998 by the Medical Research Council collecting individual data of 2128 patients from nine trials.[33] PORT was associated with significant detrimental effect on survival (HR = 1.21, CI 1.08–1.34, p = 0.001) corresponding to a 7% absolute increase in the risk of death at 2 years. Subgroup analyses showed that the detrimental effect was most pronounced for patients with stages I and II whereas there was no clear evidence for patients with stage IIIN2. Higher mortality rate in patients treated with PORT could have been due to the older technology and different dosimetry parameters.

Lally et al. reported the outcome of 7465 stage II or III NSCLC patients who underwent a lobectomy or pneumonectomy, selected from within the SEER database.[34] Overall, the use of PORT was not found to improve OS. However, subgroup analysis showed that PORT increased survival in patients with N2 disease (HR = 0.85, p < 0.9977). For patients with N0 (HR = 1.176, p = 0.04) and N1 (HR = 1.097, p = 0.019) disease, PORT was associated with significantly shorter survival.

The use of PORT in the adjuvant setting is not routinely recommended for N0–N1 patients in whom complete resection has been achieved. For patients with inadequate mediastinal lymph node dissection, close margins or extracapsular extension, PORT use should be considered.

Further evaluation of the potential role of PORT in the context of modern radiotherapy techniques is warranted. At present, a large ongoing European phase III trial (Lung ART) is comparing three-dimensional conformal PORT *versus* no-PORT in completely resected patients with pathologically proven N2 disease.[35]

NEOADJUVANT SETTING
Neoadjuvant Chemotherapy

Neoadjuvant chemotherapy is an attractive treatment option which is employed in different tumors. Neoadjuvant chemotherapy may well be associated with certain advantages such as being effective in treating occult microscopic systemic disease, downstaging mediastinal lymph node, and improving the success of surgery by tumor reduction. Furthermore, chemotherapy compliance prior to surgery is generally better than after surgery. The potential disadvantages are treatment-related toxicities and the delay of surgery. At present, neoadjuvant chemotherapy is still considered an experimental treatment modality in early stage disease and its role should be more clearly defined.

Two small randomized trials comparing neoadjuvant platinum-based chemotherapy followed by surgery *versus* surgery alone in stage IIIA had considerable impact on clinical practice.

Roth et al. evaluated the efficacy of three cycles of cisplatin-etoposide and cyclophosphamide followed by surgery *versus* a surgery-alone control arm in patients with potentially resectable clinical stage IIIA.[36,37] An additional three cycles of chemotherapy were administered after surgery to patients who achieved radiological response. Following an interim analysis, the trial was closed after a total of 60 patients had been randomized because of survival benefit in favor of the experimental arm, resulting in a 64-month median survival *versus* 11 months for the control arm.

Rosell et al. conducted a similar trial to evaluate the efficacy of three cycles of mitomycin, ifosfamide, and cisplatin followed by surgery *versus* surgery alone in patients with clinical stage IIIA.[38] The study was closed after recruitment of 60 patients when an interim analysis after a 24-month follow-up was performed. It showed survival benefit for the experimental arm with a median survival of 26 months *versus* 8 months in the surgery-alone arm

In 2001, Depierre et al. reported the results of a phase III randomized trial to evaluate the efficacy of induction course of mitomycin, ifosfamide, and cisplatin chemotherapy in resectable stage IB, II, and IIIA.[39] A total of 355 patients were randomized to surgery alone or combined modality therapy consisting of two cycles of induction chemotherapy followed by surgery, and then two additional cycles of adjuvant chemotherapy for patients who achieved benefit from the induction treatment. Postoperative mortality was 7% in the chemotherapy arm and 5% in the surgery-alone arm (p = 0.38). Median survival was 37 months in the chemotherapy group and 26 months in the control arm (p = 0.15). The results of this study were maintained with long-term follow-up.

The Southwest Oncology Group trial S9900 was a phase III randomized trial designed to evaluate the efficacy of neoadjuvant paclitaxel and carboplatin chemotherapy in early stage NSCLC.[40] It was closed prematurely in 2004 due to evidence in favor of adjuvant chemotherapy. A total of 354 patients with clinical stage IB, II, and IIIA NSCLC (excluding superior sulcus and N2 disease) were included and randomly assigned to receive three cycles of chemotherapy followed by surgery, or surgery alone. Mediastinoscopy was performed whenever the mediastinal lymph node size exceeded 1 cm. Of the patients randomized to chemotherapy, 79% completed three cycles of chemotherapy and 41% achieved radiographic response. Complete resection was possible in 94% of patients in chemotherapy group *versus* 89% in the control arm. With a median follow-up of 53 months, median survival was 62 months for the chemotherapy arm *versus* 41 months, for the surgery-alone arm (HR = 0.79, CI 0.60–1.06, p = 0.11). Although the use of chemotherapy was associated with a 19 % reduction in the risk of death, this difference did not achieve statistical significance.

In the recently published CHEST trial, chemotherapy-naïve patients with stage IB–II–IIIA NSCLC were randomized to surgery alone or neoadjuvant chemotherapy with cisplatin and gemcitabine followed by surgery.[41] This trial was closed earlier than planned with a total of 270 patients accrued (55 % stage IB/IIA). Response rate to neoadjuvant chemotherapy was 35%. The results of this trial seemed to favor the neoadjuvant arm with an HR for OS of 0.63.

The European Intergroup trial MRC-LU22/EORTC-08012/NVALT-2 was another study designed to test the efficacy of the neoadjuvant approach.[42] A total of 519 patients with resectable early stage NSCLC were randomized to either surgery alone or three cycles of platinum-based chemotherapy followed by surgery. Choice of chemotherapy regimen was decided by each participating center. This trial was also prematurely closed for slowing accrual. Of the patients randomized to chemotherapy, 75% completed three treatment cycles and 49% had radiographic response. The rate of complete resection was similar in both groups: 81% in the neoadjuvant arm *versus* 79% in the control arm. With a median follow-up of 41 months, median survival was 54 months for the neoadjuvant groups *versus* 55 months for the surgery-alone group (HR = 1.02, p = 0.86).

The NATCH study was designed to evaluate the potential role of neoadjuvant chemotherapy in resectable NSCLC *versus* an adjuvant approach.[43] This three-arm study included a total of 624 patients with stage IA (tumor size > 2 cm), IB, II, or T3N1 who were randomized to surgery alone, *versus* neoadjuvant chemotherapy followed by surgery, *versus* surgery followed by adjuvant chemotherapy. Chemotherapy schedule consisted of carboplatin and paclitaxel for three cycles. Although a trend for improved 5-year DFS rates with neoadjuvant therapy was observed (38.3% with neoadjuvant chemotherapy, 36.6% with adjuvant chemotherapy, and 34.1% with surgery alone), there were no statistical differences (p = 0.71) among the three arms. It is noteworthy that the majority of patients had stage I disease. A greater proportion (90%) of patients in the neoadjuvant group received the planned three cycles of neoadjuvant chemotherapy compared with the adjuvant group in which only 66% of the patients started adjuvant treatment. Table 9.3 summarizes the main results obtained in the SWOG 9900, the European Intergroup MRC-LU22/EORTC-08012/NVALT-2, and the NATCH neoadjuvant trials.

Two meta-analyses from data of randomized trials in early stage NSCLC are of interest. Berghmans et al. reported data from six randomized trials, published between 1990 and 2003, including 590 patients.[44] The addition of neoadjuvant chemotherapy to surgery was associated with a non-significant improvement in OS (HR = 0.65, CI 0.41–1.04).

Burdett et al. examined data from seven randomized trials, published between 1990 and 2005, including 988 patients.[45] Neoadjuvant chemotherapy improved survival (HR = 0.82, CI 0.69–0.97), with an absolute benefit of 6% at 5 years.

Finally, recently presented preliminary results from a systematic review and meta-analysis of individual patient data from 13 randomized trials reported that neoadjuvant chemotherapy was associated with an improvement in survival in operable patients with 5% absolute benefit at 5 years (HR = 0.88, p = 0.025).[46]

Neoadjuvant Radiotherapy

Reports of long-term survival in patients with superior sulcus tumors after preoperative radiotherapy prompted interest in this approach. The US Veterans Administration conducted a randomized trial including patients with central-located tumors who were assigned to preoperative radiotherapy *versus* immediate

Table 9.3 Summary of the Results of SWOG S9900, European Intergroup MRC-LU22/EORTC-08012/NVALT-2 and NATCH Neoadjuvant Trials

	SWOG 9900		European intergroup trial		Natch trial	
	Immediate surgery	Neoadjuvat CT	Immediate surgery	Neoadjuvant CT	Immediate surgery	Neoadjuvant CT
No of patients	167	169	261	258	210	199
Chemotherapy regimens		CBP-PCT		CDDP-VNR (45%) CDDP-GM (25%) CBP-DOC (12%) MIT-VIND-CDDP (12%) MIT-IFO-CDDP (7%)		CBP-PCT
CT compliance (%)		79		75		85
Stage I (%)	67	68	59	64	73	74
Stage II (%)	32	33	35	28	25	23
Stage IIIA (%)	NA	NA	6	8	2	2
Pathological complete response (%)		<10		4		10
Postoperative mortality (%)	2.3	4	2	2	6	5
Median PFS (mo)	21	33	25	26	25.1	31.5
Median OS (mo)	46	75	55	54	49	55
Overall survival at 5 years (%)	43	50	45	44	44	46.6
HR (95%CI)	0.81 (0.6–1.1)		1.02 (0.8–1.3)		0.96 (0.84–1.1)	

Table 9.4 Summary of Ongoing Phase III Trials Evaluating Novel Therapies

Study	Therapy	Stage	Primary endpoint	Planned enrollment
RADIANT	Erlotinib	IB–IIIA	DFS	945
ECOG 1505	Bevacizumab plus cisplatin-based chemotherapy	IB–IIIA	OS	1500
MAGRIT	MAGE-A3 vaccine	IB–IIIA	DFS	2270

surgery.[47] OS was 12.5% in the preoperative arm compared with 21% in the surgery arm. Given these negative results, preoperative radiotherapy cannot be recommended for patients with potentially resectable NSCLC.

TARGETED THERAPY

It is clear that adjuvant chemotherapy is beneficial for certain patients with resectable NSCLC, but its impact on survival is limited. Thus there is a need to find other strategies to further improve survival outcomes.

In recent years there has been a marked increase in the development of novel therapeutic strategies targeting signaling pathways that are implicated in lung cancer, such as epidermal growth factor receptor (EGFR) and angiogenesis. One challenge for present research is to integrate new active agents into the adjuvant setting. Table 9.4 summarizes ongoing phase III trials evaluating novel therapies in the adjuvant setting.

EGFR Inhibitors

Several strategies have been developed to target EGFR, including monoclonal antibodies that block extracellular ligand binding and tyrosine-kinase inhibitors (TKIs) that block intracellular signaling pathways. Inhibition of EGFR causes cell-cycle arrest, promotes apoptosis, and inhibits angiogenesis.

Gefitinib and erlotinib are EGFR-TKIs that have been tested in advanced NSCLC and are currently being tested in the adjuvant setting.

Tsuboi et al. conducted a phase III study designed to evaluate the potential role of adjuvant gefitinib in completely resected stage IB-IIIA NSCLC.[48] Patients were randomized to gefitinib 250 mg/day for 2 years or placebo. Recruitment was stopped after inclusion of 38 patients because of the association of interstitial-lung disease (ILD) with gefitinib use in patients with advanced NSCLC. ILD-type events were reported in one patient in the gefitinib arm who died and in two patients receiving placebo.

The NCIC BR19 trial was a phase III trial originally designed to evaluate the efficacy of gefitinib *versus* placebo in patients with resected stage IB–IIIA NSCLC.[49] It was planned to include more than 1000 patients but was prematurely closed after the inclusion of 503 patients due to the negative results from the ISEL[50] and SWOG 0023[51] studies. Overall no survival benefit was detected with adjuvant gefitinib treatment, and surprisingly a trend toward poorer survival was seen in those patients with EGFR mutations.

The RADIANT (Randomized Double-Blind Trial in Adjuvant NSCLC with Tarceva) trial is an ongoing study designed to evaluate the efficacy of erlotinib for 2 years after adjuvant platinum-based chemotherapy in patients with stage IB–IIIA NSCLC and positive for EGFR expression evaluated by immunohistochemistry and/or FISH.[52]

Angiogenesis Inhibitors

Bevacizumab is a monoclonal antibody against vascular endothelial growth factor that inhibits tumor angiogenesis and that has been approved in combination with a platinum-based doublet in first-line treatment of advanced non-squamous NSCLC.

The ongoing ECOG 1505 study is a phase III trial designed to evaluate the potential benefit of the addition of bevacizumab to adjuvant cisplatin-based chemotherapy and maintenance for up to 1 year in patients with completely resected stage IB–IIIA NSCLC.[53]

Immunotherapy

There is growing interest in cancer immunotherapy, since it has been documented to have some naturally occurring antitumor immune responses in patients with cancer.[54,55] The requirements for therapeutic vaccine development are different than those of prophylactic vaccines. Therapeutic vaccines are divided into cell-based vaccines and subunit vaccines. Whereas cellular vaccines are designed from whole tumor cells, subunit vaccines are based on the selection of antigens as potential targets. The rational for the use of lung cancer vaccines is the generation of a T-cell response against antigens which are expressed by tumors. Some of the immunosuppression observed in cancer patients is due to a circulating subpopulation of T cells called suppressor T cells, and it has been observed that low-dose chemotherapy often enhances responses to immunotherapy by reducing the number of these suppressive cells.

MAGE-A3 is a cancer immunotherapy that is being developed in the adjuvant setting in patients with resected NSCLC. MAGE-A3 is expressed by testicular germ cells in normal conditions although it is also aberrantly expressed in some tumors, including approximately one-third of stage IB–IIIA NSCLC.[56–59]

The interest in MAGE-A3 as a target has also been strengthened by its likely association with poor prognosis and the ability to identify and select patients with MAGE-A3 tumors for treatment.

MAGE-A3 vaccine combines the recombinant protein MAGE-A3 and an immunostimulant system AS02B. This recombinant protein approach allows for the potential to induce both CD8+ killer T-cell and CD4+ helper T-cell immune responses. MAGE-A3 vaccine has been associated with clinical response in patients with metastatic melanoma in phase II studies. In a double-blind, placebo-controlled phase II study in 182 patients with resected stage IB–II NSCLC and MAGE-A3-positive tumors, MAGE-A3 vaccine was associated with improved OS (HR = 0.81, CI 0.47–1.40) and DFS (HR = 0.76, CI 0.48–1.21) after a median follow-up of 44 months.[60] MAGE-A3 vaccine was also well tolerated, with high compliance of treatment, and no serious toxicities were attributed to the treatment.

MAGE-A3 vaccine is being further evaluated in the phase III trial called MAGRIT (MAGE-A3 as adjuvant non-small cell lung cancer immunotherapy) as an adjuvant therapy after surgery or after surgery and adjuvant chemotherapy in patients with stage IB–IIIA NSCLC and positive for expression of MAGE A3 by immunohistochemistry.

Initial results confirm that MAGE-A3 is expressed in approximately 30% of patients and that expression is higher in squamous cell carcinomas compared with adenocarcinomas tumors.[61]

BIOMARKERS

In advanced NSCLC the choice of chemotherapy is based on histology, stage, and clinical features. One way to improve the effectiveness and to reduce the toxicity of chemotherapy is to identify which patients are likely to benefit and which may be exposed to unnecessary toxicity in order to select appropriate treatment. As biomarkers that are indicative of prognosis and chemo-sensitivity or chemo-resistance are emerging, molecular biology is an increasingly important consideration when choosing therapy for patients with NSCLC. One challenge for present research is to use molecular biological markers to identify patients for more individualized treatment.

Signatures are being developed to select appropriate adjuvant therapy for individual patients, but proving improved outcomes with this approach is extremely difficult, especially in the adjuvant setting because of the delay of recurrence events as opposed to immediate feedback regarding tumor responses in advanced disease. In a relevant study, gene expression profiling was conducted on tissue samples prospectively collected from patients who participated in the NCIC-BR10 study.[62] It was identified that the first gene signature for prognosis is a potentially predictive marker for benefit with adjuvant chemotherapy in patients with resected NSCLC, although independent confirmation is awaited.

Technological advances now allow identification and measurement of biomarkers such as expression of the thymidylate synthase (TS), excision repair cross-complementation group 1 (ERCC1), class III -tubulin, BRCA1, and ribonucleotide reductase M1 (RRM1) genes at the RNA or protein level, which may be predictive of response to cytotoxic agents and useful for designing tailor-made chemotherapeutic strategies.[63–65]

In the study published by Olaussen et al., an immunohistochemical analysis was performed to determine ERCC1 protein expression in surgical specimens from NSCLC patients enrolled in the IALT trial.[63] Among 761 tumors, ERCC1 expression was positive in 335 (44%) and negative in 426 (56%). Adjuvant chemotherapy, as compared with observation, significantly prolonged survival among patients with ERCC1-negative tumors but not among those with ERCC1-positive tumors. In the group of patients with ERCC1-negative tumors who received cisplatin-based adjuvant chemotherapy, the risk of death decreased by 35% (HR = 0.66, CI 0.49–0.90). By contrast, no such decrease was found among patients with ERCC1-positive tumors who received cisplatin-based adjuvant chemotherapy (HR = 1.14, CI 0.84–1.55). Furthermore, among patients who did not receive chemotherapy, those with ERCC1-positive tumors survived longer than those with ERCC1-negative tumors. Additionally, the presence of EGFR-activating mutations has been associated with ERCC1 expression, and may result in greater response to chemotherapy, although this remains to be determined.[66]

The potential prognostic role of BRCA1 was investigated in chemotherapy-naïve patients with early stage NSCLC, analyzed by RT-qPCR.[65] Among a panel of nine candidate biomarkers including ERCC1, BRCA1 was found to be the only independent factor affecting OS, with overexpression predicting a poor outcome.

Four prospective multicenter trials of customized adjuvant chemotherapy are currently underway. The SWOG-S0720 trial is a phase II feasibility study in patients with pathologic stage I NSCLC, for whom adjuvant chemotherapy is currently not the standard of care. Based on ERCC1 and RRM1 levels assessed by AQUA, patients with tumors highly expressing both biomarkers are assigned to observation, while those with tumors expressing low levels of either of the two biomarkers are offered adjuvant cisplatin and gemcitabine chemotherapy. The ITACA trial is a phase III study that employs ERCC1 and TS mRNA expression levels as decision points to select regimen. The Spanish Lung Cancer Group SCAT trial is a phase III trial in which patients with completely resected N1–N2 disease are randomized to receive either cisplatin plus docetaxel as control arm or to one of three combinations based on BRCA1 levels (cisplatin plus gemcitabine for patients with tumors expressing low BRCA1 levels, single agent docetaxel for those with high BRCA1 expression, and cisplatin plus docetaxel for those with intermediate BRCA1 expression). Lastly, the TASTE trial is a phase II/III study accruing resected patients with non-squamous histology and pathologic stages II–IIIA, in which the patients in the control arm are being treated with cisplatin plus pemetrexed, whereas those on the genotype arm are being assigned to either one of three modalities according to EGFR mutation status and ERCC1 immunohistochemistry expression levels; erlotinib for patients with EGFR mutation, ciplatin plus pemetrexed for those EGFR-wild-type/ERCC1-negative tumors; and observation for those with EGFR-wild-type/ERCC1-positive tumors. The results of these randomized trials will define the role of customized treatment in the adjuvant setting.

CONCLUSIONS

In this review we summarized the adjuvant and neodjuvant approaches in NSCLC. The standard of care for early-stage NSCLC is adjuvant platinum- based doublet chemotherapy after surgical resection.[18] The benefit is evident for patients with stage II and IIIA and less clear for IB stage.[29–30] The most active chemotherapy agent in combination with platinum is not known. PORT has a role in N2 disease after surgery and adjuvant chemotherapy.[10] Neoadjuvant setting is still controversial and although it has shown improvement in survival, this approach must not be taken as the standard of care.[46] Despite all efforts, survival rates are still poor so there is a need to improve strategies of treatment. In this way, directed therapies remain a field of interest, particularly those targeting important pathways in tumorogenesis such as EGFR by erlotinib or angiogenesis by bevacizumab, and also inmunotherapy with different vaccines.[52-55] Pharmacogenomic and gene-expression profiling are expected to improve patient selection and potentially offer a more directed treatment.[62-65]

REFERENCES

1. Parkin DM, Bray F, Ferlay J, et al. Global cancer statistics, 2002. CA Cancer J Clin 2005; 55: 74–108.
2. Nesbitt JC, Putnam JB Jr, Walsh GL, et al. Survival in early-stage non-small cell lung cancer. Ann Thorac Surg 1995; 60: 466–72.
3. Crinò L, Weder W, van Meerbeeck J, et al. Early stage and locally advanced (non-metastatic) non-small-cell lung cancer: ESMO Clinical Practice Guidelines for diagnosis, treatment and follow-up. Ann Oncol 2010; 21(Suppl 5): v103–15.
4. Pisters KM, Evans WK, Azzoli CG, et al. Cancer Care Ontario and American Society of Clinical Oncology adjuvant chemotherapy and adjuvant radiation therapy for stages I–IIIA resectable non small-cell lung cancer guideline. J Clin Oncol 2007; 25: 5506–18.
5. Feld R, Rubenstein I, Weisenberger T, et al. Sites of recurrence in resected stage I non-small cell lung cancer: a guide for future studies. J Clin Oncol 1984; 2: 1352–8.
6. Martini N, Flehinger B, Zaman M, et al. Prospective study of 445 lung carcinomas with mediastinal lymph node metastases. J Thorac Cardiovasc Surg 1980; 80: 390–7.
7. Pairolero P, Williams D, Bergstralh M, et al. Post-surgical stage I bronchogenic carcinoma. Morbid implications of recurrent disease. Ann Thorac Surg 1984; 38: 331–8.
8. Thomas P, Rubenstein I. The Lung Cancer Study Group. Cancer recurrence after resection T1N0 non-small cell lung cancer. Ann Thorac Surg 1990; 48: 242–7.
9. Gu CD, Osaki T, Oyama T, et al. Detection of micrometastatic tumor cells in pN0 lymph nodes of patients with completely resected non small cell lung cáncer: impact on recurrence and survival. Ann Surg 2002; 235: 133–9.
10. Ikeda N, Nagase S, Ohira T. Individualized adjuvant chemotherapy for surgically resected lung cancer and the roles of biomarkers. Ann Thorac Cardiovasc Surg 2009; 15: 144–9.
11. Molina JR, Yang P, Cassivi SD, et al. Non-small cell lung cancer: epidemiology, risk factors, treatment, and survivorship. Mayo Clin Proc 2008; 83: 584–94.
12. Holmes EC, Bleehen NM, Le Chevalier T, et al. Postoperative adjuvant treatments for non-small cell lung cancers: a consensus report. Lung Cancer 1991; 7: 11–13.
13. The Lung Cancer Study Group. The benefit of adjuvant treatment for resected locally advanced non-small cell lung cancer. J Clin Oncol 1986; 4: 710–15.
14. Niiranen A, Niitamo-Korhonen S, Kouri M, et al. Adjuvant chemotherapy after radical surgery for non-small cell lung cancer: a randomized study. J Clin Oncol 1992; 10: 1927–32.
15. Feld R, Rubinstein L, Thomas PA. Adjuvant chemotherapy with cyclophosphamide, doxorubicin and cisplatin in patients with completely resected stage I non-small cell lung cancer. The Lung Cancer Study Group. J Natl Cancer Inst 1993; 85: 229–306.
16. Ohta M, Tsuchiya R, Shimoyama M, et al. Adjuvant chemotherapy for completely resected stage III non-small cell lung cancer. Results of a randomized prospective study. The Japan Clinical Oncology Group. J Thorac Cardiovasc Surg 1993; 106: 703–8.
17. Figlin RA, Piantodosi S. A phase III randomized trial of immediate combination of chemotherapy versus delayed combination chemotherapy in patients with completely resected stage II and III non-small cell carcinoma of the lung. Chest 1994; 106(6 Suppl): S310–12.
18. Non-small Cell Lung Cancer Collaborative Group. Chemotherapy in non-small cell lung cancer: a meta-analysis using updated data on individual patients from 52 randomised clinical trials. BMJ 1995; 311: 899–909.
19. Keller SM, Adak S, Wagner H, et al. A randomized trial of postoperative adjuvant therapy in patients with completely resected stage II or IIIA non-small-cell lung cancer. Eastern Cooperative Oncology Group. N Engl J Med 2000; 343: 1217–22.
20. Scagliotti GV, Fossati R, Torri V, et al. Randomized study of adjuvant chemotherapy for completely resected stage I, II, or IIIA non-small-cell lung cancer. J Natl Cancer Inst 2003; 95: 1453–61.
21. Waller D, Peake MD, Stephens RJ, et al. Chemotherapy for patients with nonsmall cell lung cancer: the surgical setting of the Big Lung Trial. Eur J Cardiothorac Surg 2004; 26: 173–1782.
22. Arriagada R, Bergman B, Dunant A, et al. Cisplatin-based adjuvant chemotherapy in patients with completely resected non-small-cell lung cancer. N Engl J Med 2004; 350: 351–60.
23. Arriagada R, Dunant A, Pignon JP, et al. Long-term results of the international adjuvant lung cancer trial evaluating adjuvant cisplatin-based chemotherapy in resected lung cancer. J Clin Oncol 2010; 28: 35–42.
24. Douillard JY, Rosell R, De Lena M, et al. Adjuvant vinorelbine plus cisplatin vs. observation in patients with completely resected stage IB–IIIA non-small-cell lung cancer (Adjuvant Navelbine International Trialist Association [ANITA]): a randomised controlled trial. Lancet Oncol 2006; 7: 719–27.
25. Douillard JY, Rosell R, De Lena M, et al. Impact of postoperative radiation therapy on survival in patients with complete resection and stage I, II, or IIIA non-small-cell lung cancer treated with adjuvant chemotherapy: the adjuvant Navelbine International Trialist Association (ANITA) Randomized Trial. Int J Radiat Oncol Biol Phys 2008; 72: 695–701.

26. Winton T, Livingston R, Johnson D, et al. Vinorelbine plus cisplatin vs. observation in resected non-small-cell lung cancer. N Engl J Med 2005; 352: 2589–97.

27. Butts CA, Ding K, Seymour L, et al. Randomized phase III trial of vinorelbine plus cisplatin compared with observation in completely resected stage IB and II non-small-cell lung cancer: updated survival analysis of JBR-10. J Clin Oncol 2010; 28: 29–34.

28. Pepe C, Hassan B, Winton T, et al. Adjuvant vinorelbine and cisplatin in elderly patients: National Cancer Institute of Canada and Intergroup Study JBR.10. J Clin Oncol 2007; 25: 1553–61.

29. Strauss GM, Herndon JE, Maddaus MA, et al. Adjuvant paclitaxel plus carboplatin compared with observation in stage IB non-small-cell lung cancer: CALGB 9633 with the Cancer and Leukemia Group B, Radiation Therapy Oncology Group, and North Central Cancer Treatment Group Study Groups. J Clin Oncol 2008; 26: 5043–51.

30. Pignon JP, Tribodet H, Scagliotti GV, et al. Lung adjuvant cisplatin evaluation: a pooled analysis by the LACE Collaborative Group. J Clin Oncol 2008; 26: 3552–9.

31. NSCLC Meta-analyses Collaborative Group. Arriagada R, Auperin A, Burdett S, et al. Adjuvant chemotherapy, with or without postoperative radiotherapy, in operable non-small-cell lung cancer: two meta-analyses of individual patient data. Lancet 2010; 375: 1267–77.

32. Kato H, Ichinose Y, Ohta M, et al. A randomized trial of adjuvant chemotherapy with uracil-tegafur for adenocarcinoma of the lung. N Engl J Med 2004; 350: 1713–21.

33. PORT Meta-analysis Trialists Group. Postoperative radiotherapy in non-small cell lung cancer: systematic review and meta-analysis of individual patient data from nine randomised controlled trials. Lancet 1998; 352: 257–63.

34. Lally BE, Zelterman D, Colasanto JM, et al. Postoperative radiotherapy for stage II or III non-small-cell lung cancer using the Surveillance, Epidemiology, and End Results database. J Clin Oncol 2006; 24: 2998–3006.

35. Clinical Trials. gov. Radiation therapy in treating patients with non-small cell lung cancer that has been completely removed by surgery. [Available from: http://clinicaltrials.gov/ct2/show/NCT00410683?term_lung-ART&rank_1] [Accessed 26 October 2009].

36. Roth JA, Fosella F, Komaki R, et al. A randomized trial comparing perioperative chemotherapy and surgery with surgery alone in resectable stage IIIA non-small cell lung cancer. J Natl Cancer Inst 1994; 86: 673–80.

37. Roth JA, Atkinson EN, Fosella F, et al. Long-term follow-up of patients enrolled in a randomized trial comparing perioperative chemotherapy and surgery with surgery alone in resectable stage IIIA non-small cell lung cáncer. Lung Cancer 1998; 21: 1–6.

38. Rosell R, Gomez-Codina J, Camps C, et al. A randomized trial comparing preoperative chemotherapy plus surgery with surgery alone in patients with non-small cell lung cancer. N Engl J Med 1994; 330: 153–8.

39. Depierre A, Milleron B, Moro-Sibilot D, et al. Preoperative chemotherapy followed by surgery compared with primary surgery in resectable stage I (except T1N0), II, and IIIa non-small-cell lung cancer. J Clin Oncol 2002; 20: 247–53.

40. Pisters KM, Vallieres E, Crowley JJ, et al. Surgery with or without preoperative paclitaxel and carboplatin in early-stage non-small-cell lung cancer: Southwest Oncology Group Trial S9900, an intergroup, randomized, phase III trial. J Clin Oncol 2010; 28: 1843–9.

41. Scagliotti GV, Pastorino U, Vansteenkiste JF, et al. Randomized phase III study of surgery alone or surgery plus preoperative cisplatin and gemcitabine in stages IB to IIIA non-small-cell lung cancer. J Clin Oncol 2011; JCO.2010.33.7089.

42. Gilligan D, Nicolson M, Smith I, et al. Preoperative chemotherapy in patients with resectable non-small cell lung cancer: results of the. MRC LU22/NVALT2/EORTC 08012 multicentre randomised trial and update of systematic review. Lancet 2007; 369: 1929–37.

43. Felip E, Rosell R, Maestre JA, et al. Preoperative chemotherapy plus surgery vs. surgery plus adjuvant chemotherapy vs. surgery alone in early-stage non-small-cell lung cancer. J Clin Oncol 2010; 28: 3138–45.

44. Berghmans T, Paesmans M, Meert AP, et al. Survival improvement in resectable non-small cell lung cancer with (neo) adjuvant chemotherapy: results of a metaanalysis of the literature. Lung Cancer 2005; 49: 13–23.

45. Burdett SS, Stewart LA, Rydzewska L. Chemotherapy and surgery vs. surgery alone in non-small cell lung cancer. Cochrane Database Syst Rev 2007: CD006157.

46. Burdett S, Rydzewska LH, Tierney JF. on behalf of the NSCLC Meta-analyses Collaborative Group. Pre-operative chemotherapy improves survival and reduces recurrence in operable non-small cell lung cancer: preliminary results of a systematic review and meta-analysis of individual patient data from 13 randomised trials (abstract O23.01). 14thWorld Conference on Lung Cancer. Amsterdam, The Netherlands, July 3–7, 2011.

47. Shields TW. Preoperative radiation therapy in the treatment of bronchial carcinoma. Cancer 1972; 30: 1388.

48. Tsuboi M, Kato H, Nagai K, et al. Gefitinib in the adjuvant setting: safety results from a phase III study in patients with completely resected non-small cell lung cancer. Anticancer Drugs 2005; 16: 1123–8.

49. Goss GD, Lorimer I, Tsao MS, et al. A phase III randomized, double-blind, placebo-controlled trial of the epidermal growth factor receptor inhibitor gefitinib in completely resected stage IB-IIIA non-small cell lung cancer (NSCLC): NCIC CTG BR.19. J Clin Oncol 2010; 28(Suppl): abstract LBA7005.

50. Tatcher N, Chang A, Parikh P, et al. Gefitinib plus best supportive care in previously treated patients with refractory advanced non-small cell lung cancer: results from a randomised, placebo-controlled, multicentre study (Iressa Survival Evaluation in Lung Cancer). Lancet 2005; 366: 1527–37.

51. Kelly K, Chansky K, Gaspar LE, et al. Phase III trial of maintenance gefitinib or placebo after concurrent chemora-diotherapy and docetaxel consolidation in inoperable stage III non-small-cell lung cancer: SWOG S0023. J Clin Oncol 2008; 26: 2450–6.

52. Clinical Trials. gov. RADIANT: A study of Tarceva after surgery with or without adjuvant chemotherapy in NSCLC patients who have EGFR-positive tumors (adjuvant). [Available from: http://clinicaltrials.gov/ct2/show/NCT00373425]

53. Clinical Trials Gov. Chemotherapy with or without bevacizumab in treating patients with stage IB, stage II or stage IIIA non-small lung cancer that was removed by surgery. [Available from: http://clinicaltrials.gov/ct2/show/NCT00324805erm_ecog_1505&rank_1]

54. Romero P. Current state of vaccine therapies in non-small-cell lung cancer. Clin Lung Cancer 2008; 9(Suppl 1): S28–36.

55. Boon T, Coulie PG, Eynde BJ, et al. Human T cell responses against melanoma. Annu Rev Immunol 2006; 24: 175–208.

56. Gaugler B, Van den EB, van der BP, et al. Human gene MAGE-3 codes for an antigen recognized on a melanoma by autologous cytolytic T lymphocytes. J Exp Med 1994; 179: 921–30.

57. van der Bruggen P, Traversari C, Chomez P, et al. A gene encoding an antigen recognized by cytolytic T lymphocytes on a human melanoma. Science 1991; 254: 1643–7.

58. Atanackovic D, Altorki NK, Stockert E, et al. Vaccine-induced CD4+ T cell responses to MAGE-3 protein in lung cancer patients. J Immunol 2004; 172: 3289–96.

59. Atanackovic D, Altorki NK, Cao Y, et al. Booster vaccination of cancer patients with MAGE-A3 protein reveals long-term immunological memory or tolerance depending on priming. Proc Natl Acad Sci USA 2008; 105: 1650–5.

60. Vansteenkiste J, Zielinski M, Dahabre J, et al. Multi-center, double-blind, randomized, placebo-controlled phase II study to assess the efficacy of recombinant MAGE-A3 vaccine as adjuvant therapy in stage IB/II MAGE-A3-positive, completely resected, non-small cell lung cancer (NSCLC). J Clin Oncol 2006; 24: 7019.

61. Zielinski M, Laskowski U, Bieselt R, et al. Preliminary results of MAGE-A3 expression and baseline demographic data from MAGRIT, a large phase III trial of MAGE-A3 ASCI (antigen-specific cancer immunotherapeutic) in adjuvant NSCLC. Eur J Cancer 2009; 7(Suppl): 511.

62. Zhu CQ, Ding K, Strumpf D, et al. Prognostic and predictive gene signature for adjuvant chemotherapy in resected non-small-cell lung cancer. J Clin Oncol 2010; 28: 4417–24.

63. Olaussen KA, Dunant A, Fouret P, et al. DNA repair by ERCC1 in non-small-cell lung cancer and cisplatin-based adjuvant chemotherapy. N Engl J Med 2006; 355: 983–91.

64. Bepler G, Kusmartseva I, Sharma S, et al. RRM1 modulated in vitro and in vivo efficacy of gemcitabine and platinum in non-small-cell lung cancer. J Clin Oncol 2006; 24: 4731–7.

65. Rosell R, Skrzypski M, Jassem E, et al. BRCA1: a novel prognostic factor in resected non-small-cell lung cancer. PLoS One 2007; 2: e1129.

66. Gandara DR, Grimminger P, Mack PC, et al. Association of epidermal growth factor receptor activating mutations with low ERCC1 gene expression in non-small cell lung cancer. J Thorac Oncol 2010; 5: 1933–8.

10 | Advances in surgery of lung cancer

Paul E. Van Schil, Jeroen M. Hendriks, Marjan Hertoghs, Patrick Lauwers, and Cliff K. Choong

INTRODUCTION

In this review, recent advances in the surgical treatment of lung cancer are presented and discussed. Many controversial issues remain regarding the role of surgery in the diagnosis, staging, and treatment of nonsmall cell lung cancer (NSCLC). The role of invasive staging and restaging techniques are currently debated and their present-day applications are discussed in this chapter. The different types of operative procedures that are available to the thoracic surgeon are also described. In the consideration of the surgical treatment for NSCLC, a distinction has to be made between early stage disease (stages IA/B and IIA/B), locoregionally advanced disease (stages IIIA/B), and metastatic disease (stage IV). The different indications for surgical treatment of NSCLC are discussed according to the recently introduced seventh TNM classification taking into account that surgery for locoregionally advanced disease remains a highly controversial topic. Intraoperative staging of lung cancer is extremely important to determine the extent of resection according to the intraoperative tumor (T) and nodal (N) status. Systematic nodal dissection is generally advocated to determine the precise nodal involvement which not only determines prognosis but also the application of adjuvant therapy. In 2011, a new adenocarcinoma classification was published introducing the concepts of adenocarcinoma in situ and minimally invasive adenocarcinoma. Its surgical implications including the role of limited resection are discussed. Except for very early stages of NSCLC, combined modality therapy including surgery is more frequently utilized. The impact and influence of surgery on prognosis, morbidity, and mortality are discussed in this chapter.

INVASIVE MEDIASTINAL STAGING AND RESTAGING OF LUNG CANCER

Importance of Mediastinal Lymph Node Staging

In the absence of distant metastasis, the prognosis of a patient with lung cancer and the decision to offer surgery depend on locoregional lymph node involvement. Pathological staging remains the gold standard in quantifying the extent of locoregional and mediastinal lymph node involvement. Patients with ipsilateral hilar or intrapulmonary lymph node metastases (N1), although it being a prognostic indicator, are not precluded from surgery as complete resection. Historically, in most centers, patients found to present with ipsilateral mediastinal lymph node metastases (N2) were not offered surgery due to associated poor long-term outcomes with or without surgery. In recent times, selected patients with cytologically or pathologically proven N2 disease have been treated by induction chemotherapy or chemoradiotherapy followed by restaging and surgical resection. Encouraging survival rates have recently been reported in such patients with N2 NSCLC. Patients with limited N2 disease, in whom downstaging is obtained after induction therapy, may therefore be considered for surgical resection. Patients with contralateral mediastinal or supraclavicular lymph node involvement (N3) are presently considered unsuitable surgical candidates due to poor long-term prognosis with or without surgery.

Currently available staging techniques are summarized in Table 10.1. Due to refinements in noninvasive and minimally invasive staging techniques, the role of surgical invasive staging and restaging has become a highly controversial topic and is discussed below. Intraoperative nodal staging is addressed separately in the section on intraoperative staging.

Mediastinal Staging of Lung Cancer

Noninvasive techniques include computed tomography (CT) and positron emission tomography (PET). The only useful criterion to assess malignancy on CT is size of the lymph node. Nodes that have a short axis larger than 1 cm on CT are considered abnormal. The positive predictive value (PPV) and negative predictive value (NPV) in primary staging of mediastinal lymph nodes on CT are 56% and 83%, respectively.[1]

Magnetic resonance imaging (MRI) has not been found to be useful for routine mediastinal lymph node staging.[2]

PET is more accurate than CT for the staging of mediastinal nodes as it assesses not only size but also the metabolic activity of the lymph nodes. Reportedly NPV for PET is as high as 93%, although PPV is only

Table 10.1 Currently Available Staging and Restaging Techniques for Nonsmall Cell Lung Cancer

Noninvasive techniques
    Computed tomography (CT)
    Magnetic resonance imaging (MRI)
    Positron emission tomography (PET)
    Integrated PET/CT
Minimally invasive techniques
    Transbronchial needle aspiration (TBNA)
    Transthoracic needle aspiration (TTNA)
    Endobronchial ultrasound (EBUS)
    Endoscopic ultrasound (EUS)
Invasive techniques
    (Re)mediastinoscopy
        Cervical
        Anterior
    Video-assisted mediastinal lymphadenectomy (VAMLA)
    Transcervical extended mediastinal lymphadenectomy (TEMLA)
    Video-assisted thoracic surgery (VATS), thoracoscopy

79%.[3] For that reason, a positive PET result usually would still require tissue confirmation. "Tissue will remain the issue" for the foreseeable period of time as PET avidity is not only found in malignancy but also in inflammatory and infectious diseases. Integrated PET–CT is more accurate than CT or PET alone with an overall accuracy of 90% and therefore, if available, should be routinely utilized in the staging process of NSCLC.[4]

Only a negative CT and negative PET, or a negative integrated PET–CT may render minimally invasive or invasive techniques unnecessary prior to surgery.

Minimally invasive techniques had initially shown promising results as staging modalities. Recent studies have unfortunately shown rather high false negative rates.[5,6] Cerfolio et al. published a retrospective review of 234 patients with NSCLC who were staged by endobronchial ultrasound (EBUS) or esophageal ultrasound (EUS) for suspected N2 disease on CT or PET–CT.[5] Mediastinoscopy was performed when EBUS/EUS was negative. NPVs for detecting N2 disease by EBUS, EUS, and mediastinoscopy were 79%, 80%, and 93%, respectively. EBUS was found to be false negative in 28% and EUS in 22% of the cases. In a retrospective study from a single institution by Defranchi et al., 494 patients, suspected of lung cancer, underwent EBUS.[6] A negative result was followed by mediastinoscopy. Twenty-eight percent of the patients with suspicious mediastinal lymph nodes still had N2 disease confirmed by mediastinoscopy despite a negative EBUS. In this way, negative EBUS/EUS results should be confirmed by mediastinoscopy. Rapid on-site cytological evaluation (ROSE) increases diagnostic accuracy and may facilitate the decision whether to proceed to a second, more invasive procedure in the same session.

The role of surgical mediastinal staging such as mediastinoscopy and also restaging is a matter of judgment and correct interpretation of various staging modalities and their results. None of the available techniques can be expected to provide perfect results. In that case the main question becomes: Which false negative rate one is willing to accept? The decision is influenced by the risks and morbidity of the procedures involved. Mediastinoscopy is associated with low morbidity (2%) and low mortality (0.08%) but remains an invasive procedure.[7] Right and left, high and low paratracheal nodes (stations 2R, 2L, 4R, 4L) and anterior subcarinal nodes (station 7) are accessible via this approach. The reported PPV and NPV as staging procedure in NSCLC are 100% and 96%, respectively.[8] When an extensive lymph node dissection is performed such as video-assisted mediastinal lymphadenectomy (VAMLA) or transcervical extended mediastinal lymphadenectomy (TEMLA) procedures, the false negative rate becomes extremely low.[9–11]

In patients with suspected mediastinal lymph node involvement on noninvasive techniques such as CT or PET, evaluation by EBUS/EUS followed by mediastinoscopy, in cases where no positive lymph nodes were found by EBUS/EUS, has produced excellent results with a reported increase of sensitivity in detection of mediastinal nodal disease up to 93%.[12] In the ASTER study, 241 patients with resectable, suspected, or proven NSCLC, in whom mediastinal staging was indicated based on CT or PET findings, were enrolled into a randomized controlled multicenter study. Nodal metastases were found in 35% by surgical staging alone versus 46% by endosonography (EBUS and EUS) versus 50% by endosonography followed by surgical staging. NPVs were 86, 85 (p = 0.47), and 93% (p = 0.18), respectively.[12]

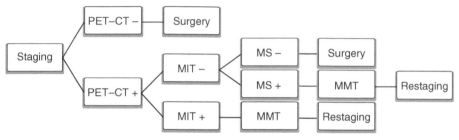

Figure 10.1 Flow chart for mediastinal staging of NSCLC in Antwerp University Hospital. *Abbreviations*: PET–CT, integrated positron emission tomography and computed tomography; MIT, minimally invasive technique (endobronchial or endoscopic ultrasound); MS, mediastinoscopy; MMT, multimodality treatment.

In concordance with the European Society of Thoracic Surgeons (ESTS) guidelines, positive CT, PET, or PET–CT findings should be cytologically or pathologically confirmed. EBUS and EUS are complementary to surgical invasive staging techniques with a high specificity but low NPV. Therefore, an invasive surgical technique is still indicated if EBUS/EUS yield a negative result. Figure 10.1 provides a flow chart of mediastinal staging in NSCLC that is used at the Antwerp University Hospital.

Mediastinal Restaging of Lung Cancer

Most patients with pathologically proven N2 disease detected during preoperative work-up will be treated by induction therapy. The mediastinum can be principally restaged by the same techniques as applied in primary staging. At the present time, neither CT, PET, or PET–CT are accurate enough to make final therapeutic decisions based on their results alone. The accuracy of CT decreases in restaging after induction therapy to 58%.[13] PET scanning is more accurate than CT for mediastinal restaging with a reported PPV to detect persisting nodal disease of 73%. To detect residual N2 disease, however, PPV was <20%.[14] The use of PET–CT fusion images significantly increases the accuracy through better localization of focal isotope uptake in mediastinal nodes. PPV varies between 75% and 93%. However, a 20% false negative and a 25% false positive rate have been reported.[15] In cases where there is a suspicion of residual mediastinal disease, invasive biopsies are still required.

Minimally invasive techniques such as EBUS and EUS comprise promising restaging modalities. However, false negative rates remain high and are approximately 20–30%.[16,17] Therefore, negative findings should still be confirmed by surgical restaging.

Repeat mediastinoscopy, although technically more difficult than the first procedure, offers the advantage of providing large biopsy samples and also allowing for detailed molecular genetic analysis. Accuracy of this procedure is between 81% and 93%.[18,19] In recent times, restaging has been the most frequent indication for remediastinoscopy but it can safely be performed for other indications as well. In contrast to imaging or functional studies, remediastinoscopy offers the advantage of not only providing a definite diagnosis of various thoracic diseases involving the mediastinal lymph nodes, but also pathological evidence of response after induction therapy.

In our combined Antwerp–Barcelona series of 104 repeat mediastinoscopies after induction therapy, patients with positive remediastinoscopy had a median survival time of 14 months, in contrast to 28 months in those with negative remediastinoscopies.[20] This difference was highly significant (p = 0.001). We also reported a median survival time for false negative remediastinoscopies of 24 months. This may indicate that, although micrometastases were found at thoracotomy, surgery may prolong survival when a complete resection can be obtained. In a multivariate analysis, only nodal status was confirmed to be a significant independent prognostic factor for survival.

The reason for false negative rates has to be determined. Conventional histological sections may not be sufficiently sensitive to detect small numbers of tumor cells in regional lymph nodes. Several studies have suggested that micrometastatic disease may be efficiently detected by immunohistochemistry. Implementation of this specific technique in the staging and restaging of NSCLC is yet to be investigated.[21,22]

The ESTS guidelines for restaging after induction treatment for NSCLC have cautioned that neither CT, PET nor PET–CT are accurate enough to make final further therapeutic decisions based on their results. A minimally invasive or invasive technique providing cytological or pathological information is recommended. For restaging, endoscopic techniques or surgical invasive techniques can be utilized. The choice may be dependent on the availability of the technique and expertise of the center.[1] For thoracic surgeons having only

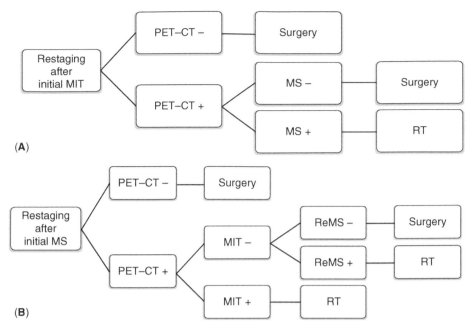

Figure 10.2 Flow chart for mediastinal restaging of NSCLC in Antwerp University Hospital. Depending on whether initially a minimally invasive procedure or mediastinoscopy was performed. *Abbreviations*: PET–CT, integrated positron emission tomography and computed tomography; MIT, minimally invasive technique (endobronchial or endoscopic ultrasound); MS, mediastinoscopy; RT, radiotherapy.

minimal or no experience with remediastinoscopy, an alternative approach consists of the initial use of minimally invasive staging procedures as EBUS or EUS to obtain a cytological proof of mediastinal nodal involvement. After induction therapy, patients are subsequently restaged by mediastinoscopy. In this way, a technically more demanding remediastinoscopy can be avoided. This approach was also found to be the most accurate in a recent review by de Cabanyes Candela and Detterbeck.[23]

Figure 10.2 provides a flow chart of mediastinal restaging in NSCLC that is used at the Antwerp University Hospital depending on whether initial proof was obtained by a minimally invasive technique or mediastinoscopy.

LUNG CANCER RESECTION
Complete R0 Resection
The final aim of surgical treatment for NSCLC is complete (R0) resection. In this respect, specific criteria have been established by a working group of the International Association for the Study of Lung Cancer (IASLC).[24] Complete resection is defined as complete removal of the primary tumor with no residual macroscopic or microscopic tumor left behind. Moreover, a systematic or lobe-specific nodal dissection must have been performed, and the highest mediastinal lymph node must be negative. Resectability and operability of a primary NSCLC depend on the staging of the tumor, the clinical fitness of the patient to undergo surgery, and the intraoperative staging. After definitive pathological examination, a distinction can be made postoperatively between R0 resections when there is no residual tumor, R1 with microscopic and R2 with macroscopic residual tumor. Detailed cardiopulmonary evaluation to determine the functional status of the patient is equally important as this might impact on the extent of resection.[25]

Types of Lung Cancer Resection
Lung cancer resections can be divided into three major groups as listed in Table 10.2.

Group 1: Standard Resections
Standard resections include lobectomy (removal of a lobe), bilobectomy (removal of two lobes on the right side), and pneumonectomy (removal of an entire lung). Pneumonectomy was initially considered as the

treatment of choice for lung cancer in the early days while lobectomy was reserved for patients with diminished pulmonary or cardiac reserve. In later years, lobectomy was found to provide a similar survival rate as pneumonectomy if the lesion could be totally resected by lobectomy.

Group 2: Conservative or Lung Parenchyma Saving Operations

These operations can be divided in proximal and distal procedures. The proximal procedures comprise all bronchoplasty and tracheoplasty operations. The most frequently performed bronchoplastic procedure is a sleeve resection of the right upper lobe for lung cancers invading the upper lobe orifice. The distal procedures include segmentectomies and wedge resections. Regarding the extent of resection, lobectomy is generally considered the procedure of choice in cancers confined to a single lobe. This includes peripheral T1aN0 NSCLC. This rationale resulted from a prospective randomized trial from the Lung Cancer Study Group comparing lobectomy to lesser resections for peripheral clinical T1N0 lesions.[26] Patients were randomized to standard lobectomy or lesser resection during standard thoracotomy. Noteworthy in this study was that nearly half of the patients had a contraindication to randomization, mostly because of location of the tumor or unexpected N1 or N2 disease. Patients who underwent a limited resection were found to have a tripling of local recurrence rate, a 30% increase in overall death rate and a 50% increase in cancer-related death rate in comparison to lobectomy patients. These results were, however, only significant at a p-value level of 0.10.

The role of sublobar resection, anatomical segmentectomy, or wide wedge resection is being reconsidered for very early lung cancer following large screening programs for lung cancer. This is due to the findings of nonsolid or part solid ground glass opacities, so-called GGO.[27] These topics will be further discussed in the section on the new adenocarcinoma classification.

Group 3: Extended Operations

Extended operations involve resection of lung parenchyma with an adjacent organ or structure invaded by the tumor. Examples include resection of chest wall, diaphragm, pericardium, left atrium, superior vena cava, and apex of the chest in superior sulcus tumors. En bloc resection of the locally involved extrapulmonary structure is advised to avoid tumor spillage and to ensure a complete R0 resection with negative margins.

Thoracic Incisions

A posterolateral thoracotomy incision is the most common incision performed. Some surgeons prefer a muscle-sparing thoracotomy incision. Sternotomy is sometimes utilized in patients requiring bilateral procedures, especially bilateral upper lobe lung cancers. An extended incision such as a hemi-clamshell incision is utilized in selected patients requiring an extended resection. Video-assisted thoracic surgery (VATS) is increasingly used as specific access to the thoracic cavity. In a series of 1100 VATS lobectomies, excellent

Table 10.2 Types of Operative Procedures

Standard
Lobectomy
Bilobectomy
Pneumonectomy
Conservative or lung parenchyma sparing operations
Proximal
Bronchotomy
Rotating bronchoplasty
Bronchial or tracheal wedge excision
Bronchial or tracheal sleeve resection
Distal
Segmentectomy
Wedge excision
Extended procedures (lung + other structure)
Pericardium (intrapericardial pneumonectomy)
Diaphragm
Chest wall (ribs, vertebrae)
Superior sulcus (Pancoast tumor)

results were reported with an operative mortality of 0.8%. This was, however, a nonrandomized study carried out in highly selected patients.[28] Morbidity generally appears to be lower with the VATS approach, although in a nationwide database of 13,619 patients who underwent lobectomy by thoracotomy or VATS, patients who underwent VATS lobectomy were 1.6 times more likely to have intraoperative complications.[29] A recent systematic review and meta-analysis of randomized and nonrandomized trials concluded that VATS lobectomy is an appropriate procedure for selected patients with early stage NSCLC.[30]

VATS has now become a standard approach for peripheral wedge resections. VATS segmentectomy is much less widely performed and its potential benefits and limitations still require further evaluation.[31,32]

Although VATS seems to be equal or even beneficial in terms of morbidity, length of stay, and survival in comparison to an open approach, further evaluation in large, prospective randomized trials is necessary.[33]

SEVENTH TNM CLASSIFICATION AND INDICATIONS FOR SURGICAL TREATMENT

The seventh edition of the TNM classification for lung and pleural tumors was initially proposed in 2007 and was subsequently formalized. It has been applied by most institutions since 2010.[34] This seventh edition is also utilized for the staging of neuroendocrine tumors and small cell lung cancer. Indications for surgical treatment can be subdivided into definite, investigational, and exceptional (Table 10.3).

Although no prospective, randomized trial exists to compare surgery versus radiotherapy in the treatment of early stage NSCLC, surgical resection has traditionally been considered the treatment of choice. Markedly improved survival rates are reported in the surgical series in comparison to patients who did not undergo surgical resection for a variety of reasons. The weighted average five-year survival rate for pT1N0 and pT2N0 was 74% and 61%, respectively, following surgery, and was only 23% after radiotherapy in stage I NSCLC.[35] Early stage disease and T3N1 NSCLC are considered definite indications for surgery (Table 10.3).

Surgery for locoregionally advanced disease remains controversial although many phase II studies have shown that surgical resection is feasible after induction therapy, as well as in patients with stage IIIB disease.

For locoregionally advanced stage IIIA-N2 lung cancer, the major question remains whether a better local control and survival is possible by induction therapy followed by surgery in comparison to standard chemoradiotherapy alone without surgery. This question was examined in two large phase III trials.

In the US Intergroup 0139 trial, patients with proven stage IIIA-N2 NSCLC were randomized between a full course of chemoradiotherapy or induction chemoradiotherapy followed by surgery.[36] There was no significant difference in overall survival between both arms: overall median survival time was 23.6 months in the surgical arm versus 22.2 months in the radiotherapy arm. There was, however, a difference in progression-free survival favoring the surgical arm, and patients who were downstaged to N0 disease had a better prognosis. The rate of locoregional recurrence was also significantly less in the surgical arm. In an exploratory analysis, patients undergoing lobectomy were matched to a similar group treated by chemoradiotherapy. There was a significant survival advantage for the surgical group. There was, however, no difference found for a matched group undergoing pneumonectomy.

In the EORTC 08941 phase III trial, patients with proven stage IIIA-N2 disease were randomized between surgery and radiotherapy after a response to induction chemotherapy.[37,38] There was no difference in overall and progression-free survival between both arms. The overall median survival time was

Table 10.3 Indications for Surgical Treatment of Nonsmall Cell Lung Cancer

Definite			
Stage			
IA	T1a,bN0		
IB	T2aN0		
IIA	T2bN0	T1a,bN1	T2aN1
IIB	T2bN1	T3N0	
IIIA	T3N1		
Investigational			
Stage			
IIIA	T1-3N2	T4N0,1	
IIIB	T4N2	T1-4N3	
Exceptional			
Stage			
IV	Single metastasis		
IV	Multiple metastases		

16.4 months in the surgical arm versus 17.5 months in the radiotherapy arm. In an exploratory analysis, patients who were downstaged to N0 or N1 disease had a significantly better prognosis than those with persisting N2 disease. Also, patients treated by lobectomy had a significantly better survival than those who had a pneumonectomy.

So, at the present time, surgical resection for stage IIIA-N2 is only indicated in patients with a mediastinal downstaging after induction therapy and who can preferentially be treated by a lobectomy to obtain a complete resection. Most of these patients will present with single-station nonbulky N2 disease, whereas bulky N2 disease is preferentially treated by chemoradiation.

Metastatic disease of a bronchogenic carcinoma is associated with a poor prognosis and is a contraindication for surgical resection. The exceptions are patients with a solitary brain or adrenal metastasis. In such patients, a reasonable five-year survival can be obtained after combined resection of the primary NSCLC and the isolated metastasis.[39]

INTRAOPERATIVE STAGING: SYSTEMATIC NODAL DISSECTION

Apart from resection of the lung cancer, careful intraoperative systematic lymph node dissection is performed as part of intraoperative staging. This is important to provide an accurate pathological TNM staging. The different intrathoracic lymph node stations were originally described by Naruke in 1978[40] and were recently updated in the seventh TNM classification where the concept of nodal zones was introduced.[41] The nodal zones and stations are listed in Table 10.4 and schematically represented in Figure 10.3.[34,41]

Thoracotomy provides the final investigation and determination of resectability. As previously mentioned, surgical candidates are patients with clinical stages IA/B, IIA/B, and resectable IIIA NSCLC.

Nonresectable tumors include T4 tumors with invasion into important adjacent structures or tumors with extensive mediastinal metastases. These include involvement of vital mediastinal structures or extracapsular N2 and N3 diseases. For resected N2 disease, invasion of the highest mediastinal lymph node heralds a poor prognosis. Massive involvement of hilar structures is generally a contraindication unless an intrapericardial pneumonectomy can be performed. Pleural metastases are also a contraindication to resection surgery.

When deciding on the type of operation to be performed, the surgeon should first perform a careful intraoperative exploration taking into account several strategic points. He should determine whether the tumor is peripheral or central, which lymph nodes are involved, and whether or not there is transgression of the fissure. If necessary, frozen section analysis of suspicious lymph nodes or margins should be performed. General guidelines are provided in Table 10.5.

Table 10.4 Regional Lymph Node Mapping into Zones and Stations According to the Seventh TNM Edition[41]

Supraclavicular zone
  1. Low cervical, supraclavicular, and sternal notch
Upper zone
  2. Upper paratracheal
  3. a. Prevascular
    b. Retrotracheal
  4. Lower paratracheal
Aortopulmonary (AP) zone
  5. Subaortic or Botallo's
  6. Para-aortic (ascending aorta or phrenic)
Subcarinal zone
  7. Subcarinal
Lower zone
  8. Para-esophageal (below carina)
  9. Pulmonary ligament
Hilar/interlobar zone
  10. Hilar
  11. Interlobar
Peripheral zone
  12. Lobar: upper, middle and lower lobe
  13. Segmental
  14. Subsegmental

Lobectomy is the procedure of choice whenever it is possible. Some have considered that "pneumonectomy is a disease in itself" due to its profound respiratory and hemodynamic implications, and associated higher complication rates in comparison to lobectomy. Most patients, however, have adapted to living with just one lung.[42] Pneumonectomy is avoided whenever possible, especially on the right side. A sleeve lobectomy in place of a pneumonectomy should be considered as an alternative whenever possible, provided a complete resection can be obtained.[43]

In a large series of 334 patients who were being evaluated for chest wall resection for NSCLC, the Memorial Sloan-Kettering Cancer Center in New York reported that the five-year survival rate was 32% in patients who underwent a complete resection in comparison to only 4% for incomplete resections and 0% for exploration only.[44] Long-term survival was mainly dependent on nodal involvement and complete resection, and less dependent on the depth of chest wall invasion. In some cases, it may be difficult to decide whether to perform an extrapleural dissection or to proceed with a full thickness chest wall resection. In the presence of thin, filmy adhesions or when the tumor readily detaches from the chest wall, the extrapleural plane is developed and the parietal pleura is stripped off the ribs. If there is a doubt or the presence of a positive frozen section margin, a chest wall resection should be performed to ensure complete resection.

For precise N staging during thoracotomy, a systematic nodal dissection is performed as advocated by Graham and Goldstraw.[45] In this technique, dissection of the mediastinal, hilar, and lobar lymph nodes proceeds in a systematic fashion. Graham and Goldstraw reviewed their results in 240 patients with clinical T1-3 N0-1 NSCLC.[45] Preoperative mediastinoscopy was performed when lymph nodes were larger than

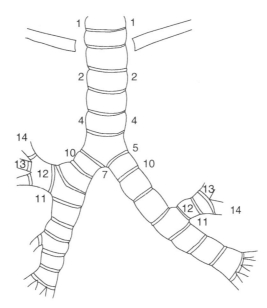

Figure 10.3 Locoregional lymph node stations according to the seventh TNM edition.[41] Lymph node station 5 lies anterior to the aortic arch.

Table 10.5 Operative Strategy According to Intraoperative Staging

T	LN	Fissure	Procedure
Peripheral	−	No transgression	Lobectomy (segmentectomy, wedge)
Peripheral	+	Transgression	(bi)Lobectomy, pneumonectomy
Central	−		Pneumonectomy, sleeve lobectomy
Central	+		Pneumonectomy (intrapericardial)
Extension or <2 cm carina			Extended procedure

Abbreviations: T, primary tumor; LN, lymph nodes.

1.5 cm on chest CT. The rate of exploratory thoracotomy without proceeding to surgical resection was only 3%. Following surgical resection, in 20% of patients, N2 disease was found. There was no subgroup with 0% incidence of N2 involvement and skip metastases were found in 34% of patients with N2 disease. Peripheral tumors <2 cm had a 24% incidence of lymph node metastases. Systematic lymph node dissection is therefore important and is now considered the gold standard for the accurate staging of nodal (N) disease.

A survival advantage of complete mediastinal lymph node dissection has only been demonstrated in one prospective randomized trial.[46] In a nonrandomized comparison of 373 patients, complete mediastinal lymph node dissection identified more levels of N2 disease in patients with stages II and IIIA NSCLC, and was associated with improved survival in *right* NSCLC in comparison to systematic nodal sampling.[47] In a recently published multicenter prospective clinical trial, patients with intraoperatively staged T1-2N0 nonhilar N1 NSCLC were randomized to lymph node sampling versus systematic nodal dissection. The latter identified occult disease in 3.8% of patients but was not associated with a benefit in overall survival.[48] It should be noted that patients in this trial were carefully staged with invasive, pathological analysis of four lymph node stations and that these results should not be generalized to higher stage tumors.

The technique of systematic lymph node dissection on the right side involves the dissection of the upper (level 2R) and lower paratracheal (level 4R) nodes, subcarinal (level 7), para-esophageal (level 8R) and inferior pulmonary ligament (level 9R) lymph node stations. On the left side, the aortopulmonary, para-aortic, and lower paratracheal nodes (levels 5, 6, 4L), and levels 7, 8L, 9L should be resected.

N1 disease also represents a heterogeneous group of diseases. This was demonstrated by Riquet who reported a series of 1174 patients with NSCLC. Twenty-two percent of the patients had N1 disease with a five-year survival of 47.5%.[49] A distinction was made between intralobar N1 (levels 12 and 13) and extralobar hilar N1 (levels 10 and 11) diseases. Five-year survival rate for intralobar N1 was 54% and for hilar N1 39%. This difference was highly significant. The prognosis of intralobar N1 is similar to N0 disease, and extralobar N1 is more closely related to N2 with single station involvement.

NEW ADENOCARCINOMA CLASSIFICATION: SURGICAL IMPLICATIONS
New Categories
In early 2011, a new adenocarcinoma classification was published by a common working group of the IASLC, American Thoracic Society (ATS) and European Respiratory Society (ERS).[50–52] This classification is listed in Table 10.6.

Table 10.6 IASLC/ATS/ERS Classification of Lung Adenocarcinoma in Resection Specimens

Preinvasive lesions
Atypical adenomatous hyperplasia
Adenocarcinoma in situ (≤3 cm formerly BAC)
Nonmucinous
Mucinous
Mixed mucinous/nonmucinous
Minimally invasive adenocarcinoma (≤3 cm lepidic predominant tumor with ≤5 mm invasion)
Nonmucinous
Mucinous
Mixed mucinous/nonmucinous
Invasive adenocarcinoma
Lepidic predominant (formerly nonmucinous BAC pattern, with >5 mm invasion)
Acinar predominant
Papillary predominant
Micropapillary predominant
Solid predominant with mucin production
Variants of invasive adenocarcinoma
Invasive mucinous adenocarcinoma (formerly mucinous BAC)
Colloid
Fetal (low and high grade)
Enteric

Abbreviation: BAC, bronchioloalveolar carcinoma.

Of special interest to thoracic surgeons are the new categories adenocarcinoma in situ (AIS) which represent small (≤3 cm), solitary adenocarcinomas consisting purely of lepidic growth without invasion, and minimally invasive adenocarcinoma (MIA) with ≤0.5 cm invasion. AIS and MIA are introduced because they should have 100% or near 100% five-year disease-free survival, respectively, if completely resected. The term bronchioloalveolar carcinoma (BAC) is no longer utilized as it applies to five different categories in the new classification which explains why this term has previously been so confusing.[50]

With the advent of helical CT and screening trials in high-risk populations, there is a renewed interest in small nodules, especially those with ground-glass opacity (GGO). Recently, results of the National Lung Screening trial were published.[53] In this trial, 53,454 persons at high risk for lung cancer were randomized between screening with low-dose CT or chest radiography. In the CT group, there was a relative reduction in mortality from lung cancer of 20.0% and a reduction in death from any cause of 6.7%.[53]

Whether some of these lesions can be treated by limited resection, so-called sublobar resection comprising of anatomical segmentectomy or wedge excision, is a prevailing question and the subject of intensive investigation.[52] For a limited resection to be oncologically valid, a precise pre- and intraoperative diagnosis becomes imperative. In terms of preoperative diagnosis, specific criteria on chest CT as percentage GGO, tumor shadow disappearance rate and histogram analysis have been shown to have a high predictive value.[54] The role of PET and integrated PET–CT scanning and specific tumor markers are currently being evaluated.[55]

Sublobar (Limited) Resection for Lung Cancer

The detection rate of smaller lung cancers in recent times is increasing and therefore the appropriateness of lobectomy for stage I lung cancer, especially those tumors ≤2 cm (cT1a disease) is again being questioned.[27,56] Recently, there have been numerous publications suggesting that sublobar resection for early lung cancers may be an adequate surgical treatment. These studies are not randomized trials and many are retrospective.[57–59] Most reports showed no difference in survival or in locoregional recurrence between lobectomy and sublobar resection for tumors 2 cm or less in size. Patients with GGO tumors on CT have been reported to have a 100% survival at five years after resection.[60–63] However, possible delayed cut-end recurrences have been described after limited resection of GGO lesions.[64]

Two recent reviews and one meta-analysis of sublobar resection concluded the well-selected use of sublobar resection, especially for pure AIS ≤2 cm, which yielded comparable survival and recurrence rates to lobectomy.[65–67] In this way, sublobar resection is generally considered acceptable for GGO lesions or adenocarcinomas with minimal invasion. Lobectomy is still considered the standard surgical treatment for tumors 2 cm or less in size that have a solid appearance on CT because such tumors are invasive carcinomas. Any change in this standard care awaits the results of two randomized trials (JCOG 0802 in Japan, CALGB 140503 in North America) that randomize such patients to either lobectomy or sublobar resection.

Whether a purely anatomical segmentectomy provides a similar or better result to a wide wedge resection has not been clearly determined yet. In general, when performing sublobar resections, several important factors affect the appropriateness of this intervention. These include the location (peripheral vs. central), appearance (GGO vs. solid), and size (T1a vs. T1b vs. T2) of the tumor. CT images, especially obtained by high-resolution CT scan with thin slices, are indispensable in the evaluation of these factors. Recent studies have shown rather good image to pathological correlations.[68] When correlating CT findings of GGO with histopathology, many of these lesions, though not all, correspond to preinvasive, noninvasive, or early forms of neoplastic growth, especially those of adenocarcinoma lineage.[60–63,69,70] In a recent prospective study from Japan (JCOG 0201), radiological noninvasive peripheral lung adenocarcinoma was defined as an adenocarcinoma ≤2.0 cm with ≤0.25 consolidation.[71]

Recent guidelines and a large, randomized screening trial state that small nodules ≤10 mm or ≤500 mm^3 that are clearly 100% pure GGO lesions on chest CT, which are suspected to be AIS or MIA, be considered for close follow-up rather than immediate surgical resection.[68,72] Specific CT characteristics to be considered are size, attenuation, shape, and growth rate.

Systematic Lymph Node Dissection for Early Stage Adenocarcinoma

The necessity of systematic hilar and mediastinal lymph node dissection is based on the fact that nearly 20% of pulmonary adenocarcinomas ≤20 mm and 5% of cases ≤10 mm in size are reported to have nodal metastases.[27,73,74] Lobe-specific nodal dissection limits dissection to the primary nodal regions draining the involved lobe. Although there is no general consensus on this specific technique, this has been shown to be a potentially adequate alternative to complete systematic nodal dissection.[24,59,75]

In some specific subsets of very early stage adenocarcinoma, especially pure GGO lesions, systematic lymph node dissection may not always be required.[76] Recent analysis of the Italian COSMOS screening study showed that systematic nodal dissection can be avoided in early stage, clinically N0 lung cancer when the maximum standardized uptake value on PET scanning is <2.0 and the pathological nodule size is ≤10 mm as the risk of nodal involvement is very low in this subset of patients.[77]

In a Japanese prospective study, a specific treatment algorithm was proposed.[78] Lesions ≤10 mm of any type or pure GGO nodules were initially observed and discussed with the patients. When size or density increased, they were subsequently resected. GGO lesions between 11 and 15 mm were treated by segmentectomy and lymph node sampling. Solid lesions between 11 and 15 mm and GGO lesions between 16 and 20 mm were removed by segmentectomy combined with lymph node dissection. Solid lesions between 16 and 20 mm were resected by lobectomy with lymph node dissection. Applying this algorithm, an excellent five-year disease-free survival rate of 98% was observed for limited resection.[78]

Multiple Lesions
Synchronous Lesions
Multifocal GGOs are often found, especially in screening programs (18% in the ELCAP trial).[79-81] When there is no evidence of mediastinal lymph node invasion, multiple nodules are not a contraindication for surgical exploration. In the ELCAP study, nonsolitary node-negative adenocarcinomas had the same prognosis as solitary node-negative cases suggesting that these represent multiple primaries and not intrapulmonary metastases.[79]

A standard treatment algorithm for multiple lesions has not yet been established. Several factors have to be taken into consideration: number and size of the different nodules, synchronous versus metachronous lesions, ipsilateral versus contralateral, primary versus metastatic lesions, and specific nature (atypical adenomatous hyperplasia, AIS, MIA). Conservative treatment with frequent follow-up is advocated for potentially benign lesions. When it is technically not possible to remove multiple synchronous pure GGO lesions, regular follow-up with chest CT represents an alternative approach to surgical resection.[82] For malignant nodules, several options exist, for example, lobectomy for same-lobe nodules (now considered to be T3 disease), bilobectomy, lobectomy with wide wedge resection(s), multiple wide wedge resections or segmentectomies, and finally, pneumonectomy, depending on functional capacity. Some of these resections can be performed by VATS.[83] A potential strategy is to perform an anatomical resection (segmentectomy or lobectomy) for larger, more invasive or more central tumors and removing the smaller or peripheral or less invasive tumors by wedge resection. Such an approach, however, has not yet been validated in clinical studies.

Metachronous Lesions
For precise diagnosis of metachronous versus synchronous lung cancers, the classical criteria of Martini and Melamed are often utilized, and in the present time also combined with molecular genetic analysis.[84] To be considered multiple primary tumors, the interval between the two diagnoses should be >2 years. When the interval is <2 years and both tumors are detected in the same lobe, different histology should be present or they should arise from foci of carcinoma in situ. When the interval is <2 years and they are found in different lobes, there should be no carcinoma cells in lymphatics common to both, and no systemic metastases.

Currently, not much information is available on metachronous AIS or MIA. If the patient's cardiopulmonary function allows, the same surgical principles as for synchronous lesions apply. Recently, three second tumors were described that were clearly cut-end scar area recurrences.[64] One case could be defined as a metachronous primary cancer after thorough pathological and mutational analysis.

COMBINED MODALITY TREATMENT INCLUDING SURGERY
The aims of induction or neoadjuvant therapy in NSCLC are to downstage a locoregionally advanced tumor, eradication of systemic micrometastases, and to cause a diminished stimulus to cancer cells by the surgical procedure itself. The disadvantages of induction therapy include increased morbidity and mortality. There is also an increase in the technical challenge of the surgery itself as induction therapy can cause an inflamed operative field and subsequent fibrosis. Surgery is generally performed within 4–5 weeks after induction therapy before the development of extensive hilar fibrosis. The tissues during this time are, however, friable and can be difficult to deal with. In this regard, it is often stated that "thoracic surgery can be terribly simple or simply terrible." Intraoperative distinction between viable tumor and fibrotic reaction is difficult. Frozen

section analysis can also be difficult and should be used with caution. To avoid a bronchopleural fistula, only minimal skeletonization of the bronchus is performed and coverage of the bronchial stump with vascularized tissue (pericardial fat pad, intercostal muscle, or parietal pleura flap) is recommended. Following what appears to be a response to induction therapy, surgical resection remains the only way to assess a precise pathologic response.

Following induction therapy, a right pneumonectomy is associated with a higher mortality and should be avoided. In a series of 470 patients who underwent surgical resection after induction chemotherapy or chemoradiotherapy, overall mortality was 3.8%.[85] The mortality after lobectomy was 2.4%, after left pneumonectomy was 0%, but after right pneumonectomy was 24%. In the multivariate analysis, independent risk factors for major complications were *right* pneumonectomy, blood loss of >500 ml, and forced expiratory volume in one second (FEV1) of <80%. The strongest predictor for mortality was *right* pneumonectomy.

These results were confirmed by the recent Intergroup 0139 trial.[36] Overall 30-day mortality in the surgical arm was 5%, after lobectomy 1%, and after pneumonectomy 26%. Mortality was 50% after right complex pneumonectomy. All these patients had induction chemoradiotherapy which may have accounted for the high mortality rate. In the EORTC 08941 trial, induction therapy consisted of chemotherapy only and the 30-day mortality in the overall surgical arm was 4%, after lobectomy 0%, and after pneumonectomy 6.9%.[38] Postoperative complications in this trial were mainly pneumonia, respiratory insufficiency, arrhythmias, air leak, cardiac decompensation, empyema, and bronchopleural fistula. Re-operation was necessary in 8.1% of patients due to positive margins, hemothorax, empyema, and bronchopleural fistula.[38] However, in a recent series of pneumonectomies performed after induction therapy for stage III NSCLC, excellent results were obtained with a mortality rate of only 3% and a five-year survival rate of 38%.[86] These results were confirmed by a recent review of 549 consecutive cases of surgical resection after induction therapy with an overall inhospital mortality of 1.8%, and a mortality of 3% after pneumonectomy.[87] Overall morbidity, however, was 46% with severe complications occurring in 23% of patients. In this series, predicted postoperative pulmonary function was the strongest predictor of operative risk.[87]

The alternative interventions to pneumonectomy are bronchoplastic procedures and these can also be performed safely after induction therapy. In a series of 30 patients who underwent a variety of bronchoplasties or tracheoplasties after induction therapy, mortality was 0%.[88] Complications occurred in 43%, but there was no specific problem related to the bronchial anastomosis.

Good results were also reported in NSCLC of the superior sulcus treated by induction chemoradiation and subsequent surgical resection. In SWOG trial 9416, the results in 110 patients were excellent with a mortality of 1.8%, a five-year survival rate of 44% for all eligible patients, and 54% for patients who had a complete resection.[89]

From these recent reports, it is clear that surgery is feasible after induction therapy for NSCLC, but is often more complex and carries a higher risk, especially when a right pneumonectomy is performed.

CONCLUSION

In conclusion, the final aim of surgical treatment for nonsmall cell lung cancer is complete resection which still represents the treatment of choice in early stage and T3N1 disease due to its good long-term results. Surgery for locally advanced disease remains controversial. Combined modality treatment including surgery is more frequently utilized but induction therapy may give rise to pronounced hilar fibrosis. Surgical resection for stage IIIA-N2 is currently only indicated in patients with mediastinal downstaging after induction therapy who can preferentially be treated by lobectomy. For correct lymph node staging a systematic nodal dissection is advised. A new adenocarcinoma classification has recently been published introducing the concepts of adenocarcinoma in situ and minimally invasive adenocarcinoma. For the latter lesions a limited resection may be adequate.

REFERENCES

1. De Leyn P, Lardinois D, Van Schil PE, et al. ESTS guidelines for preoperative lymph node staging for non-small cell lung cancer. Eur J Cardiothorac Surg 2007; 32: 1–8.
2. Schaefer-Prokop C, Prokop M. New imaging techniques in the treatment guidelines for lung cancer. Eur Respir J Suppl 2002; 35: 71s–83s.
3. Toloza EM, Harpole L, McCrory DC. Noninvasive staging of non-small cell lung cancer: a review of the current evidence. Chest 2003; 123: 137S–46S.
4. Fischer BM, Mortensen J, Hansen H, et al. Multimodality approach to mediastinal staging in non-small cell lung cancer. Faults and benefits of PET-CT: a randomised trial. Thorax 2011; 66: 294–300.

5. Cerfolio RJ, Bryant AS, Eloubeidi MA, et al. The true false negative rates of esophageal and endobronchial ultrasound in the staging of mediastinal lymph nodes in patients with non-small cell lung cancer. Ann Thorac Surg 2010; 90: 427–34.

6. Defranchi SA, Edell ES, Daniels CE, et al. Mediastinoscopy in patients with lung cancer and negative endobronchial ultrasound guided needle aspiration. Ann Thorac Surg 2010; 90: 1753–7.

7. Kirschner PA. Cervical mediastinoscopy. Chest Surg Clin N Am 1996; 6: 1–20.

8. Gdeedo A, Van Schil P, Corthouts B, et al. Prospective evaluation of computed tomography and mediastinoscopy in mediastinal lymph node staging. Eur Respir J 1997; 10: 1547–51.

9. Witte B, Hurtgen M. Video-assisted mediastinoscopic lymphadenectomy (VAMLA). J Thorac Oncol 2007; 2: 367–9.

10. Leschber G, Holinka G, Linder A. Video-assisted mediastinoscopic lymphadenectomy (VAMLA)--a method for systematic mediastinal lymphnode dissection. Eur J Cardiothorac Surg 2003; 24: 192–5.

11. Zielinski M, Hauer L, Hauer J, et al. Transcervical Extended Mediastinal Lymphadenectomy (TEMLA) for staging of non-small-cell lung cancer (NSCLC). Pneumonol Alergol Pol 2011; 79: 196–206.

12. Annema JT, van Meerbeeck JP, Rintoul RC, et al. Mediastinoscopy vs endosonography for mediastinal nodal staging of lung cancer: a randomized trial. JAMA 2010; 304: 2245–52.

13. Mateu-Navarro M, Rami-Porta R, Bastus-Piulats R, Cirera-Nogueras L, Gonzalez-Pont G. Remediastinoscopy after induction chemotherapy in non-small cell lung cancer. Ann Thorac Surg 2000; 70: 391–5.

14. De Leyn P, Stroobants S, De Wever W, et al. Prospective comparative study of integrated positron emission tomography-computed tomography scan compared with remediastinoscopy in the assessment of residual mediastinal lymph node disease after induction chemotherapy for mediastinoscopy-proven stage IIIA-N2 Non-small-cell lung cancer: a Leuven Lung Cancer Group Study. J Clin Oncol 2006; 24: 3333–9.

15. Cerfolio RJ, Bryant AS, Ojha B. Restaging patients with N2 (stage IIIa) non-small cell lung cancer after neoadjuvant chemoradiotherapy: a prospective study. J Thorac Cardiovasc Surg 2006; 131: 1229–35.

16. Annema JT, Veselic M, Versteegh MI, Willems LN, Rabe KF. Mediastinal restaging: EUS-FNA offers a new perspective. Lung Cancer 2003; 42: 311–18.

17. Herth FJ, Annema JT, Eberhardt R, et al. Endobronchial ultrasound with transbronchial needle aspiration for restaging the mediastinum in lung cancer. J Clin Oncol 2008; 26: 3346–50.

18. Rami-Porta R, Mateu-Navarro M, Serra-Mitjans M, Hernandez-Rodriguez H. Remediastinoscopy: comments and updated results. Lung Cancer 2003; 42: 363–4.

19. Stamatis G, Fechner S, Hillejan L, Hinterthaner M, Krbek T. Repeat mediastinoscopy as a restaging procedure. Pneumologie 2005; 59: 862–6.

20. De Waele M, Serra-Mitjans M, Hendriks J, et al. Accuracy and survival of repeat mediastinoscopy after induction therapy for non-small cell lung cancer in a combined series of 104 patients. Eur J Cardiothorac Surg 2008; 33: 824–8.

21. Verhagen AF, Bulten J, Shirango H, et al. The clinical value of lymphatic micrometastases in patients with non-small cell lung cancer. J Thorac Oncol 2010; 5: 1201–5.

22. Gu CD, Osaki T, Oyama T, et al. Detection of micrometastatic tumor cells in pN0 lymph nodes of patients with completely resected nonsmall cell lung cancer: impact on recurrence and Survival. Ann Surg 2002; 235: 133–9.

23. de Cabanyes Candela S, Detterbeck FC. A systematic review of restaging after induction therapy for stage IIIa lung cancer: prediction of pathologic stage. J Thorac Oncol 2010; 5: 389–98.

24. Rami-Porta R, Wittekind C, Goldstraw P. Complete resection in lung cancer surgery: proposed definition. Lung Cancer 2005; 49: 25–33.

25. Brunelli A, Charloux A, Bolliger CT, et al. ERS/ESTS clinical guidelines on fitness for radical therapy in lung cancer patients (surgery and chemo-radiotherapy). Eur Respir J 2009; 34: 17–41.

26. Ginsberg RJ, Rubinstein LV. Randomized trial of lobectomy versus limited resection for T1 N0 non-small cell lung cancer. Lung Cancer Study Group. Ann Thorac Surg 1995; 60: 615–22; discussion 22–3.

27. Asamura H, Suzuki K, Watanabe S, et al. A clinicopathological study of resected subcentimeter lung cancers: a favorable prognosis for ground glass opacity lesions. Ann Thorac Surg 2003; 76: 1016–22.

28. McKenna RJ Jr, Houck W, Fuller CB. Video-assisted thoracic surgery lobectomy: experience with 1,100 cases. Ann Thorac Surg 2006; 81: 421–5; discussion 5–6.

29. Gopaldas RR, Bakaeen FG, Dao TK, et al. Video-assisted thoracoscopic versus open thoracotomy lobectomy in a cohort of 13,619 patients. Ann Thorac Surg 2010; 89: 1563–70.

30. Yan TD, Black D, Bannon PG, McCaughan BC. Systematic review and meta-analysis of randomized and nonrandomized trials on safety and efficacy of video-assisted thoracic surgery lobectomy for early-stage non-small-cell lung cancer. J Clin Oncol 2009; 27: 2553–62.

31. Swanson SJ. Segmentectomy for lung cancer. Semin Thorac Cardiovasc Surg 2010; 22: 244–9.

32. Schuchert MJ, Pettiford BL, Pennathur A, et al. Anatomic segmentectomy for stage I non-small-cell lung cancer: comparison of video-assisted thoracic surgery versus open approach. J Thorac Cardiovasc Surg 2009; 138: 1318–25; e1.

33. Swanson SJ. Video-assisted thoracic surgery segmentectomy: the future of surgery for lung cancer? Ann Thorac Surg 2010; 89: S2096–7.

34. Goldstraw P, Crowley J, Chansky K, et al. The IASLC Lung Cancer Staging Project: proposals for the revision of the TNM stage groupings in the forthcoming (seventh) edition of the TNM Classification of malignant tumours. J Thorac Oncol 2007; 2: 706–14.

35. Reif MS, Socinski MA, Rivera MP. Evidence-based medicine in the treatment of non-small-cell lung cancer. Clin Chest Med 2000; 21: 107–20.

36. Albain KS, Swann RS, Rusch VW, et al. Radiotherapy plus chemotherapy with or without surgical resection for stage III non-small-cell lung cancer: a phase III randomised controlled trial. Lancet 2009; 374: 379–86.

37. van Meerbeeck JP, Kramer GW, Van Schil PE, et al. Randomized controlled trial of resection versus radiotherapy after induction chemotherapy in stage IIIA-N2 non-small-cell lung cancer. J Natl Cancer Inst 2007; 99: 442–50.

38. Van Schil P, Van Meerbeeck J, Kramer G, et al. Morbidity and mortality in the surgery arm of EORTC 08941 trial. Eur Respir J 2005; 26: 192–7.

39. Van Schil PE, Hendriks JM, Carp L, Lauwers PR. Surgery for oligometastatic disease in non-small-cell lung cancer. Expert Rev Anticancer Ther 2008; 8: 1931–8.

40. Naruke T, Suemasu K, Ishikawa S. Lymph node mapping and curability at various levels of metastasis in resected lung cancer. J Thorac Cardiovasc Surg 1978; 76: 832–9.

41. Rusch VW, Asamura H, Watanabe H, et al. The IASLC lung cancer staging project: a proposal for a new international lymph node map in the forthcoming seventh edition of the TNM classification for lung cancer. J Thorac Oncol 2009; 4: 568–77.

42. Deslauriers J, Ugalde P, Miro S, et al. Adjustments in cardiorespiratory function after pneumonectomy: results of the pneumonectomy project. J Thorac Cardiovasc Surg 2011; 141: 7–15.

43. Van Schil PE, Brutel de la Riviere A, Knaepen PJ, et al. Long-term survival after bronchial sleeve resection: univariate and multivariate analyses. Ann Thorac Surg 1996; 61: 1087–91.

44. Downey RJ, Martini N, Rusch VW, et al. Extent of chest wall invasion and survival in patients with lung cancer. Ann Thorac Surg 1999; 68: 188–93.

45. Graham AN, Chan KJ, Pastorino U, Goldstraw P. Systematic nodal dissection in the intrathoracic staging of patients with non-small cell lung cancer. J Thorac Cardiovasc Surg 1999; 117: 246–51.

46. Wu Y, Huang ZF, Wang SY, Yang XN, Ou W. A randomized trial of systematic nodal dissection in resectable non-small cell lung cancer. Lung Cancer 2002; 36: 1–6.

47. Keller SM, Adak S, Wagner H, Johnson DH. Mediastinal lymph node dissection improves survival in patients with stages II and IIIa non-small cell lung cancer. Eastern Cooperative Oncology Group. Ann Thorac Surg 2000; 70: 358–65; discussion 65–6.

48. Darling GE, Allen MS, Decker PA, et al. Randomized trial of mediastinal lymph node sampling versus complete lymph-adenectomy during pulmonary resection in the patient with N0 or N1 (less than hilar) non-small cell carcinoma: Results of the American College of Surgery Oncology Group Z0030 Trial. J Thorac Cardiovasc Surg 2011; 141: 662–70.

49. Riquet M, Manac'h D, Le Pimpec-Barthes F, Dujon A, Chehab A. Prognostic significance of surgical-pathologic N1 disease in non-small cell carcinoma of the lung. Ann Thorac Surg 1999; 67: 1572–6.

50. Travis WD, Brambilla E, Noguchi M, et al. International association for the study of lung cancer/american thoracic society/european respiratory society international multidisciplinary classification of lung adenocarcinoma. J Thorac Oncol 2011; 6: 244–85.

51. Travis WD, Brambilla E, Van Schil P, et al. Paradigm shifts in lung cancer as defined in the new IASLC/ATS/ERS lung adenocarcinoma classification. Eur Respir J 2011; 38: 239–43.

52. Van Schil PE, Asamura H, Rusch VW, et al. Surgical implications of the new IASLC/ATS/ERS adenocarcinoma classification. Eur Respir J 2012; 39: 478–86.

53. Aberle DR, Adams AM, Berg CD, et al. Reduced lung-cancer mortality with low-dose computed tomographic screening. N Engl J Med 2011; 365: 395–409.

54. Ikeda K, Awai K, Mori T, et al. Differential diagnosis of ground-glass opacity nodules: CT number analysis by three-dimensional computerized quantification. Chest 2007; 132: 984–90.

55. Lee HY, Han J, Lee KS, et al. Lung adenocarcinoma as a solitary pulmonary nodule: Prognostic determinants of CT, PET, and histopathologic findings. Lung Cancer 2009; 66: 379–85.

56. Henschke CI, McCauley DI, Yankelevitz DF, et al. Early Lung Cancer action project: overall design and findings from baseline screening. Lancet 1999; 354: 99–105.

57. El-Sherif A, Gooding WE, Santos R, et al. Outcomes of sublobar resection versus lobectomy for stage I non-small cell lung cancer: a 13-year analysis. Ann Thorac Surg 2006; 82: 408–15.

58. Nakamura H, Kawasaki N, Taguchi M, Kabasawa K. Survival following lobectomy vs limited resection for stage I lung cancer: a meta-analysis. Br J Cancer 2005; 92: 1033–7.

59. Okada M, Koike T, Higashiyama M, et al. Radical sublobar resection for small-sized non-small cell lung cancer: a multicenter study. J Thorac Cardiovasc Surg 2006; 132: 769–75.

60. Kodama K, Higashiyama M, Yokouchi H, et al. Prognostic value of ground-glass opacity found in small lung adenocarcinoma on high-resolution CT scanning. Lung Cancer 2001; 33: 17–25.

61. Suzuki K, Asamura H, Kusumoto M, Kondo H, Tsuchiya R. "Early" peripheral lung cancer: prognostic significance of ground glass opacity on thin-section computed tomographic scan. Ann Thorac Surg 2002; 74: 1635–9.

62. Takamochi K, Nagai K, Yoshida J, et al. Pathologic N0 status in pulmonary adenocarcinoma is predictable by combining serum carcinoembryonic antigen level and computed tomographic findings. J Thorac Cardiovasc Surg 2001; 122: 325–30.

63. Sakurai H, Maeshima A, Watanabe S, et al. Grade of stromal invasion in small adenocarcinoma of the lung: histopathological minimal invasion and prognosis. Am J Surg Pathol 2004; 28: 198–206.

64. Yoshida J, Ishii G, Yokose T, et al. Possible delayed cut-end recurrence after limited resection for ground-glass opacity adenocarcinoma, intraoperatively diagnosed as Noguchi type B, in three patients. J Thorac Oncol 2010; 5: 546–50.
65. Rami-Porta R, Tsuboi M. Sublobar resection for lung cancer. Eur Respir J 2009; 33: 426–35.
66. Blasberg JD, Pass HI, Donington JS. Sublobar resection: a movement from the Lung Cancer Study Group. J Thorac Oncol 2010; 5: 1583–93.
67. Fan J, Wang L, Jiang GN, Gao W. Sublobectomy Versus Lobectomy for stage I non-small-cell lung cancer, a meta-analysis of published studies. Ann Surg Oncol 2012; 19: 661–8.
68. Godoy MC, Naidich DP. Subsolid pulmonary nodules and the spectrum of peripheral adenocarcinomas of the lung: recommended interim guidelines for assessment and management. Radiology 2009; 253: 606–22.
69. Adler B, Padley S, Miller RR, Muller NL. High-resolution CT of bronchioloalveolar carcinoma. AJR Am J Roentgenol 1992; 159: 275–7.
70. Aoki T, Tomoda Y, Watanabe H, et al. Peripheral lung adenocarcinoma: correlation of thin-section CT findings with histologic prognostic factors and survival. Radiology 2001; 220: 803–9.
71. Suzuki K, Koike T, Asakawa T, et al. A prospective study to evaluate radiological diagnostic criteria by thin-section computed tomography to predict pathological non-invasiveness in peripheral clinical IA lung cancer (JCOG 0201). J Thor Oncol 2011; 6: 751–6.
72. van Klaveren RJ, Oudkerk M, Prokop M, et al. Management of lung nodules detected by volume CT scanning. N Engl J Med 2009; 361: 2221–9.
73. Ginsberg RJ, Rubinstein LV. Randomized trial of lobectomy versus limited resection for T1 N0 non-small cell lung cancer. Lung Cancer Study Group. Ann Thorac Surg 1995; 60: 615–22.
74. Miller DL, Rowland CM, Deschamps C, et al. Surgical treatment of non-small cell lung cancer 1 cm or less in diameter. Ann Thorac Surg 2002; 73: 1545–50; discussion 50–1.
75. Ishiguro F, Matsuo K, Fukui T, et al. Effect of selective lymph node dissection based on patterns of lobe-specific lymph node metastases on patient outcome in patients with resectable non-small cell lung cancer: A large-scale retrospective cohort study applying a propensity score. J Thorac Cardiovasc Surg 2010; 139: 1001–6.
76. Nomori H, Iwatani K, Kobayashi H, Mori A, Yoshioka S. Omission of mediastinal lymph node dissection in lung cancer: its techniques and diagnostic procedures. Ann Thorac Cardiovasc Surg 2006; 12: 83–8.
77. Veronesi G, Maisonneuve P, Pelosi G, et al. Screening-detected lung cancers: is systematic nodal dissection always essential? J Thorac Oncol 2011; 6: 525–30.
78. Kodama K, Higashiyama M, Takami K, et al. Treatment strategy for patients with small peripheral lung lesion(s): intermediate-term results of prospective study. Eur J Cardiothorac Surg 2008; 34: 1068–74.
79. Vazquez M, Carter D, Brambilla E, et al. Solitary and multiple resected adenocarcinomas after CT screening for lung cancer: histopathologic features and their prognostic implications. Lung Cancer 2009; 64: 148–54.
80. Nakata M, Sawada S, Yamashita M, et al. Surgical treatments for multiple primary adenocarcinoma of the lung. Ann Thorac Surg 2004; 78: 1194–9.
81. Hiramatsu M, Inagaki T, Matsui Y, et al. Pulmonary ground-glass opacity (GGO) lesions-large size and a history of lung cancer are risk factors for growth. J Thorac Oncol 2008; 3: 1245–50.
82. Kim HK, Choi YS, Kim J, et al. Management of multiple pure ground-glass opacity lesions in patients with bronchioloalveolar carcinoma. J Thorac Oncol 2010; 5: 206–10.
83. Mun M, Kohno T. Efficacy of thoracoscopic resection for multifocal bronchioloalveolar carcinoma showing pure ground-glass opacities of 20 mm or less in diameter. J Thorac Cardiovasc Surg 2007; 134: 877–82.
84. Pfannschmidt J, Dienemann H. Surgical treatment of oligometastatic non-small cell lung cancer. Lung Cancer 2010; 69: 251–8.
85. Martin J, Ginsberg RJ, Abolhoda A, et al. Morbidity and mortality after neoadjuvant therapy for lung cancer: the risks of right pneumonectomy. Ann Thorac Surg 2001; 72: 1149–54.
86. Weder W, Collaud S, Eberhardt WE, et al. Pneumonectomy is a valuable treatment option after neoadjuvant therapy for stage III non-small-cell lung cancer. J Thorac Cardiovasc Surg 2010; 139: 1424–30.
87. Barnett SA, Rusch VW, Zheng J, et al. Contemporary results of surgical resection of non-small cell lung cancer after induction therapy: a review of 549 consecutive cases. J Thorac Oncol 2011; 6: 1530–6.
88. Veronesi G, Solli PG, Leo F, et al. Low morbidity of bronchoplastic procedures after chemotherapy for lung cancer. Lung Cancer 2002; 36: 91–7.
89. Rusch VW, Giroux DJ, Kraut MJ, et al. Induction chemoradiation and surgical resection for superior sulcus non-small-cell lung carcinomas: long-term results of Southwest Oncology Group Trial 9416 (Intergroup Trial 0160). J Clin Oncol 2007; 25: 313–18.

11 | Recent advances in radiotherapy for lung cancer

Dirk K. M. De Ruysscher and José S.A. Belderbos

INTRODUCTION

Lung cancer remains one of the most lethal and frequent malignancies in the world.[1] After diagnosis, most patients with both non-small cell lung cancer (NSCLC) and small cell lung cancer (SCLC) still succumb to their disease. Nevertheless, the rate of survival has been increased, although slowly. Increasingly, it has been realized that even in the metastatic setting, long-term survivorship in selected patients with a few brain- or adrenal metastases may be achieved with radical systemic and local treatment.[2] In SCLC, the integration of chemotherapy and thoracic radiotherapy has been elucidated and prophylactic cranial irradiation (PCI) has shown to prolong survival in patients with extensive disease (ED) SCLC.

In this review, we will focus on recent advances made in radiotherapy. In our view, most significant is the use of stereotactic ablative body radiation (SABR) for stage I NSCLC, concurrent chemo-radiation for stage III NSCLC, the implementation of 4D CT and PET and adaptive radiotherapy strategies, the better integration of chest radiotherapy and chemotherapy for limited disease (LD) SCLC and PCI for ED-SCLC.

STEREOTACTIC ABLATIVE BODY RADIATION FOR STAGE I NSCLC

In stereotactic ablative body radiation (SABR), a limited number of very high doses of radiation are delivered to small tumors that are located in selected lung regions, for example, those remote from the more susceptible central mediastinal structures such as the main bronchi and the esophagus.[3] It is a new treatment option for early stage NSCLC in inoperable patients. The advantages of SABR compared to conventional irradiation are: overall less treatment time (1–2 weeks), and a high biological effective dose. The possibility to minimize the number of treatment sessions is an obvious benefit for medical inoperable patients suffering from cardiopulmonary disease and/or other co-morbidities or simply because of their old age. SABR requires highly specialized radiotherapy treatment preparation and execution techniques including 4D respiration correlated CT-scans and image-guided radiotherapy (IGRT) with on-line set-up corrections based on tumor guidance.

When 54–60 Gy in three fractions are delivered to patients with medically inoperable and peripherally located stage I NSCLC, local tumor control rates exceed 85% at two years, with approximately 5% subsequent estimated risk of pulmonary complications. The fractionation schedule of SABR is adapted by delivering eight fractions (7.5 Gy each); analogous outcomes as with the three fraction regimen have been described.[4] However, long-term follow-up needs to be awaited for final conclusions. It was demonstrated that a low pretreatment, FEV1 and/or DLCO, alone should not be used to exclude patients with NSCLC from treatment with SABR.[5] Although no phase III trials have been published comparing surgery with SABR, the introduction of SABR improved the survival of medically inoperable stage I NSCLC patients in a population-based analysis.[6]

In the follow-up after treatment of these patients, CT and FDG-PET (^{18}F-deoxyglucose-positron emission tomography) scans appear different than after conventional radiotherapy, with the development of a mass like consolidation on CT or persistent FDG uptake being described as long as three years and more post-therapy.[7,8]

CONCURRENT CHEMO-RADIATION FOR STAGE III NSCLC

After the superiority of induction chemotherapy followed by radiotherapy (RT) over RT alone was shown,[9] several randomized studies and one meta-analysis based on updated individual patient data have demonstrated a significant survival gain with concurrent chemo-radiation compared to the sequential schedule.[10] The survival at five-years increased from about 10% with sequential chemo-radiation to approximately 15% with the concurrent approach. This improved survival has been attributed to improved local tumor control (LC) without affecting the incidence of distant metastases.[10] This improved survival is at the expense of a higher incidence of severe (though reversible) esophagitis, occurring in 20–30%. No increased lung toxicity was observed in the concurrent regimens. All the trials have been performed in the pre-PET era however and current state-of-the-art staging examinations (brain imaging and FDG-PET scanning) were not performed. Even in these, according to current standards, suboptimal staged patients the influence of improved local control positively affected the overall survival. The radiotherapy techniques used in the reported trials were essentially 2D-based without higher-level dose calculation algorithms and adaptive protocols, all of which were not available at the time when the studies were performed. The absolute long-term survival rates are thus likely to be higher in more recent series.

Because of the still high local tumor recurrence rates in non-surgical series, two large phase III studies have addressed the role of surgical resection after induction treatment.[11,12] In the Lung Intergroup trial 0139, patients with resectable N2 disease were randomized between surgery or definitive chemo-radiation after induction concurrent chemo-radiation.[11] In the EORTC (European Organisation for Research and Treatment of Cancer) trial, patients with irresectable N2 disease who showed at least a minimal tumor response after three cycles of induction chemotherapy were randomized between RT and surgery.[12] Both trials found identical five-year survival rates in the surgical and the non-surgical arms: approximately 25% in the Intergroup study (resectable tumors) and 15% in the EORTC trial (irresectable cancers). Although vigorously debated,[13] the results of these two randomized trials are in line with previous phase II studies.[14,15] Moreover, in patients with resectable N2 disease receiving only chemotherapy followed by surgical resection, several single-institution phase II studies showed five-year survival rates of about 20%, although subgroups may have a better outcome.[16–18]

Also in concurrent chemo-radiation, it is of the utmost importance to avoid treatment delays. In a large series of the Radiation Therapy Oncology Group (RTOG), it was demonstrated that each day of treatment prolongation beyond about 6.5 weeks resulted in a 2% decrease of survival.[19] It is therefore logical that the RTOG found a positive association between higher biological radiotherapy doses and improved long-term survival rates.[20]

It should also be stressed that concurrent chemotherapy and radiotherapy are only safe in patients with no or limited co-morbidities, who are relatively young and have adequate organ functions. In a prospective, population-based study, we could estimate that only about 40% of the patients with stage III lung cancer are suitable for the concurrent approach.[21] For the remainder, sequential chemotherapy and radiotherapy remains a reasonable alternative. Moreover, the search for improvements in the radiotherapy component of both sequential and concurrent chemo-radiotherapy continues. Apart from the combination of targeted drugs and radiotherapy and technical advances, altered fractionation schedules that move away from the classical 2 Gy per day, 5 days a week regimen, have been tested.

HYPERFRACTIONATION

The basis of hyperfractionation (HFX) is to exploit the different capacity of cancer cells and late responding normal tissues to recover from sublethal radiation damage, given that the time interval between the two fractions is sufficiently long. An adequate interfraction interval is not trivial as the estimated recovery half-time in human tissues is in the order of 4–8 hours.[22] That HFX might be useful to improve the therapeutic ratio of radiotherapy is based on the difference in fractionation sensitivity between tumors and late responding tissues. Hyperfractionation with increased total dose compared to conventional fractionation may thus be an option to improve local control and survival in NSCLC, without increasing the risk of late normal tissue damage.

The combination of hyperfractionation with accelerated fractionation, leading to a short overall treatment time, resulted in the CHART schedule (continuous hyperfractionated accelerated radiotherapy).[23] In this schedule, 54 Gy is delivered in 12 days (three times 1.5 Gy per day). In a large phase III trial, CHART was compared to the conventional schedule of 60 Gy in 30 fractions.[7] In the CHART arm, the three-year local tumor control was 17% versus 13% in the conventional arm, with corresponding three-year survival rates of 20% versus 13% (p = 0.008). The CHART trial supported the hypothesis that accelerated proliferation of cancer cells is an important reason for treatment failure.

In the ECOG trial 2597, patients were randomized after induction chemotherapy to conventional fractionation (64 Gy/6.5 weeks) or hyperfractionated accelerated radiotherapy (HART) (57.5 Gy in 2.5 weeks).[24] In the experimental arm, patients received three fractions of 1.5 Gy per day, 5 days a week. The HART trial closed prematurely after recruiting 144 of the planned 388 patients, due to low patient accrual and logistical issues. The study was therefore underpowered to detect the hypothesized improvement in median survival from 14 to 21 months. The actual observed median survival was 14.9 months after conventional fractionation and 20.3 months after HART (p = 0.28), which is close to the a priori study hypothesis.

A phase II trial investigated induction chemotherapy combined with CHART in locally advanced NSCLC, in which 56 Gy was delivered in 36 fractions in 12 days. Toxicity observed was mild and the median overall survival was 15.7 months.[25]

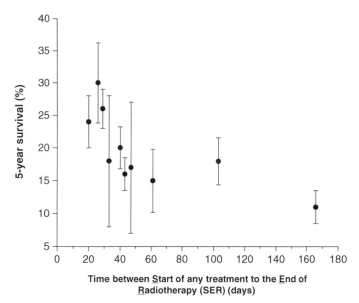

Figure 11.3 Survival at five-years as a function of the SER (start of *any* treatment to the end of radiotherapy). Each dot represents a single trial ± SE.

increase in median disease-free survival from 12.0 to 14.7 weeks and in median overall survival from 5.4 to 6.7 months after randomization. The one-year survival rate was 27.1% (95% CI, 19.4–35.5) in the PCI group and 13.3% (95% CI, 8.1–19.9) in the control group. Irradiation had side effects (fatigue) but did not seem to have a clinically significant effect on global health status, although the long-term toxicity was not examined.

CONCLUSION

Besides indisputable advances in systemic treatment and better surgical techniques, the ways to deliver radiotherapy have also significantly improved over recent years. Among the most significant evolution are the more wide-spread use of stereotactic ablative body radiation (SABR) for stage I NSCLC, concurrent chemo-radiation for stage III NSCLC, the timing of chest radiotherapy for LD SCLC and PCI for ED-SCLC, which all contributed to the better survival of patients with lung cancer. The respiration correlated 4D CT treatment planning and image-guided techniques, like cone beam CT scanning, open a completely new episode of high geometrical precision radiotherapy.

REFERENCES

1. Siegel R, Ward E, Brawley O, Jemal A. Cancer statistics, 2011: The impact of eliminating socioeconomic and racial disparities on premature cancer deaths. CA Cancer J Clin 2011; 61: 212–36.
2. Rubin P, Brasacchio R, Katz A. Solitary metastases: illusion versus reality. Semin Radiat Oncol 2006; 16: 120–30.
3. Timmerman R, Paulus R, Galvin J, et al. Stereotactic body radiation therapy for inoperable early stage lung cancer. JAMA 2010; 303: 1070–6.
4. Lagerwaard FJ, Haasbeek CJ, Smit EF, et al. Outcomes of risk-adapted fractionated stereotactic radiotherapy for stage I non-small-cell lung cancer. Int J Radiat Oncol Biol Phys 2008; 70: 685–92.
5. Henderson M, McGarry R, Yiannoutsos C, et al. Baseline pulmonary function as a predictor for survival and decline in pulmonary function over time in patients undergoing stereotactic body radiotherapy for the treatment of stage I non-small-cell lung cancer. Int J Radiat Oncol Biol Phys 2008; 72: 404–9.
6. Palma D, Visser O, Lagerwaard FJ, et al. Impact of introducing stereotactic lung radiotherapy for elderly patients with stage I non-small-cell lung cancer: a population-based time-trend analysis. J Clin Oncol 2010; 28: 5153–9.
7. Hoopes DJ, Tann M, Fletcher JW, et al. FDG-PET and stereotactic ablative body radiation (SABR) for stage I non-small-cell lung cancer. Lung Cancer 2007; 56: 229–34.
8. Dahele M, Palma D, Lagerwaard F, et al. Radiological changes after stereotactic radiotherapy for stage I lung cancer. J Thorac Oncol 2011; 6: 1221–8.
9. Non-small Cell Lung Cancer Collaborative Group. Chemotherapy in non-small cell lung cancer: a meta-analysis using updated data on individual patients from 52 randomised clinical trials. Br Med J 1995; 311: 899–909.

10. Aupérin A, Le Péchoux C, Rolland E, et al. Meta-analysis of concomitant versus sequential radiochemotherapy in locally advanced non-small-cell lung cancer. J Clin Oncol 2010; 28: 2181–90.

11. Albain KS, Swann RS, Rusch VW, et al. Radiotherapy plus chemotherapy with or without surgical resection for stage III non-small-cell lung cancer: a phase III randomised controlled trial. Lancet 2009; 374: 379–86.

12. van Meerbeeck JP, Kramer GW, Van Schil PE, et al. European Organisation for Research and Treatment of Cancer-Lung Cancer Group. Randomized controlled trial of resection versus radiotherapy after induction chemotherapy in stage IIIA-N2 non-small-cell lung cancer. J Natl Cancer Inst 2007; 99: 442–50.

13. Vansteenkiste J, Betticher D, Eberhardt W, et al. Randomized controlled trial of resection versus radiotherapy after induction chemotherapy in stage IIIA-N2 non-small cell lung cancer. J Thorac Oncol 2007; 2: 684–5.

14. Albain KS, Rusch VW, Crowley JJ, et al. Concurrent cisplatin/etoposide plus chest radiotherapy followed by surgery for stages IIIA (N2) and IIIB non-small-cell lung cancer: mature results of Southwest Oncology Group phase II study 8805. J Clin Oncol 1995; 13: 1880–92.

15. Pöttgen C, Eberhardt W, Bildat S, et al. Induction chemotherapy followed by concurrent chemotherapy and definitive high-dose radiotherapy for patients with locally advanced non-small-cell lung cancer (stages IIIa/IIIb): a pilot phase I/II trial. Ann Oncol 2002; 13: 403–11.

16. Lorent N, De Leyn P, Lievens Y, et al.; Leuven Lung Cancer Group. Long-term survival of surgically staged IIIA-N2 non-small-cell lung cancer treated with surgical combined modality approach: analysis of a 7-year prospective experience. Ann Oncol 2004; 15: 1645–53.

17. Betticher DC, Hsu Schmitz SF, Tötsch M, et al.; Swiss Group for Clinical Cancer Research (SAKK). Prognostic factors affecting long-term outcomes in patients with resected stage IIIA pN2 non-small-cell lung cancer: 5-year follow-up of a phase II study. Br J Cancer 2006; 94: 1099–106.

18. Garrido P, González-Larriba JL, Insa A, et al. Long-term survival associated with complete resection after induction chemotherapy in stage IIIA (N2) and IIIB (T4N0-1) non small-cell lung cancer patients: the Spanish Lung Cancer Group Trial 9901. J Clin Oncol 2007; 25: 4736–42.

19. Machtay M, Hsu C, Komaki R, et al. Effect of overall treatment time on outcomes after concurrent chemoradiation for locally advanced non-small-cell lung carcinoma: analysis of the Radiation Therapy Oncology Group (RTOG) experience. Int J Radiat Oncol Biol Phys 2005; 63: 667–71.

20. Machtay M, Bae K, Movsas B, et al. Higher biologically effective dose of radiotherapy is associated with improved outcomes for locally advanced non-small cell lung carcinoma treated with chemoradiation: an analysis of the Radiation Therapy Oncology Group. Int J Radiat Oncol Biol Phys 2012; 82: 425–34.

21. De Ruysscher D, Botterweck A, Dirx M, et al. Eligibility for concurrent chemotherapy and radiotherapy of locally advanced lung cancer patients: a prospective, population-based study. Ann Oncol 2008; 20: 98–102.

22. De Ruysscher D, Khoo V, Bentzen SM. Biological basis of fractionation and timing of radiotherapy. In: Harvey I, Pass MD, David P, Carbone MD, David H, Johnson MD, John D, Minna MD, Andrew T, Turrisi MD, Giorgio V, Scagliotti MD. eds Lung Cancer: Principles and Practice. 4th edn. Philadelphia, USA: Lippincott Williams & Wilkins, 2009.

23. Saunders M, Dische S, Barrett A, et al. Continuous, hyperfractionated, accelerated radiotherapy (CHART) versus conventional radiotherapy in non-small cell lung cancer: mature data from the randomised multicentre trial. CHART Steering committee. Radiother Oncol 1999; 52: 137–48.

24. Belani CP, Wang W, Johnson DH, et al. Eastern Cooperative Oncology Group. Phase III study of the Eastern Cooperative Oncology Group (ECOG 2597): Induction chemotherapy followed by either standard thoracic radiotherapy or hyperfractionated accelerated radiotherapy for patients with unresectable stage IIIA and B non-small-cell lung cancer. J Clin Oncol 2005; 23: 3760–7.

25. Jenkins P, Anderson S, Wronski S, Ashton A. A phase II trial of induction chemotherapy followed by continuous hyperfractionated accelerated radiotherapy in locally advanced non-small-cell lung cancer. Radiother Oncol 2009; 93: 396–401.

26. Baumann M, Herrmann T, Koch R, et al. On behalf of the CHARTWEL-Bronchus Study Group. Final results of the randomized phase III CHARTWEL-trial (ARO 97–1) comparing hyperfractionated-accelerated versus conventionally fractionated radiotherapy in. non-small cell lung cancer (NSCLC). Radiother Oncol 2011; 100: 76–85.

27. Stuschke M, Pottgen C. Altered fractionation schemes in radiotherapy. Front Radiat Ther Oncol 2010; 42: 150–6.

28. van Baardwijk A, Bosmans G, Bentzen SM, et al. Radiation dose prescription for non-small-cell lung cancer according to normal tissue dose constraints: an in silico clinical trial. Int J Radiat Oncol Biol Phys 2008; 71: 1103–10.

29. van Baardwijk A, Wanders S, Boersma L, et al. Mature results of an individualized radiation dose prescription study based on normal tissue constraints in stages I to III non-small-cell lung cancer. J Clin Oncol 2010; 28: 1380–6.

30. van Baardwijk A, Wanders R, Reymen B, et al. First Results of a Phase II Trial Investigating Individualized Dose-escalation Based on Normal Tissue Constraints in Concurrent Chemo-radiation for Locally Advanced Non-small Cell Lung Cancer (NSCLC) (NCT00572325). Int J Radiat Oncol Biol Phys 2010; 78: S108.

31. Kong FM, Ao X, Wang L, Lawrence TS. The use of blood biomarkers to predict radiation lung toxicity: a potential strategy to individualize thoracic radiation therapy. Cancer Control 2008; 15: 140–50.

32. De Ruysscher D, Houben A, Aerts HJ, et al. Increased (18)F-deoxyglucose uptake in the lung during the first weeks of radiotherapy is correlated with subsequent radiation-induced lung toxicity (RILT): a prospective pilot study. Radiother Oncol 2009; 91: 415–20.

33. Hamill JJ, Bosmans G, Dekker A. Respiratory-gated CT as a tool for the simulation of breathing artifacts in PET and PET/CT. Med Phys 2008; 35: 576–85.

34. Keall P. Four-dimensional computed tomography imaging and treatment planning. Semin Radiat Oncol 2004; 14: 81–90.

35. Underberg RW, Lagerwaard FJ, Slotman BJ, Cuijpers JP, Senan S. Benefit of respiration-gated stereotactic radiotherapy for stage I lung cancer: an analysis of 4DCT datasets. Int J Radiat Oncol Biol Phys 2005; 62: 554–60.

36. Bosmans G, van Baardwijk A, Dekker A, et al. Time trends in nodal volumes and motion during radiotherapy for patients with stage III non-small-cell lung cancer. Int J Radiat Oncol Biol Phys 2008; 71: 139–44.

37. Nestle U, Kremp S, Grosu AL. Practical integration of [18F]-FDG-PET and PET-CT in the planning of radiotherapy for non-small cell lung cancer (NSCLC): the technical basis, ICRU-target volumes, problems, perspectives. Radiother Oncol 2006; 81: 209–25.

38. van Der Wel A, Nijsten S, Hochstenbag M, et al. Increased therapeutic ratio by 18FDG-PET CT planning in patients with clinical CT stage N2-N3M0 non-small-cell lung cancer: a modeling study. Int J Radiat Oncol Biol Phys 2005; 61: 649–55.

39. De Ruysscher D, Wanders S, van Haren E, et al. Selective mediastinal node irradiation based on FDG-PET scan data in patients with non-small-cell lung cancer: a prospective clinical study. Int J Radiat Oncol Biol Phys 2005; 62: 988–94.

40. Belderbos JS, Heemsbergen WD, De Jaeger K, Baas P, Lebesque JV. Final results of a Phase I/II dose escalation trial in non-small-cell lung cancer using three-dimensional conformal radiotherapy. Int J Radiat Oncol Biol Phys 2006; 66: 126–34.

41. Steenbakkers RJ, Duppen JC, Fitton I, et al. Observer variation in target volume delineation of lung cancer related to radiation oncologist-computer interaction: a 'Big Brother' evaluation. Radiother Oncol 2005; 77: 182–90.

42. van Baardwijk A, Bosmans G, Boersma L, et al. PET-CT-based auto-contouring in non-small-cell lung cancer correlates with pathology and reduces interobserver variability in the delineation of the primary tumor and involved nodal volumes. Int J Radiat Oncol Biol Phys 2007; 68: 771–8.

43. Aerts HJ, Bosmans G, van Baardwijk AA, et al. Stability of (18)F-deoxyglucose uptake locations within tumor during radiotherapy for nsclc: a prospective study. Int J Radiat Oncol Biol Phys 2008; 71: 1402–7.

44. Aerts HJ, van Baardwijk AA, Petit SF, et al. Identification of residual metabolic-active areas within individual NSCLC tumours using a pre-radiotherapy (18)Fluorodeoxyglucose-PET-CT scan. Radiother Oncol 2009; 91: 386–92.

45. Cui Y, Dy JG, Sharp GC, Alexander B, Jiang SB. Robust fluoroscopic respiratory gating for lung cancer radiotherapy without implanted fiducial markers. Phys Med Biol 2007; 52: 741–55.

46. Keall PJ, Todor AD, Vedam SS, et al. "On the use of EPID-based implanted marker tracking for 4D radiotherapy". Med Phys 2004; 31: 3492–9.

47. Mageras GS, Yorke E. Deep inspiration breath hold and respiratory gating strategies for reducing organ motion in radiation treatment. Semin Radiat Oncol 2004; 14: 65–75.

48. Keall PJ, Joshi S, Vedam SS. Four-dimensional radiotherapy planning for DMLC-based respiratory motion tracking. Med Phys 2005; 32: 942–51.

49. Wolthaus JW, Schneider C, Sonke JJ. Mid-ventilation CT scan construction from four-dimensional respiration-correlated CT scans for radiotherapy planning of lung cancer patients. Int J Radiat Oncol Biol Phys 2006; 65: 1560–71.

50. Grills IS, Yan D. Martinez AA. otential for reduced toxicity and dose escalation in the treatment of inoperable non-small-cell lung cancer: a comparison of intensity-modulated radiation therapy (IMRT), 3D conformal radiation, and elective nodal irradiation. Int J Radiat Oncol Biol Phys 2003; 7: 75–890.

51. Schwarz M, Alber M, Lebesque JV. Dose heterogeneity in the target volume and intensity-modulated radiotherapy to escalate the dose in the treatment of non-small-cell lung cancer. Int J Radiat Oncol Biol Phys 2005; 62: 561–70.

52. Berbeco RI, Hacker F, Ionascu D, amon HJ. Clinical feasibility of using an EPID in CINE mode for image-guided verification of stereotactic body radiotherapy. Int J Radiat Oncol Biol Phys 2007; 9: 258–66.

53. Sonke JJ, Zijp L, Remeijer P, van Herk M. Respiratory correlated cone beam CT. Med Phys 2005; 2: 176–1186.

54. Cho B, Suh Y, Dieterich S, Keall PJ. A monoscopic method for real-time tumour tracking using combined occasional x-ray imaging and continuous respiratory monitoring. Phys Med Biol 2008; 3: 837–2855.

55. Purdie TG, Bissonnette J-P, Franks K, et al. Cone-beam computed tomography for on-line image guidance of lung stereotactic radiotherapy: localization, verification, and intrafractiontumor position. Int J Radiat Oncol Biol Phys 2007; 8: 43–252.

56. Sonke JJ, Lebesque J, van Herk M. Variability of four-dimensional computed tomography patient models. Int J Radiat Oncol Biol Phys 2008; 0: 90–598.

57. Schaake E, Belderbos J, Rit S, et al. Detailed analysis of tumor regression during radical radiotherapy in lung cancer patients. J Thorac Oncol 2011; 6: 430–1.

58. Fried DB, Morris DE, Poole C, et al. Systematic review evaluating the timing of thoracic radiation therapy in combined modality therapy for limited-stage small-cell lung cancer. J Clin Oncol 2004; 22: 4837–45; Review. Erratum in: J Clin Oncol 2005; 3: 48.

59. Pijls-Johannesma M, De Ruysscher D, Vansteenkiste J, et al. Timing of chest radiotherapy in patients with limited stage small cell lung cancer: a systematic review and meta-analysis of randomised controlled trials. Cancer Treat Rev 2007; 3: 61–473.

60. Turrisi AT 3rd, Kim K, Blum R, et al. Twice-daily compared with once-daily thoracic radiotherapy in limited small-cell lung cancer treated concurrently with cisplatin and etoposide. N Engl J Med 1999; 40: 265–371.

61. De Ruysscher D, Pijls-Johannesma M, Bentzen SM, et al. Time between the first day of chemotherapy and the last day of chest radiation is the most important predictor of survival in limited-disease small-cell lung cancer. J Clin Oncol 2006; 4: 057–1063.
62. De Ruysscher D, Bremer RH, Koppe F, et al. Omission of elective node irradiation on basis of CT-scans in patients with limited disease small cell lung cancer: a phase II trial. Radiother Oncol 2006; 80: 307–12.
63. van Loon J, De Ruysscher D, Wanders R, et al. Selective nodal irradiation on basis of [18]FDG-PET scans in limited disease small cell lung cancer: a phase II trial. Int J Radiat Oncol Biol Phys 2010; 7: 29–36.
64. Shirvani SM, Komaki R, Heymach JV, Fossella FV, Chang JY. Positron emission tomography/computed tomography-guided intensity-modulated radiotherapy for limited-stage small-cell lung cancer. Int J Radiat Oncol Biol Phys 2012; 82: e91–7.
65. Slotman B, Faivre-Finn C, Kramer G, et al. ORTC Radiation Oncology Group and Lung Cancer Group. Prophylactic cranial irradiation in extensive small-cell lung cancer. N Engl J Med 2007; 57: 64–72.

12 | Treatment of small cell lung cancer

Aleksandar Aleksic and Sanjay Popat

INTRODUCTION

Lung cancer is the most common cause of cancer-related deaths in Europe, accounting for 334,800 individuals dying from the disease in 2006. Small cell lung cancer (SCLC) accounts for 15–18% of prevalent cases, and is strongly associated with smoking. While increased public awareness of harmful effects of smoking has resulted in a decreased lung cancer-specific mortality in the Western world, and a likely future fall in incidence due to successful smoking cessation programs, smoking is an increasing problem in Asia, and will still result in a significant number of patients in years to come. The SCLC incidence in the United States between 1973 and 2000 decreased due to fewer smokers and the use of low-tar filter cigarettes. However, only a modest improvement in survival has been observed in the last 30 years.[1]

SEVENTH EDITION OF THE UICC STAGING SYSTEM

SCLC has previously traditionally been staged according to the Veterans' affairs system into limited and extensive stage contingent on the ability to deliver radical thoracic radiotherapy (TRT). The fifth edition of the International Association for the Study of Lung Cancer (IASLC) lung cancer staging system, previously described limited-stage SCLC (LS-SCLC) as "disease restricted to one hemithorax with regional lymph node metastases, including hilar, ipsilateral and contralateral mediastinal, and ipsilateral and contralateral supraclavicular nodes and should also include patients with ipsilateral pleural effusion independent of whether cytology is positive or negative," with disease not fulfilling this criteria defined as extensive-stage SCLC (ES-SCLC). This classification was published in 1997 and remained unaltered for the sixth edition in 2002, which was based on outcomes of 5319 North American lung cancer patients, the majority of whom had non-small cell lung cancer (NSCLC) and underwent surgery between 1975 and 1988.

The current IASLC seventh revision of tumor classification has now been adopted by the UICC and is based on a more comprehensive dataset including 45 different international databases with 100,869 lung cancer patients treated from 1990 to 2000, from more than 20 countries in Asia, Australia, Europe, and North America.[2] Of the 81,015 patients that fulfilled the inclusion criteria for analysis of survival outcomes by the extent of disease, 13,290 had SCLC, and of these 8,088 were TNM classified: clinical TNM (cTNM)—3125 patients, pathological TNM (pTNM)—128 patients, both cTNM and pTNM—215 patients and clinical M1—4,530 patients. Stratifiers of T, N, and M descriptors previously identified from the IASLC version 7 NSCLC staging test dataset were investigated in SCLC and found to be robust, with a clear correlation between disease stage grouping and five-year survival (Table 12.1).[3] Analysis of the N component (independent of T) showed that N0 and N1 had similar survival that was improved over N2 and N3. This TNM stratification allowed grouping into clinical stages: IA with five-year survival of 38%, IB 21%, IIA 38% (this group had small number of patients), IIB 18%, IIIA 13%, IIIB 9%, and IV 1%. Data on patients presenting with pleural effusion were limited, but indicated a worse prognosis with survival rate intermediate between LS and ES-SCLC.

Similar observations of survival were reported by Ignatius Ou and colleagues in a review of outcomes of 10,660 SCLC patients from the California Cancer Registry between 1991 and 2005, confirming that patients with N0–N1 had better survival rate than patients with mediastinal lymph node involvement.[4]

TREATMENT OF LS-SCLC
Chemotherapy

Since publication of *Lung Cancer Therapy Annual 6*, there have been minimal updates to the recommendations for the management of SCLC (Table 12.2). The current 2010 European Society for Medical Oncology (ESMO) recommendation is that the UICC version 7 staging system for NSCLC be applied to SCLC staging, and that the Veterans system is no longer used. For first-line treatment in LD-SCLC, patients should be treated with both etoposide and a platinum-based agent (preferably etoposide/cisplatin), in combination with TRT. Radiotherapy should be administered early and concurrently. The total dose and radiation fractionation regime is not agreed, but may range from 45 Gy twice daily to 55–70 Gy once daily. Surgical resection can be

Table 12.1 Survival Analysis of Patients with Small Cell Lung Cancer Based on T and N Component

T component with any N category	5-Year survival (%)	N component with any T Category	5-Year survival (%)
T1	29	N0	24
T2	15	N1	20
T3	11	N2	12
T4	10	N3	9

Table 12.2 Current Guidelines for Limited Stage-Small Cell Lung Cancer Treatment

	ACCP	ESMO	NCCN	NICE
Publication year	2007	2010	2010	2011
First line	Cisplatin/etoposide Altenative: CAV Carboplatin/etoposide	Platinum/etoposide	Platinum/etoposide	Platinum/etoposide
Thoracic radiotherapy	Accelerated hyperfractionated concurrent with platinum-based chemotherapy	Early, concurrent with platinum-based chemo. Optimal dose is still to be established	Early, concurrent	1. Concurrent 2. Sequential Early (with 1st or 2nd cycle) (2011 update).
PCI	Complete remission or patients with stage I disease who have had resection	Any response to first-line chemotherapy irrespective of stage	25 Gy in 10 fractions or 30 Gy in 10–15 fractions	25 Gy in 10 fractions, PS of 2 or less, No disease progression

Abbreviations: ACCP, American College of Chest Physicians; ESMO, European Society for Medical Oncology; NCCN, National Comprehensive Cancer Network; NICE, National Institute of Clinical Excellence.

considered for T0–1, N0 patients after confirmatory mediastinal pathological staging, after which adjuvant chemotherapy and prophylactic cranial irradiation (PCI) is recommended, and adjuvant radiotherapy considered for N1 and unforeseen N2 disease. The updated 2011 UK National Institute of Clinical Excellence (NICE) guidelines recommended concurrent thoracic irradiation with the first or second cycle of chemotherapy in good performance status patients, or sequentially after completion of chemotherapy if there has been a response. NICE 2011, however, does not recommend surgery for node-positive SCLC.

The general principles and changing trends of delivering therapy in SCLC were described in a recent Dutch study.[5] The authors retrospectively analyzed Netherlands Cancer Registry data on patient trends in delivering treatments, defined as chemoradiation, chemotherapy, or best supportive care only (CTRT, CT, BSC) from 1997–2004 to 2005–2007. This study of 13,007 SCLC patients demonstrated that more CT was delivered in 2005–2007 than in 1997–2004 across all age groups other than those ≥80 years, which translated to an increase in one-year survival for those with LS-SCLC from 40% in 1997–2004 to 51% in 2005–2007 ($p < 0.05$), but this improvement was only seen among those <80 years. In addition, while more CT was delivered in 2005–2007 compared to 1997, older patients were less likely to receive CT (only 15% of ≥80-year-old patients received therapy).

Chemoradiation

Unfortunately, since the landmark trial of concurrent CTRT in LS-SCLC- (SWOG S8269),[6] median overall survival (OS) has not significantly changed in further SWOG trials by modifying systemic therapy (results borne out by other trials). Targeting hypoxic tumor cells in addition to standard CTRT using tirapazamine (TPZ, a benzotriazine di-N-oxide with selective cytotoxicity for hypoxic cells), initially held promise with the results of SWOG 0004 (a phase I study of TPZ) demonstrating tolerability and promising activity of concurrently administered TPZ with once daily RT and cisplatin–etoposide (PE) chemotherapy, with median OS of 22 versus 17 months reported in S9713 (a trial of carboplatin-paclitaxel consolidation).[7,8] However, this was not validated in the subsequent phase II study of this agent (SWOG 0222).[9] Here, eligible patients were treated with PE (cisplatin 50 mg/m^2/day on days 1, 8, 29, and 36 and etoposide 50 mg/m^2/day IV days 1–5 and 29–33) with concurrent once-daily RT. Additionally, 260 mg/m^2 of TPZ was given on days 1 and 29, and 160 mg/m^2 on days 8, 10, 12, 36, 38, and 40 (1–3 hours before TRT). Patients received TRT once daily for 6.5 weeks to 45 Gy at 1.8 Gy/fraction/day and 16 Gy boost was delivered in eight fractions of 2 Gy daily to the gross target volume (GTV). Patients with stable and responding disease were offered consolidation CT consisting of cisplatin 60 mg/m^2 on day 1 and etoposide 120 mg/m^2 on days 1–3 of weeks 11 and 14. Finally patients who had complete response after consolidation CT also had PCI. Unfortunately S0222 was closed early due to excess observed toxicity for TPZ in a head and neck cancer trial reported elsewhere. Of the 68 assessable patients, investigators reported 25% grade 3–4 esophagitis, and 12% grade 3 febrile neutropenia. With a median follow-up of 35 months, median progression-free survival (PFS) was 11 months and median OS was 21 months.

The role of radical treatment in SCLC presenting with pleural effusion has long been debated. In a Japanese dataset, Niho et al. retrospectively investigated outcomes of 373 LS-SCLC patients from a single institution, 17% of whom presented with ipsilateral pleural effusion (62 patients).[10] Standard of care at their institution from 1998 was to offer radical TRT in patients with disappearance of effusion after CT. They reported outcomes in these 62 patients receiving induction CT. These patients were subsequently divided into three groups: group A received CT and TRT (26 patients), group B did not receive TRT after disappearance of pleural effusion following first-line chemotherapy (8 patients), and group C were only treated with CT and whose pleural effusion was present after first-line chemotherapy (28 patients). Of 62 patients in 34 (55%) pleural effusion fully disappeared after induction chemotherapy, and overall, median OS was 11.8 months, two-year survival 21%, and three-year survival 10%. However, significant differences in efficacy were observed in patients receiving TRT compared with those devoid of TRT (groups A, B, and C; median OS 19.2, 10.5, and 9.2 months, respectively; two-year survival rates 38%, 25%, and 7%, respectively), suggesting a possible benefit to radical TRT in this group of patients.

Radiotherapy

Early concurrent TRT with chemotherapy is standard of care in LS-SCLC for good performance status patients. However, overall outcomes still remain poor, and several trials have reported different RT regimens in isolation of CT, in order to optimally determine the effect of RT.

One such strategy has been to increase total dose of radiotherapy. RTOG 97–12, was a phase I trial evaluating increasing doses of concomitant CRT, with large field TRT given initially at 1.8 Gy/fraction once daily, five days a week, followed by 14.4 Gy (1.8 Gy/fraction twice daily boost) during the last three treatment days to a total dose of 50.4 Gy ranging to 64.6 Gy. Maximum tolerated dose (MTD) was defined as grade 3–4 toxicity observed in >50% of patients. Komaki and colleagues identified a MTD of 61.2 Gy with a 68% complete response rate, translating to an 18-month survival rate of 25% for 50.4 Gy and 82% for 61.2 Gy.[11] Despite this promising efficacy, toxicities were marked.

However, one possible option for escalating radiation doses without increasing toxicity is to diminish radiation fields by omitting routine elective nodal irradiation (ENI) of the mediastinum using positron emission tomography/computed tomography (PET/CT).[12] A retrospective analysis reported outcomes from a single U.S. center, 60 patients staged PET/CT that had received intensity-modulated radiotherapy (IMRT) in which ENI was intentionally omitted from the planning target volume (median 45 Gy in 30 fractions; range 40.5 Gy in 27 fractions to 63.8 Gy in 35 fractions and concurrent platinum-based chemotherapy). Here, 94% of patients had nodal disease at the time of treatment, and approximately one-third of patients had N3 involvement. Outcomes were a two-year OS and relapse-free survival (RFS) rate of 58% and 43%, respectively, with only one elective nodal failure (defined as recurrence in initially uninvolved hilar, mediastinal, or supraclavicular nodes), and toxicities of 23% grade 3 esophagitis and 7% pneumonitis.

This low rate of relapse was prospectively validated in a study of 60 patients receiving 45 Gy in twice-daily fractions reported by van Loon et al. Here, only the primary tumor and the mediastinal lymph nodes, involved on the pre-treatment PET scan, were irradiated to a dose of 45 Gy in twice-daily fractions of 1.5 Gy. A difference in the involved nodal stations seen on the pre-treatment PET/CT scan and CT scan was observed in 30% of patients. Of the 60 patients, 39 developed recurrence, with 2 experiencing isolated regional failure (3%), and overall, grade 3 esophagitis rate was 11%.[13] These results therefore support the use of PET/CT in planning TRT over that of invasively pathologically staging the mediastinum.

Surgery

Historically, while surgery was the initial treatment for SCLC, the poor survival reported by the Medical Research Council trial in the 1960s demonstrated superiority for radical radiotherapy over surgery (199 days compared to 300 days mean survival for surgery vs. radical radiotherapy).[14] No trials of surgery have ever been performed, particularly in the modern era, and the evidence base is predominantly limited to retro-spective single-institutional series. While surgery is not recommended as routine for patients with LS-SCLC, it may be acceptable for patients with very limited stage disease. Indeed, the NCCN does recommend surgery followed by adjuvant chemotherapy as standard management for T1-T2N0 disease, with chemoradiation as standard treatment for all other stages (excluding M1). Lim et al. retrospectively reviewed patients who underwent surgery at their institution between 1980 and 2006.[15] Fifty-nine patients, staged according to UICC version 6 staging, underwent complete resection with systematic nodal dissection. Of those, 53 had clinical staging information available: IA (9), IB (21), IIA (0), IIB (13), IIIA (9), and IIIB (1). This study showed excellent survival figures; the median time to follow-up was 2.8 years and one-year OS was 76%, with five-year OS of 52%. This is one of several recent reviews that highlight the potential role of surgery as primary treatment and use of clinical TNM criteria in the selection of patients with LS-SCLC.

Another U.S. study reviewed clinical outcomes after surgery for stage 1 SCLC through analysis of the National Cancer Institute (NCI) Surveillance Epidemiology and End Results (SEER) database.[16] It was assumed that all patients received systemic treatment, as SEER does not provide systemic therapy details. A total of 1,560 patients were identified with stage 1 SCLC (median age 70, range 27–94 years). Of these, 247 were treated with lobectomy, 121 with local tumor excision/ablation, pneumonectomy,[10] and 21 with unde-fined procedure. The remaining 1,161 patients did not have any cancer-directed surgery. Of 247 patients who underwent lobectomy, 205 (83%) did not receive RT, 38 (15%) did receive RT, and use of RT was unknown in 4 (2%). The authors concluded that surgery without RT offered reasonable OS outcomes, reporting three- and five-year OS in those who had lobectomy without RT of 58.1% and 50.3%, respectively; whereas those received RT had three- and five-year OS of 64.9% and 57.1%, respectively.

SEER data were additionally analyzed by Schreiber et al. who identified 14,179 patients with LS-SCLC diagnosed between 1988 and 2002 and coded as localized disease (T1-T2, Nx-N0) or regional disease (either T3-T4, Nx-N0 or T1-T4, N1-N2).[17] Of those, 863 patients (6.1%) underwent surgical resection that was associated more commonly with T1/T2 disease (p < 0.001). Median survival of the whole cohort was 28 months in the surgery group and 13 months in no-surgery group, with an improved survival reported for both localized and regional disease (median survival improved from 15 to 42 months, p < 0.001, and 12 to 22 months, p < 0.001, respectively, for surgery vs. no surgery). Patients with localized disease who underwent lobectomy had a median survival of 65 months and a five-year OS rate of 52.6%, whereas patients who had regional disease had a median survival of 25 months and a five-year OS rate of 31.8%. Subgroup analysis, performed to assess surgical outcomes based on N status, demonstrated that patients with N0 disease that underwent surgery had better median survival (40 vs. 15 months) than without surgery (p < 0.001). A simi-lar benefit was seen in N1 disease (29 vs. 14 months, p < 0.001) and N2 disease (19 vs. 12 months, p < 0.001).

In addition, the role of postoperative radiotherapy (PORT) was investigated. As expected, the majority of patients treated with PORT had regional disease (72.2%), but median survival was better after surgery alone than with additional radiotherapy in the entire group. Subset analysis on lymph node status demonstrated that while N0/N1 disease did not benefit from PORT, patients with N2 disease did markedly benefit (16 months, surgery alone vs. 22 months, PORT, p = 0.011). Naturally, this study has several limitations, including lack of data on delivered chemotherapy, and its impact. However, it does suggest a strong benefit for surgery and that in more locally advanced disease a strategy using all three modalities of treatment might be optimal.

Finally, Tashi et al. reported retrospective analysis of the Veterans Affairs Central Cancer Registry (VACCR) identifying 915 patients who had surgery alone out of 8,791 patients diagnosed with LS-SCLC between 1995 and 2008.[18] Patients with stage 1–3 SCLC were treated mostly with lobectomy and systematic LN dissection (46.3%) followed by local excision, simple lobectomy, and pneumonectomy (21.1%, 20.5%, and 6.9%, respec-tively). The median survival in stage 1 was 45.9 months for surgical versus 15.9 months for non-surgical treat-ment, in stage 2 median survival was 39.4 versus 13.7 months, and in stage 3 it was 21.8 versus 11.5 months (p < 0.0001). There was a significant survival benefit if CTRT was administered after surgery (30.9 vs. 14.7 months, p < 0.0001). Furthermore, there is a survival advantage for surgery per se (38.7 months compared to 12.4 months in the non-surgical group, p < 0.0001).

Thus, the evidence from individual centers and registry data does tend to suggest improved outcomes for LS-SCLC treated by surgery, although this will ideally need to be prospectively confirmed in a clinical trial. However, feasibility of such a trial is a critical factor, and remains questionable.

Prophylactic Cranial Irradiation

The optimal radiotherapy regime for PCI has been investigated by Le Péchoux et al. who reported the results of a large, international phase III trial of PCI, comparing 25 Gy once a day versus 36 Gy once or twice a day in patients with SCLC in complete remission.[19] This study of 720 patients demonstrated no difference in the total incidence of brain metastases between groups: 29% and 23%, respectively. While two-year overall survival was 42% in 25 Gy group versus 37% in 36 Gy group, these excess deaths were not due to brain metastases. Common toxicities reported included fatigue (most commonly reported, 30% vs. 34%, respectively) followed by headache (24% vs. 28%, respectively) and nausea and vomiting (23% vs. 28%, respectively). Further analyses of difference in mid-term and long-term neurocognitive functions and quality of life (QoL) were evaluated and recently reported.[20] Here, these outcomes were shown to be similar in both groups, with a mild communication deficit, weakness of legs, intellectual and memory deficits (all p < 0.005) observed in both groups. Further analysis of this trial[21] demonstrated that 12 months after PCI patients in the 36 Gy arm had a significant deterioration in neurocognitive function (p = 0.02), and therefore 25 Gy has been recommended as the standard of care in this setting.

TREATMENT OF ES-SCLC
First-Line Therapy
Platinum-based chemotherapy is the cornerstone of management in extensive stage (ES-) SCLC. The optimum platinum agent has been extensively investigated, with, four phase III trials comparing efficacy of each of these agents demonstrating no significant difference in anti-tumor activity[22–25] and the recently presented COCIS individual patient data meta-analysis confirming this. Here, the median OS was 9.5 months for both drugs.[26] However, since only 363 patients (from Greek and Japanese trials) actually had the same combination of chemotherapy (carboplatin/cisplatin with etoposide) in COCIS, power to demonstrate a moderate-small effect has been questioned.

Over recent years there have been considerable efforts to improve on the efficacy of platinum–etoposide, by either adding targeted therapy to standard chemotherapy, or modifying the cytotoxic chemotherapy backbone with a novel cytotoxic. These trials are reviewed in the following section.

Targeted Therapy
The efficacy and safety of bevacizumab when added to cisplatin and etoposide were investigated in a single-arm phase II trial (ECOG3501)[27] and concurrently investigated potential predictive biomarkers, including changes from baseline vascular endothelial growth factor (VEGF), soluble cell adhesion molecules (i.e., VCAM, ICAM, and E-selectin), and basic fibroblast growth factor (bFGF). Sixty-three patients with previously untreated ES-SCLC were treated. Median PFS was 4.7 months and OS 10.9 months, potentially improved compared with historical controls. Similar to other trials of bevacizumab, no biomarker was identified, although high baseline VCAM was associated with a significantly higher risk of progression or death.

Bevacizumab in addition to combination irinotecan and carboplatin was further investigated in a single-arm phase II trial, and demonstrated promising efficacy: objective response rate (ORR) 84%, median OS 12.1 months, one- and two-year OS were 51 and 14%, respectively. No new safety concerns were identified.[28] Subsequently a double blind, randomized, placebo-controlled phase II study of bevacizumab in combination with chemotherapy in previously untreated patients with ES-SCLC (SALUTE trial) was reported.[29] Here, 102 patients were randomized to cisplatin or carboplatin with etoposide and bevacizumab (BV) or the same chemotherapy with placebo. However, despite improved median PFS (5.5 months for BV vs. 4.4 months for placebo), and improved ORR, similar median OS was observed for both groups (9.4 months for BV vs. 10.9 months for placebo). Outcomes did, however, vary by platinum use, with an improved PFS for carboplatin versus cisplatin in combination with bevacizumab (HR 0.82, 0.41–1.64), and benefit from BV for OS also (HR = 1.99 for cisplatin vs. 0.82 for carboplatin).

Given the neuroendocrine pathobiology of SCLC and the in vitro evidence of efficacy of sunitinib against neuroendocrine tumors, the role of sunitinib has been investigated further in SCLC. A trial of sunitinib, as maintenance treatment, was reported by Schneider and colleagues.[30] In a small, single arm, exploratory phase II study, 16 non-progressing patients after at least four cycles of PE were offered sunitinib. Unfortunately no objective responses were observed, and drug was discontinued in up to half of the patients due to toxicities or patients' request. A further Korean small open label single-arm phase II trial in relapsed or refractory SCLC was presented at ASCO 2011,[31] demonstrating minimal efficacy, with an ORR of 9% which was below the pre-specified threshold for full accrual, resulting in premature closure. While two responses were observed in sensitive patients, most patients did not tolerate therapy. Another trial of sunitinib in ES-SCLC as either first or subsequent lines has been performed by the European Organization for Research and Treatment of Cancer (EORTC). Unfortunately, this trial also closed after poor accrual.

Chemotherapy

Several studies investigated the role of pemetrexed in treatment of SCLC in past few years but most have shown minimal activity.[32–35] One of the first encouraging results came from a small randomized phase II trial of combination pemetrexed, with either carboplatin or cisplatin that demonstrated median OS of 10.4 months, which compared favorably to 7.6 months for cisplatin/pemetrexed.[36] These early studies led to the GALES (Global Analysis of Pemetrexed in SCLC Extensive Stage) trial, a phase III, randomized, non-inferiority trial comparing pemetrexed and carboplatin (PC) with etoposide and carboplatin (EC) in chemotherapy-naïve patients with ES-SCLC.[37] Unfortunately, this study was closed following protocol-specified interim analysis demonstrating significantly lower PFS in PC arm. The final analysis confirmed inferiority of this treatment arm: OS 8.1 versus 10.6 months, and PFS 3.8 versus 5.4 months. Evidence from preclinical studies now demonstrates that due to over-expression of the pemetrexed primary target, thymidylate synthase (TS) correlates with reduced sensitivity to pemetrexed, and that SCLC has the highest TS expression levels of the neuroendocrine tumor spectrum.[38–41]

To investigate this further, exploratory expression and pharmacogenomic analysis of tumor and blood samples collected during GALES were performed and presented at ASCO 2009.[42] Tumors with low TS nuclear expression by immunohistochemistry achieved better OS in the EC arm compared to PC arm (12.9 vs. 7.5 months). Interestingly, however, there was no difference in treatment effect in patients treated for PC based on TS levels. The pharmacogenomic analyses indicated better OS for patients with two germline single-nucleotide polymorphisms in regions including *FPGS* and *SLC19A1*.

Contrasting results for irinotecan were demonstrated in two previous landmark studies. Here, encouraging data for irinotecan were reported by JCOG 9511 in a trial that was terminated early, as early stopping criteria for efficacy had been met,[43] whereas the North American/Australian Study failed to confirm this superiority.[44] Subsequently, Lara et al. reported SWOG S0124.[45] This trial enrolled 651 patients (324 in the irinotecan–cisplatin (IP) and 327 patients in etoposide–cisplatin (EP) arms, respectively), using exactly the same chemotherapy schedule as JCOG 9511. Irinotecan ($60\,mg/m^2$) was delivered on days 1, 8, and 15 with cisplatin ($60\,mg/m^2$ on day 1 every four weeks). Patients on EP were treated with $100\,mg/m^2$ of etoposide (days 1–3) and cisplatin $80\,mg/m^2$, q21. Median PFS for IP and EP was unfortunately similar (5.8 and 5.2 months, respectively) as was median OS (9.9 and 9.1 months, respectively). Severe (grade 3–4) diarrhea was more frequent with IP (19% vs. 3%) and severe neutropenia and thrombocytopenia were more frequent with EP (68% vs. 33% and 15% vs. 4%, respectively). Compared to JCOG 9511 hematological toxicity was similar in both arms. Gastrointestinal (GI) toxicity seen in JCOG 9511 (grade 3 or 4 diarrhea occurred in 16.0% of the IP patients and in none of the EP group) was similar to that observed in SWOG S0124 trial (19% in IP arm vs. 3% in EP arm). Finally there were 12 treatment-related deaths reported in the IP arm as compared to 8 in the EP arm.

SWOG S0124 failed to show superiority of IP over EP, and confirmed an excess of toxicity with IP over EP. Whether the discrepant results between S0124 and JCOG 9511 were due to ethnic differences, due to the premature protocol mandated closure of 9511, or other factors such as imbalance in smokers, since smoking can affect irinotecan metabolism, remains an open question.[46]

In a further phase III trial of cisplatin and irinotecan or etoposide, patients were randomly assigned to receive cisplatin $80\,mg/m^2$ with irinotecan $65\,mg/m^2$ days 1 and 8 or etoposide $100\,mg/m^2$ days 1–3, q21.[47] Here, median OS was not significantly improved for patients receiving IP versus EP (median 10.2 vs. 9.7 months, p = 0.06). However, non-inferiority of IP versus EP was established, with upper bound of the 95% CI of HR 1.01 (pre-specified margin IP/EP < 1.25).

The role of irinotecan in combination with carboplatin was investigated in a randomized phase III German study.[48] Chemotherapy-naïve patients with ES-SCLC received carboplatin AUC 5 with irinotecan $50\,mg/m^2$ on days 1, 8, and 15 (IP) or etoposide $140\,mg/m^2$ on days 1–3 (EP). Differences in PFS and OS between two arms were not statistically significant, with median PFS the same in both arms (6 months) and median OS 10 months for IP and 9 months for EP (p = 0.06).

A further Swedish trial of combination irinotecan with carboplatin has been reported.[49] Here, carboplatin (AUC 4) and irinotecan ($175\,mg/m^2$) IV, both on day 1, improved survival and quality of life over carboplatin (AUC 4) and etoposide ($120\,mg/m^2$/day) orally days 1–5. Median OS for IP group was improved over EP (8.5 vs. 7.1 months, respectively, p = 0.02) and this survival difference remained statistically significant following stratification by age, sex, and performance status. No differences in any of the variables of QoL between two groups were observed.

In order to improve irinotecan-associated toxicities, a split course, three-weekly regime of irinotecan ($50\,mg/m^2$ on days 1 and 8) and carboplatin (AUC5) was reported in phase II U.S. study.[50] This single-arm study of 56 patients demonstrated reasonable irinotecan activity (ORR 58%, median PFS 5.3 months, and one-year OS of 28.7%). This same regime was also investigated in a Japanese single-arm phase II trial reported by Murata et al. in patients 70 years and older.[51] Here, an ORR of 84% was demonstrated, with a median OS of 14 months, and acceptable toxicities.

Amrubicin hydrochloride is a novel synthetic 9-aminoanthracycline derivative prodrug, and a potent inhibitor of topoisomerase II. Structurally it is similar to doxorubicin. However, its anti-tumor activity is superior to doxorubicin and has little appreciable cardiotoxicity. It is currently approved for the treatment of SCLC in Japan where the majority of phase I and II studies have been completed. Later phase studies were recently completed in the United States and Europe, and are reported next.

The EORTC 08062 study compared amrubicin monotherapy, combination cisplatin–amrubicin, and cisplatin–etoposide.[52] This was a phase II, multicenter, open label, randomized study of 88 patients with chemotherapy-naïve ES-SCLC who were randomized to three-weekly amrubicin (45 mg/m^2 days 1–3), three-weekly cisplatin (60 mg/m^2) and amrubicin (40 mg/m^2 days 1–3), or three-weekly cisplatin (75 mg/m^2) and etoposide (100 mg/m^2 day 1 followed by oral 200 mg/m^2 days 2–3, or 100 mg/m^2 IV days 1–3). The primary endpoint was ORR. Unfortunately, no significantly superior efficacy was observed for amrubicin, but the cisplatin–amrubicin arm demonstrated the best overall response rate (77%), compared with that for amrubicin alone (61%) and cisplatin–etoposide (63%). However, grade 3–4 toxicities were more frequent in amrubicin arms, especially febrile neutropenia (18%, 13%, 6%, for cisplatin–amrubicin, amrubicin monotherapy, cisplatin–etoposide, respectively).

In order to investigate an optimal schedule for the elderly, a single-arm Japanese phase II study investigating amrubicin with carboplatin in elderly patients has been completed.[53] In this study, 36 chemotherapy-naïve patients were treated with amrubicin (35 mg/m^2 days 1–3) and carboplatin AUC4 (q21). The primary endpoint was ORR. An ORR of 89% was reported with median PFS of 5.8 months and median OS of 18.6 months. However, grade 3–4 neutropenia observed in 97% of patients, and a 17% febrile neutropenia rate will likely limit this regime's utility. In a similar study of amrubicin monotherapy in 27 first-line patients aged >75 and with PS2,[54] the febrile neutropenia rate was 15% and ORR was 70%, with PFS of 6.6 months, and median OS 9.3 months.

Topotecan is active against SCLC and has been investigated in a number of settings both as monotherapy and in combination. The role of intravenous (IV) topotecan in addition to cisplatin (TP) as first-line treatment for ES-SCLC was compared with standard treatment (EP) in a large German/Austrian randomized phase III study of topotecan (1 mg/m^2 IV, days 1–5) and cisplatin (75 mg/m^2 IV, day 5) compared to etoposide (100 mg/m^2 IV, days 1–3) with cisplatin (75 mg/m^2, day 1) in 795 chemotherapy-naïve patients.[55] The trial was powered for superiority and non-inferiority for TP. Efficacy data demonstrated no superiority for TP, but non-inferiority criteria for OS was met (10.3 vs. 9.4 months, p = 0.40) along with superior time to tumor progression (TTP, 6.9 vs. 5.9 months, p = 0.004) and ORR (55.5% vs. 45.5%, p = 0.01, all results TP vs. PE, respectively). However, grade 3–4 thrombocytopenia was more frequent for TP (18.7% vs. 4.8%), limiting the utility of this regime.

Relapsed SCLC

Over recent years, several randomized trials have investigated topotecan, anthracycline-based chemotherapy, gemcitabine, and irinotecan with or without BSC, aiming to improve treatment options in this difficult clinical setting.[56–60] In addition there remains considerable scepticism on the patient benefit of chemotherapy in the relapsed setting.

In order to benchmark current efficacy of chemotherapy in the relapsed setting, a recent multi-institutional retrospective analysis of 161 patients treated with platinum-based re-challenge, anthracycline-based therapy, or topotecan demonstrated an ORR of 22.9% with median PFS of 4.3 months and median OS of 5.8 months[61] for the whole group. Within this, the platinum-based regimen achieved better RR, PFS, and OS, with ECOG-PS and response to first-line treatment the only independent prognostic factors in a multi-variable model. Amrubicin has been extensively investigated in relapsed SCLC, both in the Far East and in the West. In a Western single-arm phase II trial of amrubicin (40 mg/m^2 days 1–3, q21) in platinum-refractory SCLC, Ettinger et al. reported encouraging activity, with an ORR of 21.3% (primary endpoint), median PFS of 3.2 months, and OS of 6.0 months.[62]

A Japanese phase II single-arm study in both sensitive and refractory relapsed SCLC investigated combination carboplatin and amrubicin.[63] Here, 25 patients, 48% with sensitive and 52% with refractory relapse received amrubicin 35 mg/m^2 days 1–3 and carboplatin AUC4 day 1. The ORR was 36%, with 58% and 15% for sensitive and refractory relapsed disease, respectively. Consistent with other combination trials, myelosuppression was common, and grade 3–4 neutropenia was observed in 88% of patients.

The efficacy of amrubicin monotherapy in the second-line setting compared with topotecan was evaluated in North Japan Lung Cancer Study Group Trial 0402.[64] This was a randomized phase II study of 60 patients randomized to either amrubicin (40 mg/m^2 days 1–3) or topotecan (1.0 mg/m^2 IV days 1–5). Patients were stratified by ECOG performance status (0, 1, or 2) and type of relapse (chemotherapy sensitive, or refractory). ORR for amrubicin was 38%, and superior to 13% for topotecan. In both chemotherapy-sensitive and refractory strata, ORRs were improved for amrubicin compared to topotecan: ORR 53% versus 21% for amrubicin versus topotecan, respectively, in sensitive relapse, and 17% versus 0% for amrubicin versus topotecan, respectively, in refractory relapse. These translated to an overall median PFS of 3.5 months for amrubicin arm and 2.2 months for topotecan arm. Again myelosuppression was a notable toxicity, with grade 4 neutropenia observed in 79% of amrubicin patients and 43% for topotecan. There was one toxic death due to sepsis. A recent Japanese phase II study has investigated combination amrubicin and topotecan in a small single-arm phase II study in relapsed or ED-SCLC (Okayama Lung Cancer Group Study trial 0401).[65] Fifty-nine patients (31 chemotherapy-naïve and 28 relapsed SCLC) received topotecan 0.75 mg/m^2 (days 1–5) and amrubicin 35 mg/m^2 (days 3–5). An ORR of 74% and 43% in chemotherapy-naïve and relapsed SCLC was observed, with a 27% ORR in refractory patients. However, a 97% grade 3–4 neutropenia rate was observed, which translated to 41% grade 3–4 febrile neutropenia, and two toxic deaths.

In the West, Jotte and colleagues reported a phase II trial of amrubicin monotherapy versus topotecan in the second-line setting for sensitive relapse.[66] Seventy-six patients were randomized to amrubicin arm at 40 mg/m^2/day days 1–3 and topotecan 1.5 mg/m^2/day days 1–5, q21. The primary endpoint was ORR, and this was met, with an ORR for amrubicin of 44%, significantly higher than that for topotecan 15%. Median PFS and OS were 4.5 and 9.2 months for amrubicin, respectively, and 3.3 and 7.6 months with topotecan, respectively. By contrast to the Japanese data, grade 3–4 neutropenia and thrombocytopenia was more frequent for topotecan compared to amrubicin (78% vs. 61% and 61% vs. 39%, respectively).

This body of Japanese data with similar Western data led to a randomized phase III trial of amrubicin versus topotecan (ACT1).[67] Here, 637 patients were accrued, and identical treatment as per the phase II was administered. The primary endpoint was OS. While PS2 patients were initially eligible, these were subsequently excluded and GCSF mandated, after protocol amendment due to excess toxic deaths. Although the ORR significantly favored amrubicin (31% vs. 17%) as did PFS (4.1 vs. 3.5 months, p = 0.02), OS was not superior (median OS 7.5 vs. 7.8 months, amrubicin vs. topotecan, respectively). However, superior efficacy for amrubicin was suggested by subgroup analysis of refractory patients (median OS 6.2 vs. 5.7 months, amrubicin vs. topotecan, respectively). Hemtological toxicities were similar in both arms (grade 3–4 neutropenia 41 vs. 53% amrubicin vs. topotecan), but an excess of grade 3–4 febrile neutropenia was observed for amrubicin 9.3% vs. 3.6%.

The role of sorafenib monotherapy in relapsed SCLC was investigated in a recently reported single-arm phase II trial (SWOG 0435).[68] Here, 89 PS 0–1 patients, who relapsed after a previously single-line platinum-based chemotherapy received sorafenib at a dose of 400 mg orally BID. Patients were stratified by platinum sensitivity, and an ORR of 11% was observed in the platinum-sensitive group, but 2% in platinum-refractory group, translating to a median OS of 6.7 months in the platinum-sensitive stratum and 5.3 months in the platinum-refractory stratum.

Picoplatin is a novel platinum, designed to overcome thiol-mediated resistance. Following encouraging results from a single-arm phase II trial that reported modest efficacy of picoplatin (median PFS of 9.1 weeks, and OS 26.9 weeks),[69] a randomized phase III trial has been completed, and was reported by Ciuleanu et al. at ASCO 2010 (SPEAR).[70] Here, 401 patients, either non-responsive or progressive within six months of first-line platinum-based therapy, were randomized to picoplatin (150 mg/m^2 IV, q21) with BSC or BSC alone. The primary endpoint was OS. Unfortunately, in the ITT population, superiority of picoplatin was not demonstrated, with median OS of 21 weeks with picoplatin versus 20 weeks with BSC alone. Secondary outcomes demonstrated some activity for picoplatin, with an ORR of 4.3 versus 0%, and both TTP and PFS favoring picoplatin (TTP, HR = 0.6, 0.47–0.79, p = 0.002; PFS HR = 0.783, 0.64–0.98, p = 0.0281). Toxicities were principally hematological: grade 3–4 thrombocytopenia 43% (no incidences of bleeding), grade 3–4 neutropenia 19% (two patients had febrile neutropenia). However, a posthoc analysis of refractory patients or those who relapsed within 45 days demonstrated some possible benefit of picoplatin, with an improvement in median OS from 18 to 21 weeks. Exactly why some benefit was observed for this population and not in the ITT group remains unexplained, as postprogression therapy was not presented, and correlative translational analyses were not performed. In summary, therefore, picoplatin appears modestly active but not superior to other available treatments.[71]

BCL2 dysregulation has long been identified as contributing to chemo-resistance in SCLC. Novel therapeutic approaches to target this have been recently reported. Navitoclax (ABT263) is a BH3 mimetic, that has been investigated in a phase I study including 29 SCLC or pulmonary carcinoid patients, identified that dose-dependant thrombocytopenia as the dose-limiting toxicity (DLT), and pro-gastrin releasing peptide was identified as a surrogate marker of BCL-2 amplification and changes correlated with changes in tumor volume.[72] A phase II study of this compound was further investigated in ED-SCLC. Although ABT263 was well tolerated, activity was modest.[73]

Obatoclax mesylate is another small molecule BH3-mimetic that enhances activity of cisplatin and etoposide in vitro, with scheduling optimized over three hours.[74] A randomized phase II study of 155 chemotherapy-naïve ES-SCLC patients treated with carboplatin and etoposide with or without 30 mg of obatoclax over three hours followed by obatoclax maintenance has been recently reported.[75] The primary endpoint was ORR, and a non-significant improvement in this (64.9% vs. 53.8%, $p = 0.11$) was observed, with a trend to improvement in one-year survival (45.5% vs. 37.2%, $p = 0.08$) and median OS (11.9 vs. 10.1 months, $p = 0.051$). In addition, the refractory rate (death or progression during initial six cycles of chemotherapy) was reduced from 40.0% for chemotherapy alone to 25.4% in obatoclax arm. The drug was well tolerated, and the only grade 3–4 non-hem toxicity reported was mood effect: somnolence (8% vs. 0%). By contrast, an open label single-arm phase II trial of obatoclax (14 mg/m^2 days 1–3) with IV topotecan (1.25 mg/m^2 days 1–5, q21), in relapsed SCLC with a primary end-point of overall response rate did not identify any objective responses.[76]

CONCLUSION

Despite many high quality trials reported over recent years, treatment of SCLC is still extremely challenging. This review has highlighted current attempts to improve clinical outcomes across all stages of SCLC. Drug development is generally moving toward personalized therapy, and many trials in other tumor types have now started to report drug efficacy stratified by molecular phenotype. However, such studies have been rare in SCLC and future advances in SCLC pathobiology coupled to advances in somatic genetics and molecular technologies will likely result in significant therapeutic advances in the years ahead.

ACKNOWLEDGMENTS

SP is in receipt of a Clinical Senior Lectureship Award from the Higher Education Funding Council for England. We also acknowledge NHS funding to the Royal Marsden Hospital/Institute of Cancer Research NIHR Biomedical Research Centre.

REFERENCES

1. Govindan R, Page N, Morgensztern D, et al. Changing epidemiology of small-cell lung cancer in the United States over the last 30 years: analysis of the surveillance, epidemiologic, and end results database. J Clin Oncol 2006; 24: 4539–44.
2. Rami-Porta R, Crowley JJ, Goldstraw P. The revised TNM staging system for lung cancer. Ann Thorac Cardiovasc Surg 2009; 15: 4–9.
3. Vallieres E, Shepherd FA, Crowley J, et al. The IASLC Lung Cancer Staging Project: proposals regarding the relevance of TNM in the pathologic staging of small cell lung cancer in the forthcoming (seventh) edition of the TNM classification for lung cancer. J Thorac Oncol 2009; 4: 1049–59.
4. Ignatius OSH, Zell JA. The applicability of the proposed IASLC staging revisions to small cell lung cancer (SCLC) with comparison to the current UICC 6th TNM Edition. J Thorac Oncol 2009; 4: 300–10.
5. Janssen-Heijnen ML, Maas HA, Siesling S, et al. Treatment and survival of patients with small-cell lung cancer: small steps forward, but not for patients >80. Ann Oncol 2012; 23: 954–60.
6. McCracken JD, Janaki LM, Crowley JJ, et al. Concurrent chemotherapy/radiotherapy for limited small-cell lung carcinoma: a Southwest Oncology Group Study. J Clin Oncol 1990; 8: 892–8.
7. Le QT, McCoy J, Williamson S, et al. Phase I study of tirapazamine plus cisplatin/etoposide and concurrent thoracic radiotherapy in limited-stage small cell lung cancer (S0004): a Southwest Oncology Group study. Clin Cancer Res 2004; 10: 5418–24.
8. Edelman MJ, Chansky K, Gaspar LE, et al. Phase II trial of cisplatin/etoposide and concurrent radiotherapy followed by paclitaxel/carboplatin consolidation for limited small-cell lung cancer: Southwest Oncology Group 9713. J Clin Oncol 2004; 22: 127–32.
9. Le QT, Moon J, Redman M, et al. Phase II study of tirapazamine, cisplatin, and etoposide and concurrent thoracic radiotherapy for limited-stage small-cell lung cancer: SWOG 0222. J Clin Oncol 2009; 27: 3014–19.

10. Niho S, Kubota K, Yoh K, et al. Clinical outcome of chemoradiation therapy in patients with limited-disease small cell lung cancer with ipsilateral pleural effusion. J Thorac Oncol 2008; 3: 723–7.
11. Komaki R, Swann RS, Ettinger DS, et al. Phase I study of thoracic radiation dose escalation with concurrent chemotherapy for patients with limited small-cell lung cancer: Report of Radiation Therapy Oncology Group (RTOG) protocol 97-12. Int J Radiat Oncol Biol Phys 2005; 62: 342–50.
12. Shirvani SM, Komaki R, Heymach JV, Fossella FV, Chang JY. Positron emission tomography/computed tomography-guided intensity-modulated radiotherapy for limited-stage small-cell lung cancer. Int J Radiat Oncol Biol Phys 2012; 82: e91–7.
13. van Loon J, De Ruysscher D, Wanders R, et al. Selective nodal irradiation on basis of (18)FDG-PET scans in limited-disease small-cell lung cancer: a prospective study. Int J Radiat Oncol Biol Phys 2010; 77: 329–36.
14. Fox W, Scadding JG. Medical Research Council comparative trial of surgery and radiotherapy for primary treatment of small-celled or oat-celled carcinoma of bronchus. Ten-year follow-up. Lancet 1973; 2: 63–5.
15. Lim E, Belcher E, Yap YK, Nicholson AG, Goldstraw P. The role of surgery in the treatment of limited disease small cell lung cancer: time to reevaluate. J Thorac Oncol 2008; 3: 1267–71.
16. Yu JB, Decker RH, Detterbeck FC, Wilson LD. Surveillance epidemiology and end results evaluation of the role of surgery for stage I small cell lung cancer. J Thorac Oncol 2010; 5: 215–19.
17. Schreiber D, Rineer J, Weedon J, et al. Survival outcomes with the use of surgery in limited-stage small cell lung cancer: should its role be re-evaluated? Cancer 2010; 116: 1350–7.
18. Tashi T, Aldoss I, Gonsalves W. Surgical resection in early limited-stage small cell lung cancer: time to rethink? A retrospective analysis of the VA Central Cancer Registry. J Clin Oncol 2011; 29(Suppl): abstract 7021.
19. Le Péchoux C, Dunant A, Senan S, et al. Standard-dose versus higher-dose prophylactic cranial irradiation (PCI) in patients with limited-stage small-cell lung cancer in complete remission after chemotherapy and thoracic radiotherapy (PCI 99-01, EORTC 22003-08004, RTOG 0212, and IFCT 99-01): a randomised clinical trial. Lancet Oncol 2009; 10: 467–74.
20. Le Pechoux C, Laplanche A, Faivre-Finn C, et al. Clinical neurological outcome and quality of life among patients with limited small-cell cancer treated with two different doses of prophylactic cranial irradiation in the intergroup phase III trial (PCI99-01, EORTC 22003-08004, RTOG 0212 and IFCT 99-01). Ann Oncol 2011; 22: 1154–63.
21. Wolfson AH, Bae K, Komaki R, et al. Primary analysis of a phase II randomized trial Radiation Therapy Oncology Group (RTOG) 0212: impact of different total doses and schedules of prophylactic cranial irradiation on chronic neurotoxicity and quality of life for patients with limited-disease small-cell lung cancer. Int J Radiat Oncol Biol Phys 2011; 81: 77–84.
22. Skarlos DV, Samantas E, Kosmidis P, et al. Randomized comparison of etoposide-cisplatin vs. etoposide-carboplatin and irradiation in small-cell lung cancer. A Hellenic Co-operative Oncology Group study. Ann Oncol 1994; 5: 601–7.
23. Joss RA, Alberto P, Hurny C, et al. Quality versus quantity of life in the treatment of patients with advanced small-cell lung cancer? A randomized phase III comparison of weekly carboplatin and teniposide versus cisplatin, adriamycin, etoposide alternating with cyclophosphamide, methotrexate, vincristine and lomustine. Swiss Group for Clinical Cancer Research (SAKK). Ann Oncol 1995; 6: 41–8.
24. Okamoto H, Watanabe K, Kunikane H, et al. Randomised phase III trial of carboplatin plus etoposide vs split doses of cisplatin plus etoposide in elderly or poor-risk patients with extensive disease small-cell lung cancer: JCOG 9702. Br J Cancer 2007; 97: 162–9.
25. Lee SM, James LE, Qian W, et al. Comparison of gemcitabine and carboplatin versus cisplatin and etoposide for patients with poor-prognosis small cell lung cancer. Thorax 2009; 64: 75–80.
26. Rossi A, Di Maio M, Chiodini P. Carboplatin- Or CISplatin-based chemotherapy as first-line treatment of small-cell lung cancer (SCLC): the COCIS individual patient data meta-analysis. J Clin Oncol 2011; 29(Suppl): abstract 7022.
27. Horn L, Dahlberg SE, Sandler AB, et al. Phase II study of cisplatin plus etoposide and bevacizumab for previously untreated, extensive-stage small-cell lung cancer: Eastern Cooperative Oncology Group Study E3501. J Clin Oncol 2009; 27: 6006–11.
28. Spigel DR, Greco FA, Zubkus JD, et al. Phase II trial of irinotecan, carboplatin, and bevacizumab in the treatment of patients with extensive-stage small-cell lung cancer. J Thorac Oncol 2009; 4: 1555–60.
29. Spigel DR, Townley PM, Waterhouse DM, et al. Randomized phase II study of bevacizumab in combination with chemotherapy in previously untreated extensive-stage small-cell lung cancer: results from the SALUTE trial. J Clin Oncol 2011; 29: 2215–22.
30. Schneider BJ, Gadgeel SM, Ramnath N, et al. Phase II trial of sunitinib maintenance therapy after platinum-based chemotherapy in patients with extensive-stage small cell lung cancer. J Thorac Oncol 2011; 6: 1117–20.
31. Han J, Lim K, Kim H. Phase II study of sunitinib in patients with relapsed or refractory small cell lung cancer (SCLC). J Clin Oncol 2011; 29(Suppl): abstract 7084.
32. Socinski MA, Raju RN, Neubauer M, et al. Pemetrexed in relapsed small-cell lung cancer and the impact of shortened vitamin supplementation lead-in time: results of a phase II trial. J Thorac Oncol 2008; 3: 1308–16.
33. Jalal S, Ansari R, Govindan R, et al. Pemetrexed in second line and beyond small cell lung cancer: a Hoosier Oncology Group phase II study. J Thorac Oncol 2009; 4: 93–6.
34. Gronberg BH, Bremnes RM, Aasebo U, et al. A prospective phase II study: high-dose pemetrexed as second-line chemotherapy in small-cell lung cancer. Lung Cancer 2009; 63: 88–93.

35. Jett J, Bernath A, Foster N. Phase II trial of pemetrexed (P) and carboplatin (C) in previously untreated extensive stage disease small cell lung cancer (ED-SCLC): A NCCTG study. J Clin Oncol 2008; 26(Suppl): abstract 8066.

36. Socinski MA, Weissman C, Hart LL, et al. Randomized phase II trial of pemetrexed combined with either cisplatin or carboplatin in untreated extensive-stage small-cell lung cancer. J Clin Oncol 2006; 24: 4840–7.

37. Socinski MA, Smit EF, Lorigan P, et al. Phase III study of pemetrexed plus carboplatin compared with etoposide plus carboplatin in chemotherapy-naive patients with extensive-stage small-cell lung cancer. J Clin Oncol 2009; 27: 4787–92.

38. Sigmond J, Backus HH, Wouters D, et al. Induction of resistance to the multitargeted antifolate Pemetrexed (ALIMTA) in WiDr human colon cancer cells is associated with thymidylate synthase overexpression. Biochem Pharmacol 2003; 66: 431–8.

39. Giovannetti E, Mey V, Nannizzi S, et al. Cellular and pharmacogenetics foundation of synergistic interaction of pemetrexed and gemcitabine in human non-small-cell lung cancer cells. Mol Pharmacol 2005; 68: 110–18.

40. Scagliotti GV, Parikh P, von Pawel J, et al. Phase III study comparing cisplatin plus gemcitabine with cisplatin plus pemetrexed in chemotherapy-naive patients with advanced-stage non-small-cell lung cancer. J Clin Oncol 2008; 26: 3543–51.

41. Ceppi P, Volante M, Ferrero A, et al. Thymidylate synthase expression in gastroenteropancreatic and pulmonary neuroendocrine tumors. Clin Cancer Res 2008; 14: 1059–64.

42. Smit EF, Socinski MA, Mullaney B. Pharmacogenomic analysis from a phase III study of pemetrexed plus carboplatin (PC) versus etoposide plus carboplatin (EC) in chemonaive patients (pts) with extensive-stage disease small cell lung cancer (ED-SCLC). J Clin Oncol 2009; 27(15 Suppl): abstract 8030.

43. Noda K, Nishiwaki Y, Kawahara M, et al. Irinotecan plus cisplatin compared with etoposide plus cisplatin for extensive small-cell lung cancer. N Engl J Med 2002; 346: 85–91.

44. Hanna N, Bunn PA Jr, Langer C, et al. Randomized phase III trial comparing irinotecan/cisplatin with etoposide/cisplatin in patients with previously untreated extensive-stage disease small-cell lung cancer. J Clin Oncol 2006; 24: 2038–43.

45. Lara PN Jr, Natale R, Crowley J, et al. Phase III trial of irinotecan/cisplatin compared with etoposide/cisplatin in extensive-stage small-cell lung cancer: clinical and pharmacogenomic results from SWOG S0124. J Clin Oncol 2009; 27: 2530–5.

46. van der Bol JM, Mathijssen RH, Loos WJ, et al. Cigarette smoking and irinotecan treatment: pharmacokinetic interaction and effects on neutropenia. J Clin Oncol 2007; 25: 2719–26.

47. Zatloukal P, Cardenal F, Szczesna A, et al. A multicenter international randomized phase III study comparing cisplatin in combination with irinotecan or etoposide in previously untreated small-cell lung cancer patients with extensive disease. Ann Oncol 2010; 21: 1810–16.

48. Schmittel A, Sebastian M, Fischer VW, et al. A German multicenter, randomized phase III trial comparing irinotecan-carboplatin with etoposide-carboplatin as first-line therapy for extensive-disease small-cell lung cancer. Ann Oncol 2011; 22: 1798–804.

49. Hermes A, Bergman B, Bremnes R, et al. Irinotecan plus carboplatin versus oral etoposide plus carboplatin in extensive small-cell lung cancer: a randomized phase III trial. J Clin Oncol 2008; 26: 4261–7.

50. Horn L, Zhao Z, Sandler A, et al. A phase II study of carboplatin and irinotecan in extensive stage small-cell lung cancer. Clin Lung Cancer 2011; 12: 161–5.

51. Murata Y, Hirose T, Yamaoka T, et al. Phase II trial of the combination of carboplatin and irinotecan in elderly patients with small-cell lung cancer. Eur J Cancer 2011; 47: 1336–42.

52. O'Brien ME, Konopa K, Lorigan P, et al. Randomised phase II study of amrubicinubicin as single agent or in combination with cisplatin versus cisplatin etoposide as first-line treatment in patients with extensive stage small cell lung cancer - EORTC 08062. Eur J Cancer 2011; 47: 2322–30.

53. Inoue A, Ishimoto O, Fukumoto S, et al. A phase II study of amrubicinubicin combined with carboplatin for elderly patients with small-cell lung cancer: North Japan Lung Cancer Study Group Trial 0405. Ann Oncol 2010; 21: 800–3.

54. Igawa S, Ryuge S, Fukui T, et al. Amrubicinubicin for treating elderly and poor-risk patients with small-cell lung cancer. Int J Clin Oncol 2010; 15: 447–52.

55. Heigener D, Freitag L, Eschbach C. Topotecan/cisplatin (TP) compared to cisplatin/etoposide (PE) for patients with extensive disease-small cell lung cancer (ED- SCLC): final results of a randomised phase III trial. J Clin Oncol 2008; 26(Suppl): abstract 7513.

56. O'Brien ME, Ciuleanu TE, Tsekov H, et al. Phase III trial comparing supportive care alone with supportive care with oral topotecan in patients with relapsed small-cell lung cancer. J Clin Oncol 2006; 24: 5441–7.

57. von Pawel J, Schiller JH, Shepherd FA, et al. Topotecan versus cyclophosphamide, doxorubicin, and vincristine for the treatment of recurrent small-cell lung cancer. J Clin Oncol 1999; 17: 658–67.

58. Pallis AG, Agelidou A, Agelaki S, et al. A multicenter randomized phase II study of the irinotecan/gemcitabine doublet versus irinotecan monotherapy in previously treated patients with extensive stage small-cell lung cancer. Lung Cancer 2009; 65: 187–91.

59. Eckardt JR, von Pawel J, Pujol JL, et al. Phase III study of oral compared with intravenous topotecan as second-line therapy in small-cell lung cancer. J Clin Oncol 2007; 25: 2086–92.

60. Graziano SL, Herndon JE, Socinski MA, et al. Phase II trial of weekly dose-dense paclitaxel in extensive-stage small cell lung cancer: cancer and leukemia group B study 39901. J Thorac Oncol 2008; 3: 158–62.

61. Garassino MC, Torri V, Michetti G, et al. Outcomes of small-cell lung cancer patients treated with second-line chemotherapy: a multi-institutional retrospective analysis. Lung Cancer 2011; 72: 378–83.
62. Ettinger DS, Jotte R, Lorigan P, et al. Phase II study of amrubicinubicin as second-line therapy in patients with platinum-refractory small-cell lung cancer. J Clin Oncol 2010; 28: 2598–603.
63. Hirose T, Nakashima M, Shirai T, et al. Phase II trial of amrubicinubicin and carboplatin in patients with sensitive or refractory relapsed small-cell lung cancer. Lung Cancer 2011; 73: 345–50.
64. Inoue A, Sugawara S, Yamazaki K, et al. Randomized phase II trial comparing amrubicinubicin with topotecan in patients with previously treated small-cell lung cancer: North Japan Lung Cancer Study Group Trial 0402. J Clin Oncol 2008; 26: 5401–6.
65. Nogami N, Hotta K, Kuyama S, et al. A phase II study of amrubicinubicin and topotecan combination therapy in patients with relapsed or extensive-disease small-cell lung cancer: Okayama Lung Cancer Study Group Trial 0401. Lung Cancer 2011; 74: 80–4.
66. Jotte R, Conkling P, Reynolds C, et al. Randomized phase II trial of single-agent amrubicinubicin or topotecan as second-line treatment in patients with small-cell lung cancer sensitive to first-line platinum-based chemotherapy. J Clin Oncol 2011; 29: 287–93.
67. Jotte R, von Pawel J, Spigel DR. Randomized phase III trial of amrubicinubicin versus topotecan (Topo) as second-line treatment for small cell lung cancer (SCLC). J Clin Oncol 2011; 29(Suppl): abstract 7000.
68. Gitlitz BJ, Moon J, Glisson BS, et al. Sorafenib in platinum-treated patients with extensive stage small cell lung cancer: a Southwest Oncology Group (SWOG 0435) phase II trial. J Thorac Oncol 2010; 5: 1835–40.
69. Eckardt JR, Bentsion DL, Lipatov ON, et al. Phase II study of picoplatin as second-line therapy for patients with small-cell lung cancer. J Clin Oncol 2009; 27: 2046–51.
70. Ciuleanu T, Samarzija M, Demidchik Y. Randomized phase III study (SPEAR) of picoplatin plus best supportive care (BSC) or BSC alone in patients (pts) with SCLC refractory or progressive within 6 months after first-line platinum-based chemotherapy. J Clin Oncol 2010; 28(Suppl): abstract 7002.
71. William WN Jr, Glisson BS. Novel strategies for the treatment of small-cell lung carcinoma. Nat Rev Clin Oncol 2011; 8: 611–19.
72. Gandhi L, Camidge DR, Ribeiro DO, et al. Phase I study of Navitoclax (ABT-263), a novel Bcl-2 family inhibitor, in patients with small-cell lung cancer and other solid tumors. J Clin Oncol 2011; 29: 909–16.
73. Rudin CM, Garon E, De Oliveira M. Patient outcome and exploratory analysis from a phase 2A study of navitoclax (ABT-263) in patients with advanced small cell lung cancer. J Thorac Oncol 2011; 6(Suppl 2): S644–5.
74. Chiappori A, Schreeder M, Moezi M. A phase Ib trial of Bcl-2 inhibitor obatoclax in combination with carboplatin and etoposide for previously untreated patients with extensive-stage small cell lung cancer (ES-SCLC). J Clin Oncol 2009; 27(15 Suppl): abstract 3576.
75. Langer C, Albert I, Kovacs P. A randomized phase II study of carboplatin (C) and etoposide (E) with or without pan-BCL-2 antagonist obatoclax (Ob) in extensive-stage small cell lung cancer (ES-SCLC). J Clin Oncol 2011; 29(Suppl): abstract 7001.
76. Paik PK, Rudin CM, Pietanza MC, et al. A phase II study of obatoclax mesylate, a Bcl-2 antagonist, plus topotecan in relapsed small cell lung cancer. Lung Cancer 2011; 74: 481–5.

the presence or absence of NF2/Hippo pathway mutations.[58] In some of the following sections it will be highlighted how molecular pathology knowledge is implemented for new therapeutic strategies.

Diagnosis

A clinical diagnosis of MPM is not possible because symptoms such as chest pain or dyspnea are unspecific. An accurate diagnosis of MPM is made based on histopathological examination. There are three main histological subtypes according to WHO classification: the epithelioid, the sarcomatoid and a mixture of both—including at least 10% of each growth pattern—the biphasic subtype. As the diagnosis of MPM is difficult to make, the recommendation of the Guidelines of the European Respiratory Society (ERS) and the European Society of Thoracic Surgeons (ESTS)[59] strongly support thoracoscopic tissue biopsy in order to get multiple and deep tissue biopsies because cytological assessment of pleural effusion may not be sensitive and specific enough.

The two main differential diagnoses for the epithelioid subtype are adenocarcinoma, particularly from lung, and reactive mesothelial hyperplasia with atypia. Sarcomatoid MPM must be primarily separated from sarcomatoid carcinoma, sarcoma NOS, and solitary fibrous tumor (SFT). Immunohistochemistry has a central role in this diagnostic process; however, despite the availability and testing of multiple antibodies, no reliable marker exists for the sarcomatoid histotype. For example, both sarcomatoid MPM and sarcomatoid carcinoma are positive for pan-cytokeratin. Desmin and S-100 may be used as negative markers.[59] For epithelioid MPM and the differential of carcinoma, it is recommended to use a 4 to 6 marker panel: calretinin, WT1, CK5/6, D2-40 (podoplanin), and mesothelin for MPM against TTF-1, Berep4, and CEA for adenocarcinoma.

The identification of mesothelin-related proteins as serum markers of mesothelioma might be useful for patients' follow-up[60]; however for the time being, the determination is not sensitive enough[61,62] for diagnostic purposes.

Regarding prognosis factors with impact on patients' outcome regardless of the treatment, there are no strong recommendations about clinical parameters although sarcomatoid histotype is an exclusion criteria in some clinical trials[59] since it was associated with poor prognosis in most series. Data about the role of mediastinal lymph node involvement are conflicting and may be clarified as a result of the new IASLC/IMIG staging project.[63,64]

Imaging

Imaging has two central roles for the management of MPM—first for initial diagnosis and clinical staging, and second for the assessment of treatment response if patients undergo any kind of induction treatment. For both questions, there are several modalities available including computed tomography (CT), magnetic resonance imaging (MRI), positron emission tomography (PET), and PET/CT. CT scan is the primary imaging modality. The main CT findings in mesothelioma patients include pleural thickening and pleural effusion. There are some features which might help to differentiate MPM from benign pleural plaques in contrast-enhanced thoracic CT: "rind-like pleural involvement," "mediastinal pleural involvement," "pleural nodularity," and "pleural thickness more than 1 cm." These findings allow a differentiation malignant from benign pleural disease with sensitivity/specificity values of 54/95%, 70/83%, 38/96%, and 47/64%, respectively.[65] For further treatment and operation planning, the clinical T stage assessment is mandatory, but unfortunately, CT tends to underestimate the extent of MPM. But still, there are some unresectability criteria which can be visualized by CT: invasion of extrapleural or even extrathoracic soft tissue or fat, infiltration or even fracture of ribs, a loss of the fat plan in the mediastinal tissue, and tumor encasing the hemidiaphragm with a loss of the regular infradiaphragmatic surface.[66] For the cN stage, CT plays a limited role because enlargement is the only criteria and is not reliable to predict lymph node involvement.

MRI adds more information about chest wall and diaphragmatic involvement because of its excellent resolution and may increase the precision of clinical T staging. MPM has intermediate or slightly higher signal intensity on T1-weighted (T1-W) and moderately high signal intensity on T2-weighted images (T2-W).[66] In comparison to CT scan, MRI seems to be superior in clinical T staging as it was found by Heelan et al. that MRI was more accurate in showing endothoracic fascia or solitary resectable foci of chest wall invasion (46% for CT vs. 69% for MRI).[67]

FDG-PET-CT diagnoses MPM with high sensitivity (88%), specificity (92.9%), and accuracy (88.9%), but with a low sensitivity for stage N2 (38%) and T4 (67%).[68] Besides this, PET-CT can detect occult distant metastases and permits to assess the tumor metabolism with FDG-activity, which may also help to interpret tumor response. To complete the staging investigations for patients qualifying for a multimodality treatment, a video-mediastinoscopy for accurate mediastinal lymph node staging should be considered whenever possible. According to institutional practice, laparoscopy and contralateral VATS may be performed if clinically indicated.[59]

Response assessment in malignant mesothelioma remains difficult because of the rind-like growth pattern of MPM. Modified RECIST is the standard currently,[69] but was criticized for a high inter-observer variability.[70] More sophisticated methods such as computerized analysis of CT scans measuring the tumor volume[71] or PET-CT based algorithms—such as assessment of total glycolytic volume or total lesion glycolysis or decrease in SUV-max, which have been demonstrated to have prognostic value as well—are under evaluation.[72]

SURGERY AS PART OF A MULTIMODALITY TREATMENT

Currently, there are no widely accepted guidelines for a standard surgical approach for the management of MPM. The extent of procedures available ranges from thoracoscopic pleurodesis or tumor debulking as palliative measures, to pleurectomy/decortication (P/D) and extrapleural pneumonectomy (EPP) as more radical procedures with the aim of a maximum cytoreduction. While the surgical technique of EPP has been well standardized with en bloc resection of the parietal and visceral pleura with the ipsilateral lung, pericardium, and diaphragm,[73] the technique of P/D is not standardized in all centers as demonstrated during the ongoing staging project of the International Mesothelioma Interest Group (IMIG) and the International Association for the Study of Lung Cancer (IASLC).[74] Although some surgeons define P/D as macroscopic tumor removal with pleurectomy of the parietal pleura and decortication of the visceral pleura, others include resection of partial pericardium and diaphragm involved by the tumor (now recommended by the working group to be nominated as "extended" P/D). These results demonstrate that besides the "natural" difficulty of mesothelioma studies because of a low incidence resulting in, for example, long observation periods with heterogeneous patient cohorts, even the procedure of P/D itself is not equally performed everywhere, and therefore a decision for a "standard" surgical approach is difficult. Accordingly, to correctly interpret the outcome of P/D studies a clear definition of surgical operation is necessary.

Even EPP has been recently a matter of controversy despite an increasing amount of phase II studies reporting favorable results (Table 13.1). The MARS trial[75] concluded that "EPP within trimodal therapy offers no benefit and possibly harms patients" although the trial was not designed to answer the question of benefit or not of EPP but rather the feasibility of such a trial. A definitive answer to this question would need an accrual of 670 patients to identify a survival benefit.[76] Also the criticism of too high morbidity and mortality rates is not supported by recently reported trials for trimodality therapy including EPP (Table 13.1) showing that mortality can be reduced to 0–5% in experienced centers, while taking into account all studies published between 1985 and 2010, it is reduced to 0 to a maximum of 11.8 %.[77] Morbidity stays high (22–82%) but seems to be manageable in terms of improvement of quality of life for all parameters at three months postoperatively.

For the time being, and because of the reasons mentioned above, there is yet no scientifically based answer as to which procedure is the more appropriate surgical technique for MPM. Most investigations have studied one or the other technique and when studied together, P/D was chosen for more early stages and EPP for more advanced stages, a decision which is often taken only in the operating theatre and not before due to a lack of reliable clinical staging. In a large multicenter comparative study combining the experience of three large centers in the United States, the outcome of 663 patients treated between 1990 and 2006 was analyzed retrospectively.[78] The authors conclude that the study emphasizes the similarities in outcome after EPP or P/D for MPM in a multicenter setting and cannot give a clear recommendation for either one or the other surgical approach, which is consistent with overall (Tables 13.1 and 13.2) comparable survival data ranging between 9 and 30 months for P/D and 12 and 35 months for EPP in a multimodal setting. One situation where P/D is clearly advised is for patients with compromised cardiac or pulmonary function, or with certain co-morbidities, in particular at early stage disease, in order preserve lung function. If all gross tumor cannot be removed macroscopically in stage IV patients, a parenchyma-sparing procedure as debulking P/D is recommended.[79] Besides these quite unambiguous situations, the decision to perform P/D or EPP in stage I, II, and III should be individually tailored to tumor load and patients performance. Currently, most high volume centers would combine EPP or P/D to another modality targeted to residual microscopic disease. Therefore, both procedures should eventually not be interpreted as rivaling but alternatives being one more adequate than the other under specific circumstances. For this reason, the implication for future protocols should be to find precise selection criteria for each procedure in an adapted staging system taking into account important prognostic factors such as tumor volume.[80]

Besides improvement on the selection criteria for multimodality treatment, the effort of future protocols should aim to improve local tumor control, as local tumor recurrence continues to be a problem ranging up to 62% after EPP and even 90% after P/D.[81] Localized intracavitary therapy is an attractive approach in this context and several studies are ongoing to refine existing successful protocols with intracavitary chemotherapy

Table 13.1 Multimodal Treatment Including Neo-/Adjuvant Chemotherapy with Extrapleural Pneumonectomy or Pleurectomy/Decortication Plus Optional Adjuvant Radiotherapy

Investigator	Chemotherapy	Surgery	RT	Mortality	MST
de Perrot	Neoadjuvant	EPP 30	+	6.7	14[a]
Krug	Neoadjuvant	EPP 40	+	3.7	16.8[a]
Van Schil[103]	Neoadjuvant	EPP 42	+	6.5	18
Weder	Neoadjuvant	EPP 45	+	2.2	19.8
Baldini	Adjuvant	EPP 49	+	4	22
Rice	Neoadjuvant	EPP 63	+	8	10.2[a], 14.2[b]
Sugarbaker	Adjuvant	EPP 183	+	3.8	19
Bolukbas	Adjuvant	PD 35	+	5.8	30
Rusch	Adjuvant	PD 27	−	3.7	17[b]
Allen	Adjuvant	EPP 40	+	7.5	13.3
		PD 56		5.4	9
Aziz	Adjuvant	EPP 51	−	9.1	35[b]
		PD 47		0	14[a]
Branscheid	Adjuvant	EPP 76	−	11.8	9.3
		Pall. PD 82		2.4	10.4
De Vries	Adjuvant	EPP 15	+/	5.8	12
		PD 29		3.8	9
Maggi	Adjuvant	EPP 23	+/	6	9.5
		PD 9			
Nakas	Adjuvant	EPP 13	+/	23	11.5
		VATS PD 42		7.1	14
Flores	Adjuvant	EPP 385	+/	7	12
		P/D 278		4	16
Rusch	Adjuvant	115 EPP	+/	5.2	14.7
		59 P/D		3.5	18.5
Schipper	Neoadjuvant	EPP 73	+/	8.2	16
		SUB PD 34		2.9	8
		rad PD 10		0	17.2

All references are summarized from several reviews,[104,105] studies before 1990 or with less than 20 patients are not considered.
[a]Intention to treat survival.
[b]Selected patient survival.
Abbreviations: RT, radiotherapy; MST, median survival time.

Table 13.2 Ongoing (September 2011) Mesothelioma Phase II Interventional Clinical Trials Including Novel Therapies

Drug	Mechanism	Combination	Clinical trial ID
CBP-501	MAPKAP-K2, C-Tak1, and CHK1 inhib	Cisplatin/pemetrexed	NCT007003w36
Cetuximab	Anti-EGFR	Cisplatin or carboplatin and pem	NCT00996567
Cediranib	VEGF tyrosine kinase inhibitor	Cisplatin/pemetrexed	NCT01064648
AMG 102	Anti-HGF	Cisplatin/pemetrexed	NCT01105390
Axitinib	VGFR, PDGFR, c-kit inhibitor	Cisplatin/pemetrexed	NCT01211275
Bortezomib	Proteasome inhib	Eloxatin	NCT00996385
K562-GM cell vaccines	Immunotherapy	Celecoxib and cyclophosphamide	NCT01143545
WT-1 vaccine	Immunotherapy	Single agent	NCT01265433
Everolimus	mTOR inhibitor	Single agent	NCT00770120 NCT01024946
Pegylated Arginine Deiminase	Growth inhibition of ASS negative tumors	Single agent	NCT01279967
GC1008	Anti-TGFbeta	Single agent	NCT01112293
IMC-A12	Anti-IGF-1R	Single agent	NCT01160458
Zoledronic Acid	Tumor associated macrophage repolarization	Single agent	NCT01204203

(as reviewed in[82,83]), photodynamic therapy,[84] or gene therapy.[85] These specific protocols aim to attack the minimal residual disease which may be left behind after surgery—P/D or EPP.

Radiotherapy

Palliative radiotherapy (RT) can be delivered locally to the chest wall in view of pain control.[59] Prophylactic RT to prevent tumor cell seeding along thoracocentesis or drainage tracts did not show a significant reduction of the relative risk of tract metastases as assessed in a metaanalysis.[86] Curative RT in a P/D setting led to median survival times of 10–18 months.[87] Promising results regarding intensity modulated radiotherapy (IMRT) after P/D with a median survival of 26 months have been reported.[88] Adjuvant RT in an EPP setting has the major advantage as the lung is removed, but other critical organs as the heart, liver, kidneys, and spinal cord as well as the contralateral lung are still at risk. The approaches available include a moderate-dose photon technique (MDRT), a high-dose matched photon/electron technique, and a high-dose IMRT. The high dose hemithoracic IMRT has been developed to improve accuracy and precision and to reduce toxicity. However, fatal pneumonitits is a critical side effect resulting from such a dose; hence, this technique is recommended in clinical trials at specialized centers only.[59] Hemithoracic radiation after EPP has been evaluated in several studies with good local tumor control in comparison to historical controls.[89] An ongoing multicenter Swiss trial (SAKK) is currently evaluating in a randomized protocol the value of curative postoperative hemithoracic radiotherapy after neoadjuvant chemotherapy and EPP (NCT00334594) (Table 13.2).

Systemic Therapy

Recent reviews[90,91] summarize milestones that brought to current gold standard first-line systemic therapy, based on antifolate pemetrexed and cisplatin, which achieves best overall survival (median 12 months with a response rate around 40%) and quality of life. The role of pemetrexed in maintenance therapy after antifolate/platinum regimen is currently evaluated (www.clinicaltrial.gov: NCT01085630) and an ongoing phase III randomized study (NCT00651456) will determine whether current gold standard therapy can be improved by anti-VEGF antibody bevacizumab.

While chemotherapy with cisplatin and pemetrexed is now accepted as standard frontline treatment, the question of second-line treatment remains. There are few ongoing/recently terminated phase III studies (status September 2011) for second-line therapy. The first tested the effect of vorinostat, a histone deacetylase inhibitor, versus placebo (NCT00128102). The results were presented at ESMO ECCO meeting 2011 by Lee Krug. The study was negative. In another phase III trial, thalidomide has also been tested with no evidence of benefit on progression-free or overall survival.[92]

In an ongoing phase III trial, patients are randomized to receive placebo plus best investigator's choice (doxorubicin or gemcitabine or vinorelbine) or NGR-hTNF, a TNF targeted to tumor vasculature antigen CD13, plus best investigator's choice (NCT01098266). NGR-hTNF has been shown in experimental models to increase tumor cell doxorubicin content[93] but has no cytotoxic activity on tumor cells per se.[94]

Currently there are 76 phase interventional phase II trials with known recruiting status: 25 of them are still open. Fourteen of the open trials (Table 13.2) test targeted therapies (reviewed in[90,91,95–97]) either in combination with chemotherapy or alone.

Although mesothelioma is not considered particularly immunogenic, immunotherapy investigation in mesothelioma has been fostered by observations (reviewed in[98]) that immune system often recognizes mesothelioma. For the time being, there is only one completed phase II trial where immunotherapy has been explored concurrently with pemetrexed and cisplatin.[97] In this trial, highly expressed antigen mesothelin, is targeted by MORAb-009, a high affinity chimeric (mouse/human) monoclonal antibody which kills mesothelin expressing cell lines via antibody-dependent cellular cytotoxicity and inhibits the binding of mesothelin to its ligand CA-125.[99]

For the time being, no validated predictive markers exist for mesothelioma chemotherapy although low thymidylate synthase protein levels were predictive for improved survival in a retrospective analysis of patients who received pemetrexed[100] and NF2, which has been recently used for targeted mTOR therapy selection in preclinical studies[101] and is currently being evaluated in an ongoing clinical trial evaluating everolimus.

CONCLUSION

Malignant pleural mesothelioma continues to be a clinical challenge and its incidence will continue to increase worldwide. Once diagnosed with pleural mesothelioma, patients nearly invariably die of the disease. While the benefit of chemotherapy for advanced disease has been firmly established, many other aspects of treatment continue to be controversial, in particular, with regard to surgery and radiotherapy. However, the best survival data are reported from groups using multimodality treatment including surgery for patients qualifying from a tumor stage and functional perspective. Therefore, efforts should focus on improving staging systems. Translational studies should be included with the final aim of finding reliable markers for response to therapy.

Despite both, the increase in basic biologic knowledge and the fact that many new agents have reached various stages of development, the number of new treatments that have been approved for patients has not increased. Being mesothelioma a rare disease, the number of patients is limiting and more innovative trial designs (such as multi-arm multi-stage trials[102]) using cooperative platforms to eliminate less effective treatments may be the best way forward.

ACKNOWLEDGMENTS
We thank Drs A. Soltermann and Frauenfelder and Prof. Weder for critical reading of the manuscript. The work is supported by the Stiftung fuer Angewandte Krebsforschung, Krebsliga Zurich, Swiss National Science Foundation, and ESMO fellowship. The contribution of all collaborators in Task Force Mesothelioma Zurich is kindly acknowledged.

REFERENCES
1. Park EK, Takahashi K, Hoshuyama T, et al. Global magnitude of reported and unreported mesothelioma. Environ Health Perspect 2011; 119: 514–18.
2. Testa JR, Cheung M, Pei J, et al. Germline BAP1 mutations predispose to malignant mesothelioma. Nat Genet 2011; 43: 1022–5.
3. Marinaccio A, Binazzi A, Cauzillo G, et al. Analysis of latency time and its determinants in asbestos related malignant mesothelioma cases of the Italian register. Eur J Cancer 2007; 43: 2722–8.
4. Baris YI, Grandjean P. Prospective study of mesothelioma mortality in Turkish villages with exposure to fibrous zeolite. J Natl Cancer Inst 2006; 98: 414–17.
5. Jaurand MC. Mechanisms of fiber-induced genotoxicity. Environ Health Perspect 1997; 105(Suppl 5): 1073–84.
6. Mossman B, Light W, Wei E. Asbestos: mechanisms of toxicity and carcinogenicity in the respiratory tract. Annu Rev Pharmacol Toxicol 1983; 23: 595–615.
7. Miserocchi G, Sancini G, Mantegazza F, Chiappino G. Translocation pathways for inhaled asbestos fibers. Environ Health 2008; 7: 4.
8. Donaldson K, Murphy FA, Duffin R, Poland CA. Asbestos, carbon nanotubes and the pleural mesothelium: a review of the hypothesis regarding the role of long fibre retention in the parietal pleura, inflammation and mesothelioma. Part Fibre Toxicol 2010; 7: 5.
9. Kamp DW. Asbestos-induced lung diseases: an update. Transl Res 2009; 153: 143–52.
10. Heintz NH, Janssen-Heininger YM, Mossman BT. Asbestos, lung cancers, and mesotheliomas: from molecular approaches to targeting tumor survival pathways. Am J Respir Cell Mol Biol 2010; 42: 133–9.
11. Sekido Y. Genomic abnormalities and signal transduction dysregulation in malignant mesothelioma cells. Cancer Sci 2010; 101: 1–6.
12. Broaddus VC, Everitt JI, Black B, Kane AB. Non-neoplastic and neoplastic pleural endpoints following fiber exposure. J Toxicol Environ Health B Crit Rev 2011; 14: 153–78.
13. Dostert C, Petrilli V, Van Bruggen R, et al. Innate immune activation through Nalp3 inflammasome sensing of asbestos and silica. Science 2008; 320: 674–7.
14. Wang NS. Anatomy of the pleura. Clin Chest Med 1998; 19: 229–40.
15. Pietruska JR, Kane AB. SV40 oncoproteins enhance asbestos-induced DNA double-strand breaks and abrogate senescence in murine mesothelial cells. Cancer Res 2007; 67: 3637–45.
16. Kuilman T, Michaloglou C, Vredeveld LC, et al. Oncogene-induced senescence relayed by an interleukin-dependent inflammatory network. Cell 2008; 133: 1019–31.
17. Mutsaers SE. Mesothelial cells: their structure, function and role in serosal repair. Respirology 2002; 7: 171–91.
18. Beachy PA, Karhadkar SS, Berman DM. Tissue repair and stem cell renewal in carcinogenesis. Nature 2004; 432: 324–31.
19. Robinson C, Walsh A, Larma I, et al. MexTAg mice exposed to asbestos develop cancer that faithfully replicates key features of the pathogenesis of human mesothelioma. Eur J Cancer 2011; 47: 151–61.
20. Lansley SM, Searles RG, Hoi A, et al. Mesothelial cell differention into osteoblast- and adipocyte-like cells. J Cell Mol Med 2011; 15: 2095–105.
21. Frei C, Opitz I, Soltermann A, et al. Pleural mesothelioma side populations have a precursor phenotype. Carcinogenesis 2011; 32: 1324–32.
22. Glinsky GV, Berezovska O, Glinskii AB. Microarray analysis identifies a death-from-cancer signature predicting therapy failure in patients with multiple types of cancer. J Clin Invest 2005; 115: 1503–21.

23. Uematsu K, Kanazawa S, You L, et al. Wnt pathway activation in mesothelioma: evidence of Dishevelled overexpression and transcriptional activity of beta-catenin. Cancer Res 2003; 63: 4547–51.

24. Abutaily AS, Collins JE, Roche WR. Cadherins, catenins and APC in pleural malignant mesothelioma. J Pathol 2003; 201: 355–62.

25. Matsuyama A, Hisaoka M, Iwasaki M, et al. TLE1 expression in malignant mesothelioma. Virchows Arch 2010; 457: 577–83.

26. Lee AY, He B, You L, et al. Expression of the secreted frizzled-related protein gene family is downregulated in human mesothelioma. Oncogene 2004; 23: 6672–6.

27. Gee GV, Koestler DC, Christensen BC, et al. Downregulated MicroRNAs in the differential diagnosis of malignant pleural mesothelioma. Int J Cancer 2010; 127: 2859–69.

28. Graziani I, Eliasz S, De Marco MA, et al. Opposite effects of Notch-1 and Notch-2 on mesothelioma cell survival under hypoxia are exerted through the Akt pathway. Cancer Res 2008; 68: 9678–85.

29. Kimura K, Toyooka S, Tsukuda K, et al. The aberrant promoter methylation of BMP3b and BMP6 in malignant pleural mesotheliomas. Oncol Rep 2008; 20: 1265–8.

30. Kratzke RA, Otterson GA, Lincoln CE, et al. Immunohistochemical analysis of the p16INK4 cyclin-dependent kinase inhibitor in malignant mesothelioma. J Natl Cancer Inst 1995; 87: 1870–5.

31. Yang CT, You L, Yeh CC, et al. Adenovirus-mediated p14(ARF) gene transfer in human mesothelioma cells. J Natl Cancer Inst 2000; 92: 636–41.

32. Cheng JQ, Jhanwar SC, Klein WM, et al. p16 alterations and deletion mapping of 9p21-p22 in malignant mesothelioma. Cancer Res 1994; 54: 5547–51.

33. Xio S, Li D, Vijg J, et al. Codeletion of p15 and p16 in primary malignant mesothelioma. Oncogene 1995; 11: 511–15.

34. Prins JB, Williamson KA, Kamp MM, et al. The gene for the cyclin-dependent-kinase-4 inhibitor, CDKN2A, is preferentially deleted in malignant mesothelioma. Int J Cancer 1998; 75: 649–53.

35. Toyooka S, Pass HI, Shivapurkar N, et al. Aberrant methylation and simian virus 40 tag sequences in malignant mesothelioma. Cancer Res 2001; 61: 5727–30.

36. Wong L, Zhou J, Anderson D, Kratzke RA. Inactivation of p16INK4a expression in malignant mesothelioma by methylation. Lung Cancer 2002; 38: 131–6.

37. Destro A, Ceresoli GL, Baryshnikova E, et al. Gene methylation in pleural mesothelioma: correlations with clinico-pathological features and patient's follow-up. Lung Cancer 2008; 59: 369–76.

38. Bianchi AB, Mitsunaga SI, Cheng JQ, et al. High frequency of inactivating mutations in the neurofibromatosis type 2 gene (NF2) in primary malignant mesotheliomas. Proc Natl Acad Sci USA 1995; 92: 10854–8.

39. Sekido Y, Pass HI, Bader S, et al. Neurofibromatosis type 2 (NF2) gene is somatically mutated in mesothelioma but not in lung cancer. Cancer Res 1995; 55: 1227–31.

40. Deguen B, Goutebroze L, Giovannini M, et al. Heterogeneity of mesothelioma cell lines as defined by altered genomic structure and expression of the NF2 gene. Int J Cancer 1998; 77: 554–60.

41. Jin H, Sperka T, Herrlich P, Morrison H. Tumorigenic transformation by CPI-17 through inhibition of a merlin phosphatase. Nature 2006; 442: 576–9.

42. Tang X, Jang SW, Wang X, et al. Akt phosphorylation regulates the tumour-suppressor merlin through ubiquitination and degradation. Nat Cell Biol 2007; 9: 1199–207.

43. Thurneysen C, Opitz I, Kurtz S, et al. Functional inactivation of NF2/merlin in human mesothelioma. Lung Cancer 2009; 64: 140–7.

44. Opitz I, Soltermann A, Abaecherli M, et al. PTEN expression is a strong predictor of survival in mesothelioma patients. Eur J Cardiothorac Surg 2008; 33: 502–6.

45. Fleury-Feith J, Lecomte C, Renier A, et al. Hemizygosity of Nf2 is associated with increased susceptibility to asbestos-induced peritoneal tumours. Oncogene 2003; 22: 3799–805.

46. Lecomte C, Andujar P, Renier A, et al. Similar tumor suppressor gene alteration profiles in asbestos-induced murine and human mesothelioma. Cell Cycle 2005; 4: 1862–9.

47. Jongsma J, van Montfort E, Vooijs M, et al. A conditional mouse model for malignant mesothelioma. Cancer Cell 2008; 13: 261–71.

48. Kinzler KW, Vogelstein B. Cancer-susceptibility genes. Gatekeepers and caretakers. Nature 1997; 386: 761–3.

49. Li W, You L, Cooper J, et al. Merlin/NF2 suppresses tumorigenesis by inhibiting the E3 ubiquitin ligase CRL4(DCAF1) in the nucleus. Cell 2010; 140: 477–90.

50. Lau YK, Murray LB, Houshmandi SS, et al. Merlin is a potent inhibitor of glioma growth. Cancer Res 2008; 68: 5733–42.

51. Zhao B, Lei QY, Guan KL. The Hippo-YAP pathway: new connections between regulation of organ size and cancer. Curr Opin Cell Biol 2008; 20: 638–46.

52. Dong J, Feldmann G, Huang J, et al. Elucidation of a universal size-control mechanism in Drosophila and mammals. Cell 2007; 130: 1120–33.

53. Slee EA, Harte MT, Kluck RM, et al. Ordering the cytochrome c-initiated caspase cascade: hierarchical activation of caspases-2, -3, -6, -7, -8, and -10 in a caspase-9-dependent manner. J Cell Biol 1999; 281–92.

54. Zhang J, Ji JY, Yu M, et al. YAP-dependent induction of amphiregulin identifies a non-cell-autonomous component of the Hippo pathway. Nat Cell Biol 2009; 11: 1444–50.

55. Striedinger K, VandenBerg SR, Baia GS, et al. The neurofibromatosis 2 tumor suppressor gene product, merlin, regulates human meningioma cell growth by signaling through YAP. Neoplasia 2008; 10: 1204–12.

56. Yokoyama T, Osada H, Murakami H, et al. YAP1 is involved in mesothelioma development and negatively regulated by Merlin through phosphorylation. Carcinogenesis 2008; 29: 2139–46.

57. Murakami H, Mizuno T, Taniguchi T, et al. LATS2 Is a tumor suppressor gene of malignant mesothelioma. Cancer Res 2011; 71: 873–83.

58. Bott M, Brevet M, Taylor BS, et al. The nuclear deubiquitinase BAP1 is commonly inactivated by somatic mutations and 3p21.1 losses in malignant pleural mesothelioma. Nat Genet 2011; 43: 668–72.

59. Scherpereel A, Astoul P, Baas P, et al. Guidelines of the European Respiratory Society and the European Society of Thoracic Surgeons for the management of malignant pleural mesothelioma. Eur Respir J 2010; 35: 479–95.

60. Hollevoet K, Nackaerts K, Gosselin R, et al. Soluble mesothelin, megakaryocyte potentiating factor, and osteopontin as markers of patient response and outcome in mesothelioma. J Thorac Oncol 2011; 6: 1930–7.

61. Luo L, Shi HZ, Liang QL, et al. Diagnostic value of soluble mesothelin-related peptides for malignant mesothelioma: a meta-analysis. Respir Med 2010; 104: 149–56.

62. Hollevoet K, Nackaerts K, Thimpont J, et al. Diagnostic performance of soluble mesothelin and megakaryocyte potentiating factor in mesothelioma. Am J Respir Crit Care Med 2010; 181: 620–5.

63. Krug LM, Pass HI, Rusch VW, et al. Multicenter phase II trial of neoadjuvant pemetrexed plus cisplatin followed by extrapleural pneumonectomy and radiation for malignant pleural mesothelioma. J Clin Oncol 2009; 27: 3007–13.

64. de Perrot M, Feld R, Cho BC, et al. Trimodality therapy with induction chemotherapy followed by extrapleural pneumonectomy and adjuvant high-dose hemithoracic radiation for malignant pleural mesothelioma. J Clin Oncol 2009; 27: 1413–18.

65. Metintas M, Ucgun I, Elbek O, et al. Computed tomography features in malignant pleural mesothelioma and other commonly seen pleural diseases. Eur J Radiol 2002; 41: 1–9.

66. Yamamuro M, Gerbaudo VH, Gill RR, et al. Morphologic and functional imaging of malignant pleural mesothelioma. Eur J Radiol 2007; 64: 356–66.

67. Heelan RT, Rusch VW, Begg CB, et al. Staging of malignant pleural mesothelioma: comparison of CT and MR imaging. AJR Am J Roentgenol 1999; 172: 1039–47.

68. Zahid I, Sharif S, Routledge T, Scarci M. What is the best way to diagnose and stage malignant pleural mesothelioma? Interact CardioVasc Thorac Surg 2011; 12: 254–9.

69. Byrne MJ, Nowak AK. Modified RECIST criteria for assessment of response in malignant pleural mesothelioma. Ann Oncol 2004; 15: 257–60.

70. Armato SG, Ogarek JL, Starkey A, et al. Variability in mesothelioma tumor response classification. AJR 2006; 186: 1000–6.

71. Frauenfelder T, Tutic M, Weder W, et al. Volumetry: an alternative to assess therapy response for malignant pleural mesothelioma? Eur Respir J 2011; 38: 162–8.

72. Ceresoli GL, Chiti A, Zucali PA, et al. Early response evaluation in malignant pleural mesothelioma by positron emission tomography with [18F]fluorodeoxyglucose. J Clin Oncol 2006; 24: 4587–93.

73. Sugarbaker DJ, Jaklitsch MT, Bueno R, et al. Prevention, early detection, and management of complications after 328 consecutive extrapleural pneumonectomies. J Thorac Cardiovasc Surg 2004; 128: 138–46.

74. Rice D, Rusch V, Pass H, et al. Recommendations for uniform definitions of surgical techniques for malignant pleural mesothelioma: a consensus report of the international association for the study of lung cancer international staging committee and the international mesothelioma interest group. J Thorac Oncol 2011; 6: 1304–12.

75. Treasure T, Lang-Lazdunski L, Waller D, et al. Extra-pleural pneumonectomy versus no extra-pleural pneumonectomy for patients with malignant pleural mesothelioma: clinical outcomes of the Mesothelioma and Radical Surgery (MARS) randomised feasibility study. Lancet Oncol 2011; 12: 763–72.

76. Weder W, Stahel RA, Baas P, et al. The MARS feasibility trial: conclusions not supported by data. Lancet Oncol 2011; 12: 1093–4; author reply 4–5.

77. Cao CQ, Yan TD, Bannon PG, McCaughan BC. A systematic review of extrapleural pneumonectomy for malignant pleural mesothelioma. J Thorac Oncol 2010; 5: 1692–703.

78. Flores RM, Pass HI, Seshan VE, et al. Extrapleural pneumonectomy versus pleurectomy/decortication in the surgical management of malignant pleural mesothelioma: results in 663 patients. J Thorac Cardiovasc Surg 2008; 135: 620–6; 6 e1–3.

79. Flores RM. Surgical options in malignant pleural mesothelioma: extrapleural pneumonectomy or pleurectomy/decortication. Semin Thorac Cardiovasc Surg 2009; 21: 149–53.

80. Pass HI, Temeck BK, Kranda K, Steinberg SM, Feuerstein IR. Preoperative tumor volume is associated with outcome in malignant pleural mesothelioma. J Thorac Cardiovasc Surg 1998; 115: 310–17; discussion 7–8.

81. David R. Surgery for malignant pleural mesothelioma. Ann Diagn Pathol 2009; 13: 65–72.

82. Tilleman TR, Richards WG, Zellos L, et al. Extrapleural pneumonectomy followed by intracavitary intraoperative hyperthermic cisplatin with pharmacologic cytoprotection for treatment of malignant pleural mesothelioma: a phase II prospective study. J Thorac Cardiovasc Surg 2009; 138: 405–11.

83. Mujoomdar AA, Sugarbaker DJ. Hyperthermic chemoperfusion for the treatment of malignant pleural mesothelioma. Semin Thorac Cardiovasc Surg 2008; 20: 298–304.

84. Friedberg JS. Photodynamic therapy for malignant pleural mesothelioma: the future of treatment? Expert Rev Respir Med 2011; 5: 49–63.
85. Sterman DH, Recio A, Vachani A, et al. Long-term follow-up of patients with malignant pleural mesothelioma receiving high-dose adenovirus herpes simplex thymidine kinase/ganciclovir suicide gene therapy. Clin Cancer Res 2005; 11: 7444–53.
86. Ung YC, Yu E, Falkson C, et al. The role of radiation therapy in malignant pleural mesothelioma: a systematic review. Radiother Oncol 2006; 80: 13–18.
87. Baldini EH. Radiation therapy options for malignant pleural mesothelioma. Semin Thorac Cardiovasc Surg 2009; 21: 159–63.
88. Zauderer MG, Krug LM. The evolution of multimodality therapy for malignant pleural mesothelioma. Curr Treat Options Oncol 2011; 12: 163–72.
89. Rusch VW, Rosenzweig K, Venkatraman E, et al. A phase II trial of surgical resection and adjuvant high-dose hemi-thoracic radiation for malignant pleural mesothelioma. J Thorac Cardiovasc Surg 2001; 122: 788–95.
90. Campbell NP, Kindler HL. Update on malignant pleural mesothelioma. Semin Respir Crit Care Med 2011; 32: 102–10.
91. van Meerbeeck JP, Scherpereel A, Surmont VF, Baas P. Malignant pleural mesothelioma: the standard of care and challenges for future management. Crit Rev Oncol Hematol 2011; 78: 92–111.
92. Baas P, Buikhuisen W, Dalesio O, et al. A multicenter, randomized phase III maintenance study of thalidomide (arm A) versus observation arm (arm B) in patients with malignant pleural mesothelioma (MPM) after induction chemotherapy. 2011 Asco Annual Meeting. Chicago. J Clin Oncol 2011. 29(Suppl): abstract 7006.
93. Curnis F, Sacchi A, Corti A. Improving chemotherapeutic drug penetration in tumors by vascular targeting and barrier alteration. J Clin Invest 2002; 110: 475–82.
94. Sacchi A, Gasparri A, Gallo-Stampino C, et al. Synergistic antitumor activity of cisplatin, paclitaxel, and gemcitabine with tumor vasculature-targeted tumor necrosis factor-alpha. Clin Cancer Res 2006; 12: 175–82.
95. Jakobsen JN, Sorensen JB. Review on clinical trials of targeted treatments in malignant mesothelioma. Cancer Chemother Pharmacol 2011; 68: 1–15.
96. Bagia M, Nowak AK. Novel targeted therapies and vaccination strategies for mesothelioma. Curr Treat Options Oncol 2011; 12: 149–62.
97. Kelly RJ, Sharon E, Hassan R. Chemotherapy and targeted therapies for unresectable malignant mesothelioma. Lung Cancer 2011; 73: 256–63.
98. Gregoire M. What's the place of immunotherapy in malignant mesothelioma treatments? Cell Adh Migr 2010; 4: 153–61.
99. Hassan R, Ebel W, Routhier EL, et al. Preclinical evaluation of MORAb-009, a chimeric antibody targeting tumor-associated mesothelin. Cancer Immun 2007; 7: 20.
100. Righi L, Papotti MG, Ceppi P, et al. Thymidylate synthase but not excision repair cross-complementation group 1 tumor expression predicts outcome in patients with malignant pleural mesothelioma treated with pemetrexed-based chemotherapy. J Clin Oncol 2010; 28: 1534–9.
101. Lopez-Lago MA, Okada T, Murillo MM, Socci N, Giancotti FG. Loss of the tumor suppressor gene NF2, encoding merlin, constitutively activates integrin-dependent mTORC1 signaling. Mol Cell Biol 2009; 29: 4235–49.
102. Parmar MK, Barthel FM, Sydes M, et al. Speeding up the evaluation of new agents in cancer. J Natl Cancer Inst 2008; 100: 1204–14.
103. Van Schil PE, Baas P, Gaafar R, et al. Trimodality therapy for malignant pleural mesothelioma: results from an EORTC phase II multicentre trial. Eur Respir J 2010; 36: 1362–9.
104. Kaufman AJ, Flores RM. Surgical treatment of malignant pleural mesothelioma. Curr Treat Options Oncol 2011; 12: 201–16.
105. Weder W, Opitz I, Stahel R. Multimodality strategies in malignant pleural mesothelioma. Semin Thorac Cardiovasc Surg 2009; 21: 172–6.

14 | Thymic tumors

Enrico Ruffini, Pier Luigi Filosso, Paolo Lausi, and Alberto Oliaro

INTRODUCTION

Thymic malignancies are rare mediastinal tumors with an incidence of 0.15 per 100,000 person-years.[1] They comprise thymomas and thymic carcinomas, which have been only recently differentiated. Studies on thymic malignancies date back to early 70s and are based upon case series or retrospective monoinstitutional reviews. Until recently, progress in research and management in thymic malignancies have been relatively slow as compared to other neoplasms. Nonetheless, the first decade of the third millennium has witnessed a tremendous momentum in the study of thymic malignancies which may be summarized in one single word: international collaboration.

The aim of this chapter is to present the state of the art and the most recent acquisitions in management and research in thymic malignancies and to give the reader an overview of the current knowledge and common efforts for the management of these rare tumors.

CLINICAL PRESENTATION AND DIAGNOSIS
Clinical Presentation

Thymomas are the most common anterior mediastinal compartment neoplasms. The disease has usually a slow-growing pattern and most patients are between 40 and 60 years of age with no difference between sexes. The age of onset differs according to the presence of myasthenia gravis (MG): thymoma patients with MG are younger (30–40 years) than thymoma patients without MG (60–70 years).[2-4] Thirty to fifty percent of the patients are asymptomatic at presentation, the most common symptoms being cough, chest pain, or signs of superior vena vava (SVC) syndrome. Various autoimmune diseases (so-called parathymic syndromes) are associated to thymic malignancies. Among these myasthenia gravis is the most common, and about 30–50% of thymomas have an associated MG, while about 10–15% of patients with MG have an associated thymoma.[5] Other associated parathymic syndromes have been described (Table 14.1) occurring in about 25–30% of the patients. Finally, about 10–15% of patients with thymoma will present a second primary malignancy, a higher percentage than in the general population.[6,7]

Diagnosis
Clinical and Imaging Techniques

Diagnosis includes clinical examination, radiologic imaging, and cyto-histologic biopsy in selected cases. Clinical examination may reveal signs and symptoms of associated parathymic syndromes (MG, red blood cell aplasia, hypogammaglobulinemia) or of local invasion (SVC syndrome). In these patients, radiologic imaging with chest X ray and CT scan (with intravenous contrast) are usually diagnostic, evidencing an anterior mediastinal mass. CT scan is still considered the imaging modality of choice in the initial assessment as well as in the follow-up of patients with thymic malignancies. New CT techniques provide a rapid acquisition of thin-section slices with the possibility of giving high-quality images and remodeling in multiple plans. CT scan characteristics[8] include a well-defined round or oval mass, anterior to the great vessels and the ascending aorta and in close proximity to the great veins (SVC and left innominate vein) (Fig. 14.1). The mass may present cystic, or with calcification (15% of the cases), which is a useful differential diagnostic sign with other anterior mediastinal lesions. A well-defined capsule is identified in early stage thymomas with a clear cleavage plan with the surrounding structures. Invasive thymomas tend to wrap all the mediastinal structures, and present signs of local invasion (abutment>50% of the involved mediastinal structure with loss of fat plan, infiltration of surrounding fat plane, adjacent lung alterations, direct vascular endoluminal invasion) and other characteristics (large size, lobulated contours, calcifications, pleural effusion) (Fig. 14.2).[9] Pleural nodules ranging from few millimeters up to several centimeters in diameters are evident in case of stage IVa thymomas with or without pleural effusion. Diaphragmatic elevation may be a sign of phrenic nerve invasion or phrenic nerve resection after surgery. Magnetic resonance imaging (MRI) is of little utility in diagnosis of thymic malignancies, except

Table 14.1 Thymic Malignancies' Associated Disorders

Neuromuscular
   Myasthenia Gravis[a], Myositis, Myotonic dystrophy
Hematologic
   Red cell aplasia/hypoplasia[b]
   Erytrocytosis
   Pancytopenia
   Acute leukemia
   Agranulocytosis
   Hemolytic anemia
   Multiple myeloma
Immune system
   Hypogammaglobulinemia[b]
   T-cell deficiency syndrome
Collagen diseases
   Systemic lupus erythematosus[b]
   Thyroiditis[b]
   Polymyositis
   Scleroderma
   Sarcoidosis
   Raynaud's disease
Endocrine
   Cushing's syndrome[c]
   Hashimoto's thyroiditis
   Addison's disease
   Multiple Endocrine Neoplasia (MEN) 1 and 2[c]
Dermatologic
   Chronic mucocutaneous candidiasis
   Pemphigus
   Alopecia
Renal
   Nephrotic syndrome
   Minimal change nephropathy

[a]Most common.
[b]Common.
[c]Associated with Neuroendocrine tumors of the thymus (NETT).

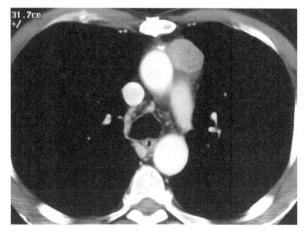

Figure 14.1 CT scan of a thymoma presenting as a well-defined oval mass in the anterior mediastinum.

in case of suspected infiltration of the heart and great vessels. Finally, positron emission tomography (PET) scan has been evaluated in its ability to differentiate thymic hyperplasia from thymoma, low-risk versus high-risk thymomas, and thymoma versus thymic carcinoma. A study on 25 consecutive patients with thymic pathology (hyperplasia, thymoma, recurrent thymoma) indicated that PET was useful in differentiating thymic hyperplasia from thymoma (but fails to recognize ectopic thymic tissue) and thymoma

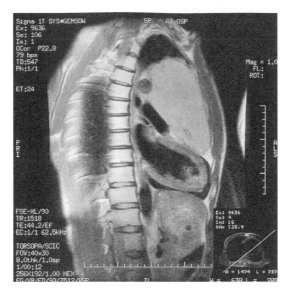

Figure 14.2 CT scan of an invasive thymoma with signs of infiltration of the mediastinal tissue.

from thymic carcinoma.[10] Two additional studies[11,12] on 36 and 46 patients with thymic malignancies suggested that a significant correlation exists between standard uptake value (SUV) and the histologic subtypes, when divided into low-risk (A, AB, B1) and high-risk (B2, B3, and thymic carcinoma) tumors. There are however negative studies which failed to differentiate between non-invasive and invasive thymomas, and between thymoma and thymic hyperplasia.[13,14] A recent survey conducted among ESTS members[15] indicates that 50% of the interviewed centers use PET or integrated PET–CT in the preoperative assessment of thymic tumors.

Finally, imaging techniques are useful in the follow-up of resected patients. Optimal technique and the frequency of follow-up imaging have not been clarified yet. A recent ITMIG consensus statement[16] proposed a yearly CT scan of the thorax for the first five years after surgery, followed by a chest X ray alternating with CT scan on a yearly basis. Advanced stage thymomas and thymic carcinomas should probably be followed-up more frequently, with a six-month CT scan for the first three years. MRI might be used instead of CT scan to reduce the radiation doses, particularly in young patients. There is no current role for routine PET scan in the follow-up patients with thymic tumors, although PET scan may be occasionally indicated in case of suspected recurrence not evidenced at CT/MRI.

Histologic Diagnosis
When imaging techniques are equivocal for a diagnosis of a thymic tumor, histological diagnosis is required. In the past it was suggested that every anterior mediastinal lesion should be biopsied before final treatment to obtain a definite diagnosis. In more recent years, however, refinements in imaging techniques resulted in an improved diagnostic yield, and the need for a mediastinal biopsy dramatically decreased. In a recent survey among ESTS members,[15] 90% of the interviewed centers stated that they do not routinely look for a histological confirmation of a suspected thymoma. There is a general agreement, however, that biopsy should be reserved in case of undefined CT findings which may suggest lymphoma, or in case of unresectable tumors before induction chemotherapy or definite chemoradiotherapy.[17]

Mediastinal biopsy may be obtained with different techniques: (1) non-surgical biopsies that include fine-needle aspiration (FNA) biopsy or needle core biopsy using transthoracic ultrasound (US) or computed tomography (CT), and (2) surgical biopsies that include anterior mediastinotomy (Chamberlain's procedure), video-assisted thoracic surgery (VATS), and minithoracotomy. Sensitivity of the different procedures is high, on average; it is lower using FNA (60%) than surgical techniques (>98%).[18,19] Complication rate is low, and pneumothorax is the most common complication in non-surgical techniques, occurring in 5–30% of the cases, depending upon the location of the mass. Complications of surgical procedures are minimal. Seeding of the pleural space or the biopsy site has been a concern in the past,[20] but there is no evidence to support that in the literature.[21]

STAGING SYSTEMS, HISTOLOGY, AND PROGNOSTIC FACTORS IN THYMIC MALIGNANCIES

By definition, a prognostic factor is a variable that can account for some of the heterogeneity associated with the expected course and outcome of a tumor. Prognostic factors are customarily divided in tumor-related, host-related, and environmental-related factors, all of which have different impact on the patient's outcome.[22]

One of the most important prognostic factors is the anatomic extent of the tumor, which is the stage. Unfortunately, stage alone is not sufficient to reliably predict prognosis and for most neoplasms a more complete prognostic model is accepted instead of the simpler TNM staging system as valid prognosticator. Other tumor-related prognostic factors include histology and tumor biology which reflect in the molecular and genetic tumor characteristics.

Staging Systems

The issue of stage in thymoma is therefore intimately connected with the search for significant and validated prognostic factors. Unlike other malignancies, a reliable staging system for thymomas is yet to be defined.

The first staging system for thymomas was proposed in 1978 by Bergh and associates[23] and comprised three stages (capsulated, invasion of the mediastinal fat, and invasion into the surrounding organs or intrathoracic metastases). In 1981, Masaoka[24] proposed the four-tiered system based upon the surgical-anatomic extent of the tumor. In 1994, the classification was revised by Masaoka and Koga[25] based on a patient population of 79 patients (Table 14.2). Modifications of the Masaoka–Koga systems were suggested, including subdivision of stage I into Ia and Ib on the basis of adherences without microscopic invasion, and subdivision of stage III by the presence/absence of great vessels invasion but in the end the system was not modified. In France, many centers have adopted the Groupe d'Etudes des Tumeurs Thymiques (GETT) staging system based upon both the anatomical extent (similar to Masaoka) and the extent and completeness of surgical resection.[26]

Unlike Masaoka and Masaoka-modified classifications which are based upon the anatomic extension of the disease, in the 90s several groups tried to adapt the standard TNM system to thymomas with conflicting results. All TNM-based staging systems basically adopted the same T descriptor (based upon the Masaoka or Masaoka–Koga system) as well as the N and M descriptors although the stage grouping was slightly different. In the most credited system from Yamakawa and Masaoka (Y–M system),[27] the T descriptor parallels that of Masaoka, and the N and M descriptors were grouped together into stage IVb (Table 14.3). Tsuchiya in 1994[28] proposed the pathologic TNM and staging NCCHJ system using a Masaoka/Koga-derived T descriptor, and N and M descriptors similar to Y–M system. The stage grouping included three IV stage subgroups (IVa, IVb, and IVc), while N1 disease resulted in one-step stage upgrade. Bedini,[29] from the National Cancer Institute in Italy, recognizes three stages (stage I, locally restricted disease, stage II locally advanced disease, and stage III, systemic disease) and further incorporated the concept of residual disease into the staging system (R0/R1, R2a, R2b). Finally, in 2004 the WHO Consensus Committee[30] proposed its TNM staging system (Table 14.3) which is similar to the Y–M system except for two points: (1) histologic invasion into mediastinal pleura is T3, and (2) N1 disease upgrades stage to stage III. Of all the aforementioned TNM systems, only the Y–M system has undergone validation studies.

Table 14.2 The Masaoka Staging System and its Update (Masaoka–Koga) for Thymic Malignancies

Masaoka Staging System (1981)	
Stage I	Macroscopically completely encapsulated and microscopically no capsular invasion
Stage II	1. Macroscopic invasion into surrounding fatty tissue or mediastinal pleura or 2. Microscopic invasion into capsule
Stage III	Macroscopic invasion into neighboring organ, i.e., pericardium, great vessels, or lung
Stage IVa	Pleural or pericardial dissemination
Stage IVb	Lymphogenous or hematogenous metastasis
Masaoka–Koga staging system (1994)	
Stage I	Grossly and microscopically completely encapsulated tumor
Stage IIa	Microscopic transcapsular invasion
Stage IIb	Macroscopic invasion into thymic or surrounding fatty tissue or Grossly adherent to but not breaking through mediastinal pleura or pericardium
Stage III	Macroscopic invasion into neighboring organ, i.e., pericardium, great vessels, or lung
Stage IVa	Pleural or pericardial metastases
Stage IVb	Lymphogenous or hematogenous metastases

The local extension of the disease (T descriptor) which forms the basis of the Masaoka and Masaoka–Koga system is an excellent descriptor in case of thymomas, where the rate of lymphatic and distant metastasis is negligible (2% for N, 1.2% for M).[31] In thymic carcinomas (including neuroendocrine thymic tumors, NETT), however, up to one-third of the patients present with lymphatic or distant metastasis (25% for N and 12% for M),[32] and for these patients a TNM system is more appropriate. The increasing number of patients with thymic carcinoma who are reported in the most recent series calls for a revision of the current staging system which would incorporate a TNM system.

ITMIG recently summarized the conclusions of consensus statements and workshops to provide clarity in the ambiguities that have emerged in the Masaoka and Masaoka–Koga systems.[33]

Histology

The second most important tumor-related prognostic factor is histology. Thymomas are tumors arising from the epithelial cells of the thymus, and the lymphocytes are usually reactive to tumor proliferation.

Table 14.3 TNM classifications of Thymic Malignancies

TNM classification by Yamakawa and Masaoka (Y–M TNM staging system)			
T factor			
T1: Macroscopically completely encapsulated and microscopically no capsular invasion			
T2: Macroscopically showing adhesion or invasion into surrounding fatty tissue or bv mediastinal pleura, or microscopic invasion into capsule			
T3: Invasion into neighboring organs such as pericardium, great vessels and lung			
T4: Pleural or pericardial dissemination			
N factor			
N0: No lymph node metastasis			
N1: Metastasis to anterior mediastinal lymph nodes			
N2: Metastasis to intrathoracic lymph nodes except anterior mediastinal lymph nodes			
N3: Metastasis to extrathoracic lymph nodes			
M factor			
M0: No hematogenous metastasis			
M1: Hematogenous metastasis			
Stage I	T1	N0	M0
Stage II	T2	N0	M0
Stage III	T3	N0	M0
Stage IVa	T4	N0	M0
Stage IVb	Any T	N1,2,3	M0
	Any T	Any N	M1
TNM classification by WHO			
T factor			
T1: Tumor completely encapsulated			
T2: Tumor invades pericapsular connettive tissue			
T3: Tumor invades into neighboring organs such as pericardium, mediastinal pleura, thoracic wall, great vessels and lung			
T4: Tumor with pleural or pericardial dissemination			
N factor			
N0: No lymph node metastasis			
N1: Metastasis to anterior mediastinal lymph nodes			
N2: Metastasis in other intrathoracic lymph nodes excluding anterior mediastinal nodes			
N3: Metastasis in scalene and/or supraclavicular lymph nodes			
M factor			
M0: No distant organ metastasis			
M1: Distant organ metastasis			
Stage I	T1	N0	M0
Stage II	T2	N0	M0
Stage III	T1, T2	N1	M0
	T3	N0,1	M0
Stage IV	T4	Any N	M0
	Any T	N2,3	M0
	Any T	Any N	M1

Many histological classifications have been proposed in the past 50 years. Bernatz[34] in 1961 proposed the first widely used histologic classification into predominantly lymphocytic, predominantly epithelial, predominantly mixed and predominantly spindle-cell type lymphoma. Unfortunately, the classification could not differentiate prognostic groups. Levine and Rosai[35] in 1978 were the first to propose a clinically relevant histologic classification. They divided thymomas into benign (non-invasive) and malignant (invasive) thymomas. The latter were further classified into Type I (no or minimal atypia) and Type II (moderate to severe atypia). Type II thymomas were considered thymic carcinomas. A major step forward occurred in 1985 when Muller-Hermelink and Marino[36] classified thymomas according to their resemblance to the architecture of the normal thymus. The system, which was subsequently confirmed by other authors,[37,38] included six subtypes: medullary, mixed, predominantly cortical, cortical, well-differentiated carcinoma, and thymic carcinoma. Finally, in 1999, the World Health Organization (WHO)[39] reached a consensus on histologic classification of thymomas based upon both morphology and the lymphocyte to epithelial cell ratio using letters and numbers and identifying six subtypes: Type A (medullary); Type AB (mixed); Type B1 (organoid); Type B2 (cortical); Type B3 (well-differentiated thymic carcinoma), and Type C (thymic carcinoma). Type A thymomas have spindle or oval cells, while Type B thymomas have dendritic or epithelioid cells, and they are further subdivided on the basis of the proportional increase in epithelial cell and atypias from B1 to B3. Despite its clarity and validation in clinical studies,[40] the overall intra- and inter-observer level of agreement have been shown to be far from satisfactory, particularly among pathologists with little experience in thymic malignancies.[41] Most of the discrepancies are related to type B thymomas and for some type AB tumors. To overcome these problems, Suster and Moran in 2008[42] proposed a simplified classification into three subtypes, thymoma (well-differentiated tumors), atypical thymomas (intermediate differentiation), and thymic carcinomas (poorly differentiated tumors), while others, maintaining the WHO classification, demonstrated that among the six subtypes, there were only three WHO prognostically significant categories: A/AB/B1, B2/B3 and C types.

The most recent credited classification, the 2004 WHO update,[43] although maintaining the subtypes A through B3, made two important points: (1) it clearly separated thymic carcinomas from thymomas because while thymomas are organotypic tumors (meaning that their morphology is unique and not found in other organs), thymic carcinomas are not (i.e., similar tumors are present in other organs and they do not have the capacity to promote the maturation of intratumoral immature T cells), and (2) thymic carcinomas were further subdivided into 11 subtypes, among which however, squamous cell carcinoma, lymphoepithelioma-like carcinomas, and neuroendocrine tumors account for the vast majority of tumors.

Other Prognostic Factors

The third prognostic factor which has received major credit is the association with myasthenia gravis.[4,44] Characteristics of patient with thymoma with and without MG seem different and some authors have claimed that the mechanism of MG in thymoma and in non-thymomatous MG is different.[45] Indeed, patients with MG and thymoma tend to be significantly younger than patients with thymoma without MG. Also, MG patients with thymoma tend to have a prevalence of B-type thymomas and they are at early stages as compared with patients with thymoma without MG.[46]

In a recent review, Detterbeck and associates conducted a search for English language articles[47] evaluating prognostic factors using as outcome measures either survival or recurrence from 1980 to 2010. The factors most consistently identified as significant are the stage according to Masaoka or Masaoka–Koga classification and the completeness of resection (R0). These are therefore the only validated prognostic factors to date. The stage was most often dichotomized in stage I–II versus stage III–IV. When stage was considered as a nominal variable (stage I through IV) or when dichotomized differently (stage I vs. II or II vs. III or III vs. IV) the significance was less evident. The histologic subtype according to the WHO classification was not identified as significant, with the exception of thymic carcinoma. The association of myasthenia gravis should be considered as a validated non-significant prognostic factor (Table 14.4).

Among other factors, age and tumor size were considered in several series. Either older or younger ages were found to be significant prognostic factors, and some studies found that tumors larger than 8 cm[48] are associated with a poorer prognosis. Of these, however, none proved to be prognostically significant in a sufficient number of reports to reach a level of validation.

In summary, the 30-year search for a management scenario to be applicable to thymic malignancies is yet to be concluded. The most important prognostic factor, the stage according to Masaoka or Masaoka–Koga system, was proved to be effective to a certain extent, but not optimal. It is plausible that an optimal staging system for thymomas will include a prognostic model composed of different variables, the anatomic stage

appeared with a sufficiently long follow-up.[76] It should be noted, however, that despite a reported reduced hospital stay and less postoperative pain, there is still a lack of evidence for a clear benefit as compared to open procedures,[77] and a prospective collaborative data collection is in progress at an international level. In a recent report from ITMIG,[78] definitions of minimally invasive surgery were agreed upon as followed: (1) any approach as long as no sternotomy (including partial sternotomy) or thoracotomy with rib spreading is involved in an "intent-to-treat" manner; (2) a significant part of the operation is conducted looking at a monitor (with the exception of the dissection of the superior thymus poles); (3) visualization of the innominate vein, phrenic nerves and any other structure suspect to be involved is required; (4) conversion to open should always be possible in case of violation of oncologic principles or intraoperative complications. In addition to that, an access incision should be provided large enough not to disrupt the specimen or create confusion for the pathologist for correct orientation. Different access incisions have been proposed, including transcervical, extended transcervical, VATS, and robotic approach (right or left, bilateral, combined right or left + cervical, subxiphoid). Although excellent results have been reported following resection of thymomas by minimally invasive approaches,[79,80] ITMIG recommendations limit its use to straightforward cases at stage I or II. Patients with stage III and IV thymomas are not candidates to resection by minimally invasive techniques.

RADIOTHERAPY

Thymic tumors are highly radiosensitive and have a tendency to grow and recur locally. This has always been considered a prerequisite for the adoption of radiotherapy (RT) in the management strategy of these tumors. Unfortunately, the rarity of these tumors and the lack of prospective, randomized trials make it difficult to draw evidence-based recommendations about the efficacy of RT in the different clinical settings.

RT may be delivered before surgery, after surgery, in patients not considered for surgery or for treatment of recurrent tumors.

The current standard technique of RT in thymic tumors is conformal radiotherapy with three-dimensional (3D) planning using linear accelerators and high-energy photons (>10 MeV). The delivered doses varied according to the clinical setting, ranging from 45 Gy as induction therapy, to 45–55 Gy as postoperative RT to 60–66 Gy as exclusive treatment. The usual fractionation scheme is adopted (1.8–2.0 Gy/day).[81] In case of hemithoracic radiotherapy to the entire hemithorax for prevention of pleural dissemination, a total dose of 10–17 Gy is delivered in stage II–III which may be increased in case of advanced (stage IVa) disease.[82,83]

Preoperative RT

Preoperative RT has been used alone[84,85] or in combination with chemotherapy (sequential or concurrent)[53] in a neoadjuvant (induction) setting to improve resectability rates. Unfortunately, with the exception of few reports most of the reported series failed to demonstrate significantly better resectability rates and survivals as compared to preoperative chemotherapy alone.

Postoperative RT

Postoperative RT is customarily performed within three months after surgery for a total dose of 40–45 Gy in 1.8–2.0 Gy fractions. Indications to postoperative RT depend upon the stage at surgery, the completeness of resection and additional prognostic factors (WHO histology, tumor size). Stage I thymomas are not irradiated postoperatively. In stage II thymomas, the largest series so far found either no differences with or without RT[32] or even a detrimental effect[73]; it should be noted, however, that more recent series suggested an improved disease-free survival using postoperative RT in high-risk WHO types (B2–B3 and thymic carcinoma).[86–88] In stage III thymic tumors the practice of using adjuvant RT is well-established although on little evidence-based premises. Several old studies report a decrease of recurrence rate after postoperative RT to 0–20% after complete resection, which was significantly lower than the recurrence rate after surgery alone.[89,90] Few recent studies demonstrated the efficacy of postoperative radiotherapy in Masaoka stage III–IV.[91,92] Unfortunately, other studies including more recent series failed to find any significant advantage in using postoperative RT.[32,93] The study based on the surveillance, epidemiology and end results (SEER) registry on 626 invasive thymomas found a similar cause-specific survival when using RT postoperatively versus surgery alone (91% vs. 86%, p = 0.12).[94] Similar results were obtained in a recent meta-analysis[95] incorporating stage II and III: out of 592 patients from 13 different studies, no significant difference (OR 1.05, p = 0.63) was observed in the two groups (surgery alone vs. surgery + RT).

Based on the current literature, therefore, it appears that there is no convincing evidence to support the use of postoperative RT in completely resected invasive thymomas. Incorporation of additional factors including high-risk WHO histologic subtypes (B2-B3-thymic carcinoma), large-sized tumors (>8 cm) and close margin sizes should be taken into account in the individual patient for indication to postoperative RT. Finally, a higher level of evidence seems to support the use of adjuvant RT in patients receiving an incomplete (R1 and R2) resection.

Definitive RT

Definite radiation therapy means a RT delivered as exclusive local modality for disease control, usually in combination with chemotherapy. It is customarily reserved for inoperable patients or patients deemed inoperable after induction chemotherapy. Chemoradiation is usually delivered in a sequential manner at a total dose of 50–70 Gy. A 70% response rate, with a five-year survival of 70–80% has been reported, paralleling the results obtained after incomplete resection.[81,96,97]

CHEMOTHERAPY AND TARGETED THERAPY IN THYMIC MALIGNANCIES
Chemotherapy

Thymomas are chemosensitive tumors, and chemotherapy is widely employed in different settings.[98] Chemotherapy strategies comprise chemotherapy used as initial treatment and as treatment in case of recurrence. Chemotherapy as initial treatment can be further divided into chemotherapy with curative intent (primary chemotherapy or postoperative chemotherapy) and chemotherapy with palliative intent.

Primary (Induction) Chemotherapy

Primary chemotherapy, as indicated in a recent document from ITMIG,[99] is a chemotherapy delivered as first treatment in case of locally advanced nonmetastatic thymic tumors deemed unresectable at preoperative work-up. The main objective is to improve resectability rates and ultimately survival. Some centers also used chemoradiotherapy before surgery, particularly when great vessels were involved.[53,84,85] On the other hand, preoperative chemoradiation increases the risks of toxicity, may alter the chemotherapeutic doses and may limit the ability to give radiation therapy postoperatively, which may be indicated in case of R+ resection. Primary chemotherapy in thymic tumors presents some advantages as compared to induction therapy in lung cancer patients: patients with thymic tumors are usually younger, fitter, show less comorbidities and in general tolerate preoperative chemotherapy regimens better; even in patients with MG or other paraneoplastic syndromes, chemotherapy is usually well tolerated. Indications to primary chemotherapy include patients with locally advanced thymic tumors (stage III and IVa) in which incomplete resection may be anticipated. In general, stage III patients are considered candidates for primary chemotherapy when there is an extended involvement of the mediastinum with no evident cleavage plans, with major involvement of the lung and chest wall and the great vessels. A limited invasion of the SVC or innominate veins should not be considered an indication to primary chemotherapy, since a complete resection may be achieved with appropriate techniques. Many series have published results of multimodality therapy, usually including a mixture of stage III and IVa patients (Table 14.5). On average, they indicated a resectability rate of 65%, a pathologic response of 24% and a pooled five-year survival of 77%.[53–60,100–103] By comparison, upfront surgery resulted in resectability rates ranging between 25% and 50%.[3,52,104] The two populations (upfront surgery vs. primary chemo + surgery) are not comparable however, since they refer to different periods and reflect the experience of different centers. Following chemotherapy, a re-evaluation with CT is usually performed. The time interval between the last cycle of chemotherapy and surgery should not exceed eight weeks. For patients who do not receive surgery after primary chemotherapy, radiotherapy is delivered with a definite intent. If radiotherapy is not feasible for the extent of the tumor or comorbidities increasing the risks of radiation-induced toxicity, definite treatment is consolidation chemotherapy. Stage IVa patients with evident pleural/pericardial dissemination are candidates to primary chemotherapy, followed by extensive surgery depending on the response (pleural implants resection, pleurectomy, or extrapleural pneumonectomy) and a consolidation therapy after surgery (chemotherapy or radiotherapy). With this multimodality approach, a survival up to 78% at 5 years and 65% at 10 years has been reported in high-volume centers.[66] On average, however, major series indicate satisfactory 5- and 10-year survival rates (Table 14.6).

Table 14.5 Multimodality Treatment in Locally Advanced (Stage III–IV) Thymomas

Study Year	Pts No.	Stage	Induction	Adjuvant	% R0	% pR	5-Yrs	10-Yrs
Macchiarini 1991	7	III	CT	RT	57%	29%	78%	
Venuta 2003	45	III	CT	RT/CT	86%	7%		78%
Rea 1993	16	III–IV	CT	RT/CT	69%	31%	57%	
Kim 2004	22	III–IV	CT	RT/CT	76%	37%	95%	
Bretti 2004	25	III–IV	CT	RT	44%	8%	57Mo[a]	
Lucchi 2006	30	III–IV	CT	RT/CT	77%			86 (III) 76 (IVa)
Yokoi 2007	17	III–IV	CT	RT	50%		81%	
Wright 2008	10	III–IV	RT/CT	CT	80%	40%	69%	
Kunitoh 2010	23	III–IV	CT	RT	43%	14%	85%	
Average					65%	24%	77%	

[a]Progression-free survival.

Table 14.6 Results of Surgical Treatment of Stage IVa Thymic Tumors

Author	Year	Pts No.	5-year survival	10-year survival
Masaoka	1991	11	50%	0%
Maggi	1991	21	59%	40%
Regnard	1996	19	60%	30%
Yagi	1996	5	67%	33%
Wilkins	1999	5	40%	40%
Kondo	2003	103	71%	48%
Nakagawa	2003	11	47%	47%
Lucchi	2005	16	NR	46%
Wright	2006	5	75%	50%
Huang	2007	18	78%	65%
Cardillo	2010	27	NR	28%
Margaritora	2010	14	76%	52%
Average			62%	40%

Postoperative Chemotherapy

Postoperative chemotherapy is defined as a chemotherapy delivered after surgery. Due to the low incidence of systemic recurrence after surgery, the rationale to use postoperative chemotherapy is limited, and usually radiotherapy is the standard of care in case of increased risk of loco-regional recurrence. Nonetheless, several series reported good results with a multimodality therapy using primary chemotherapy followed by surgery and consolidation therapy with chemotherapy and radiotherapy in complete and incomplete resections.[32,58,59,105–107] Postoperative chemotherapy should be initiated within 12 weeks after surgery.

Palliative Chemotherapy

The rationale of palliative-intent chemotherapy is to improve potential tumor-related symptoms and to achieve a tumor response. A prolonged disease control is obtainable, but tumor eradication is not expected. Many chemotherapeutic drugs have demonstrated activity in thymic malignancies either as single-agent schedule or in different platinum-based combinations. An objective response is seen in about 60% of the patients with a large variability among the different series.[96,108–111] Most of these series included advanced thymomas, and only a few patients with thymic carcinoma were included. The impact on survival is difficult to assess because of the heterogeneity of the series, the different regimens employed and the number of patients enrolled. Most studies, however, report a significant disease control and an increased time-to-progression. Promising results have been reported by some authors with the use of somatostatin analogs (octreotide) and prednisone.[112,113]

Targeted Therapy in Thymic Malignancies

Unlike lung cancer, where target-based therapy is well-recognized and approved, the search for biologic agents in thymic malingnancies has yielded disappointing results so far, although some exceptions exist.

Thymic tumors show some molecular characteristics, including oncogenes (EGFR, HER2, KIT, KRAS), tumor suppressor genes (TP53, p16), and angiogenic factors (VEGF). A clear correlation between these molecular characteristics and other factors (histology, stage, invasiveness, and prognosis) has sporadically been reported, but never validated. A brief overview of the most important molecularly targeted agents is reported.

1. *Epidermal growth factor receptor (EGFR) inhibitors.* Epidermal growth factor receptor (EGFR) is over-expressed in thymomas and thymic carcinomas (TC). The rate of overexpression varies among the different series, ranging from 33% to 100%, being higher in thymomas (70%) than thymic carcinomas (50%).[114,115] Small evidence exists of a clear correlation between EGFR staining and histology or stage. Unfortunately, the frequency of EGFR mutations (which are correlated with response to inhibitors) in thymic tumors (thymomas and TC) is very low (below 5%). This may partly explain the low response rate with the use of EGFR-tyrosine kinase inhibitors (gefitinib, erlotinib). More encouraging results were reported with the use of cetuximab, a monoclonal antibody to EGFR.

2. *KIT signaling pathway.* Kit is a transmembrane growth factor with tyrosine kinase activity which was first described in gastrointestinal stromal tumors (GIST). KIT inhibitor imatinib produced a dramatic improvement in the treatment of GIST inducing a rapid, substantial, and durable tumor response. KIT staining has been evaluated in thymic malignancies. Although KIT immunostaining is rare in thymomas (<5%), it is present in about 80% of thymic carcinoma and this represents a potential target for KIT inhibitors.[116] Some authors even proposed to use KIT as a diagnostic marker of thymic carcinoma versus thymoma, although the level of expression seems to be correlated with the histologic subtype. Scattered reports using the three available oral multikinase KIT inhibitors (imatinib, dasatinib, and sorafenib) indicate excellent, although isolated, responses. In conclusion, KIT represents an interesting biologic drug in thymic carcinomas and, despite the low frequency of activating mutation as compared to GIST, warrants further prospective trials.

3. *Histone deacetylase (HDAC) inhibitor.* Histone deacetylase are enzymes that exert an influence on DNA packaging and chromatin remodeling. HDAC inhibition can alter gene expression and induce apoptosis. The most employed HDAC inhibitor, belinostat, was tested in patients with metastatic or recurrent thymomas and thymic carcinomas. The authors found a limited response in thymomas, but no response in thymic carcinoma.[117]

4. *Angiogenesis inhibitors.* Angiogenesis is mandatory for any tumor to grow beyond the 1-cm diameter. The most powerful pro-angiogenic molecules are those of the VEGFR signaling pathway. VEGF is expressed in thymomas and thymic carcinomas. An anti-VEGF antibody is commercially available, bevacizumab, which was found to produce excellent response in renal cell carcinoma and, to a lesser extent, in non-squamous tumors of the lung. Few data are available about the efficacy of anti-VEGF therapy in thymic malignancies with no major responses so far.

5. *Octreotide.* Somatostatin receptor (SSR) subtypes, code-named sst 1–5, are heterogeneously expressed in the normal human thymus. Octreotide, a somatostatin analog, proved to be effective in the treatment of some neuroendocrine tumors. A high in vivo uptake of [111In-DTPA-D-Phe1]octreotide using Octreoscan has been reported in patients bearing thymoma. Scattered reports of response to octreotide in thymic malignancies have been published in the literature. The largest trial was conducted by the Eastern Cooperative Oncology Group[112] on 38 patients with thymoma and thymic carcinoma which received octreotide for a maximum of one year alone or with prednisone. The overall response rate was 32% with acceptable toxicity. The authors concluded that the combination of octreotide and prednisone exhibited modest activity and may be considered for the treatment of advanced or recurrent octreotide scan-positive thymomas.

In summary, there is a continuing search for a better understanding of molecular characteristics of thymic tumors. Unfortunately, the rarity of the disease and its heterogeneity make it difficult to test the target-based therapy on a large scale. What we can conclude (Table 14.7) is that in thymoma, cetuximab may be effective in selected patients with EGFR overexpression; KIT inhibitors are a promising therapy in thymic carcinomas; octreotide therapy (somatostatin analog) may be proposed in octreotide-scan positive tumors.

Table 14.7 Targeted Therapy in Thymic Malignancies

Mutation	Action	Agent	Target tumor
EGFR expression	EGFR inhibitors Erlotinib (TARCEVA) Monoclonal Ab	Gefitinib (IRESSA) Cetuximab (ERBITUX)	Thymoma
c-KIT (CD117)	c-KIT inhibitors	Imatinib (GLIVEC) Dasatinib (SPRYCEL) Sorafenib (NEXAVAR)	Thymic carcinoma
Histone deacetylase (HDACs)	HDAC inhibitors	Belinostat	Thymoma
VEGF	VEGF inhibitors	Bevacizumab (AVASTIN)	Thymoma Thymic carcinoma

Abbreviations: EGFR, epidermal growth factor receptor; VEGF, vascular endothelial growth factor.

RECURRENCE

Recurrence of thymic tumors is frequent, occurring in 30–50% of the cases after complete resection.[2,52] Average time-to-recurrence is five years, although recurrences have been recorded up to 20 years after initial resection. The recurrence rate is dependent upon the stage, being negligible after resection of stage I thymomas (<4%) and progressively increasing from stage II to stage IVa (20 to 50%).[32,72] Some confusion has occurred in the past literature regarding the exact terminology in recurrent thymic tumors. A recent report from ITMIG[16] clarified the issue. According to ITMIG proposal, the term recurrence is appropriate if it is plausible that all disease has been eradicated (R0 resection). The pattern of recurrence comprises (1) local recurrence, when the recurrent disease appears in the anterior mediastinum or lower neck, or contiguous to the initial thymoma; (2) regional recurrence, when intrathoracic recurrent disease occurs in the pleura (visceral or parietal) or pericardium not contiguous with the thymus bed; (3) distant recurrence, when the tumor recurs outside the thorax or lower neck or in the form of intrapulmonary nodules. Overall, the distribution pattern includes local recurrence in 30–35%, regional recurrence in 50–55% and distant recurrence in 5–10% of the patients.[72] A recent review[47] report 12 studies evaluating different prognostic factors for the development of recurrence. The single most important predictor of recurrence was the stage at presentation. Completeness of resection with safe surgical margins is obviously a determinant for recurrence as part of the definition of recurrence. WHO histology (thymic carcinoma), although prognostic for survival, was less prognostic when recurrence was analyzed. Among other prognostic factors, only tumor size and invasion of great vessels were occasionally reported as prognostic for recurrence.

The role of adjuvant RT in reducing recurrence rates in invasive thymomas has been discussed elsewhere in this chapter. The most recent series indicate that there is no convincing evidence that postoperatively RT is beneficial in reducing recurrence rates in completely resected stage II–IVa diseases.[17] Indeed, most of thymomas relapse in the pleura, which is outside the radiation field of postoperative RT.[118] Low-dose whole hemithorax irradiation in the prevention of pleural relapse has also been advocated by some authors.[82,83] In absence of approved guidelines, indication to RT after complete resection of invasive thymomas should be based on an individual basis, based upon different co-variates (tumor size, distance of free-margins, WHO histology, and invasion of great vessels).

Treatment of recurrence is surgical whenever possible. This occurs in 50–75% of the largest published series.[52,73,74,48,119] All series but one[120] demonstrated an improved survival if complete resection of recurrence is feasible (which occurs in about 65% of the cases), with survival rates comparable to those of the initial stages,[121] ranging from 50% to 70% at 10-years in complete resections, as compared to 0–20% in incompletely resected patients.[17] Iterative surgery in case of subsequent resectable relapses is also indicated. Surgery should be extensive and complete, particularly in case of pleural dissemination. Two recent series[65,118] report excellent survival rates after aggressive surgery including extrapleural pneumonectomy and the use of hyperthermic intrapleural chemotherapy in the management of pleural recurrence of thymic malignancies. Nonsurgical treatments of recurrence include chemotherapy or chemoradiotherapy which have been associated with reasonable outcomes (25% to 50% five-year survival).[17,52,72]

THYMIC CARCINOMA AND NEUROENDOCRINE THYMIC TUMORS

Although thymomas are by far the most common thymic malignancies, other thymic neoplasms are of increased interest and deserve a brief description: thymic carcinoma and neuroendocrine thymic tumors (NETT).

Thymic Carcinoma

Overall, thymic carcinomas are exceedingly rare (1–3 cases/10.000.000 inhabitants).[1] The 2004 update of the WHO histologic classification of thymic tumors(43) clearly differentiates thymomas from thymic carcinomas for which the term C type, previously indicated in the 1999 WHO classification, was no longer suggested. Thymic carcinomas are further subclassified in 11 types. The most frequent subtypes are the squamous cell (40%) and lymphoepithelioma-like (30%) variants. Most of the patients (50–80%) are symptomatic, reflecting the high stage (III–IV) at presentation.[5,17,32] Myasthenia Gravis is not associated with thymic carcinoma. In contrast to thymomas, lymphnodal metastases are common (up to 30% of the cases) as are distant metastases. The current staging system (Masaoka or Masaoka–Koga) is suboptimal for thymic carcinomas, and a TNM system[27,30] seems more appropriate. As in other thymic malignancies, surgical resection is the cornerstone of treatment, although a complete resection may be performed in about 30% of the patients. For this reason, many authors suggest multimodality approach including primary chemotherapy followed by surgery and postoperative radio or chemotherapy. Prognosis is generally poor with 5- and 10-year survival rates around 40% and 30% respectively in most series.[122–124] A majority of patients (75%) develop recurrences, half of which are distant. For inoperable patients, exclusive chemotherapy and radiotherapy have been employed producing response rates ranging from 20% to 60%. The recent identification of molecular markers (KIT) in thymic carcinomas provides a rationale to test biologic drugs (KIT inhibitors, imatinib) and opens new hope for these patients.

Neuroendocrine Thymic Tumors

Primary neuroendocrine tumors of the thymus (NETT) are rare, and about 250 cases have been reported in the current literature.[125] Differently from their counterpart in other organs (lung, GEtract), they show an aggressive behavior, the vast majority being atypical carcinoids. The WHO classification considers NETT as a subtype of thymic carcinoma and identifies two categories[126]: well-differentiated NETT (typical and atypical carcinoids) and poorly-differentiated NETT (small-cell and large-cell NE carcinomas). NETT express somatostatin receptors (subtypes sst 1–5). Clinically, patients with NETT have associated endocrinopathies including Cushing's syndrome and multiple endocrine neoplasia (MEN-1) syndrome. Association with MG is exceptional. At diagnosis, 50% of the patients have nodal metastases, and 30% have distant metastases. As in other thymic tumors, surgery is the preferred treatment, although the rate of complete resection is variable among the centers (28% to 100%, mean 85%). Multimodality treatment including preoperative chemotherapy followed by surgery and postoperative radiotherapy has been proposed, but the limited number of patients makes it difficult to interpret the results. Nonetheless, some series report satisfactory results with 5- and 10-year survival rates ranging from 28% to 77% and 10% to 75% respectively.[32,127] Biologic therapy using somatostatin analogs (octreotide, lantreotide) has been tested with conflicting results which cannot presently suggest its use as standard treatment.

GUIDELINES AND RECOMMENDED MANAGEMENT OF PATIENTS WITH THYMIC TUMORS

Several reviews on management of patients with thymic tumors are available in the literature.[5,17,49,50,77,128] In addition, there is also a guideline compiled by the National Cancer Institute (freely available at http:/www.cancer.org/cancertopics/pdq/treatment/thymoma/healthprofessional) which is periodically updated. Finally, two recent volumes have been published on **Thoracic Surgery Clinics (February 2011) and on a supplement of JTO (July 2011)** which give an excellent overview about all the major aspects and topics related to thymic malignancies. The interested reader is strongly advised to refer to these sources for a thorough knowledge.

The best available evidence from the literature suggests that the recommended treatment strategies in patients with thymic malignancies are dependent upon the stage according to Masaoka or Masaoka/Koga and histology according to WHO classification (Table 14.8).

1. *Stage I.* Stage I thymomas are best approached by upfront surgery. The rate of postoperative recurrence is negligible (1–4%) and postoperative radiotherapy is not indicated. Resectability rate approaches 100%. Complete resection of the thymoma and the thymus is recommended either in patients with or without MG. The role of partial thymectomy in non-MG (negative serum antiacetylcholine receptor AchR antibodies) is still experimental and should be avoided at this time. The best surgical approach is sternotomy (either partial or total). Minimally invasive resection is justified using the ITMIG criteria. Very small (<1 cm) stage I thymomas in elderly patients may be followed up without resection. Despite the early stage, long-term follow-up (>20 years) is required.

Table 14.8 Management of Thymic Malignancies by Stage (Masaoka) and recurrence

Stage	Preoperative	Surgery	Postoperative	Note
Stage I	None	Recommended	None	Long-term F-U
Stage II	None	Recommended	None	RT considered for high-risk WHO histologic subtypes (B2-B3 and TC) and high risk of recurrence
Stage III				
Resectable	None	Recommended	RT[a]	Adjuvant CT in selected cases at high-risk of recur or incomplete resection
Unresectable	CT	Recommended in case of response	RT	Induction CT+RT also possible
Stage IVa				
Resectable	CT	Recommended in case of response	CT/RT	
Unresectable	CT	Recommended in case of response	CT/RT	
Stage IVb	CT	Not recommended		
Recurrence				
Resectable		Recommended		
Unresectable		Not recommended	Exclusive RT/CT	

Abbreviations: CT, chemotherapy; RT, radiotherapy; TC, thymic carcinoma.
[a]Probably not indicated in R0 resection with adequate resection margins.

2. *Stage II.* Stage II thymomas are usually diagnosed after resection, since invasion of the capsule is seldom evident preoperatively. Stage II thymomas are best approached by upfront surgery. Resectability rates are still high (43% to 100%, average 85%). Recurrence rate is 4–14%. Postoperative radiotherapy does not add a survival advantage and is not routinely recommended. Some authors use postoperative RT in stage II thymomas on a selective basis based upon histology (for B2-B3 and thymic carcinoma) and risk of recurrence (close free surgical margins).

3. *Stage III.* Stage III thymomas are best approached by a multidisciplinary team. The surgeon's judgment is crucial in the preoperative work-up. Two scenarios may occur:

   a. Resectable stage III thymomas. If the tumor is judged resectable, upfront surgery is indicated, with the use of extended resection of neighboring organs, including SVC and innominate veins. Unilateral phrenic nerve resection is feasible even in myasthenic patients. In case of complete resection (R0) postoperative radiotherapy is recommended in almost all the published guidelines. Adjuvant chemotherapy is indicated in selected cases or in case of incomplete resection.

   b. Unresectable stage III thymomas. If the tumor is judged unresectable, then primary (induction) chemotherapy is indicated (some authors recommend chemo+ radiotherapy, although this is not universally recognized). After surgery, radiotherapy is recommended. Maximal debulking surgery is an option in case the resection is not complete.

4. *Stage IVa.* Pleural/pericardial dissemination is rarely cured. If stage IVa disease is diagnosed intraoperatively, resection of the pleural implants or pleurectomy is indicated, followed by chemo- or radiotherapy. When stage IVa disease is diagnosed preoperatively, then a multimodality approach including primary chemotherapy followed by surgery and postoperative selective radiotherapy or chemotherapy is recommended. Extensive surgery including PPE is to be considered experimental until further confirmation. Exclusive chemotherapy is recommended for inoperable disease or in case of progression after primary chemotherapy.

5. *Thymic carcinoma.* Thymic carcinomas pose additional problems, because they show a more aggressive behavior, and tend to metastasize to lymphnodes through the bloodstream. They usually present at advanced stages, and a multimodality approach including primary chemotherapy followed by surgery and postoperative radiotherapy is recommended, although yet to be validated. Overall, survival rates are far lower than those of thymomas (40% and 30% respectively at 5 and 10 years). Recurrence is common (up to 75% of the patients).

6. *Recurrence.* An aggressive approach to recurrence is recommended when feasible. Fifty to seventy percent of the recurrences are considered amenable to surgical resection, with a resectability rate of 60% on average. When complete resection is possible, long-term survival is anticipated (50% to 70% 10-year survival). In case of incomplete resection or unresectable disease, reasonable intermediate survival rates have been reported using chemotherapy and radiotherapy.

THE GLOBAL EFFORT

Advancements in thymic malignancies have been slow so far, due to the rarity of the condition and the lack of coordination among those centers which have sufficient experience to provide consistent results. In an era of globalization and ease of communication there is no excuse against the lack of cooperation which has occurred so far. In the past decade, the most important thoracic societies addressed this issue by promoting dedicated thymic groups.

In 2010, the International Thymic Malignancies Interest Group (ITMIG) was officially constituted,[129,130] supported by the most representatives medical and surgical societies around the globe. The mission of ITMIG is to promote the advancement of clinical and basic science related to thymic malignancies. It provides infrastructure for international cooperation, maintains close collaboration with other related organizations, and facilitates spread of knowledge about thymic neoplasms. ITMIG works in close cooperation with the major thymic groups of international societies (ESTS, EACTS, JART). It is a multidisciplinary organization, involving thoracic surgeons, radiation and medical oncologists, pathologists, pulmonologists, radiologists, and basic science researchers.

The first major effort of ITMIG was to create a common language in thymic malignancies. In a comprehensive set of manuscripts which were recently published in a supplement of Journal of Thoracic Oncology, ITMIG proposes a consistent set of definition covering all aspects of management of thymic malignancies. It is conceivable, therefore, that from now on all studies will comply with these definitions in order to have comparable series and results.

The second major project of ITMIG, which necessitates a close interaction with regional thymic groups, is the creation of a retrospective and a prospective database of thymic malignancies. This is essential to provide a platform for clinical and research projects, and to develop a formal, validated thymic staging system for the next eighth edition of the American Joint Commission on Cancer Staging Manual, expected in 2017.

In Europe, the ESTS thymic working group[15] is currently collecting retrospectively all thymic malignancies among its members. Almost 2000 patients have entered so far the ESTS retrospective database. The data will be forwarded to ITMIG for international projects, and will form the basis for regional projects in collaboration with ETOP, the best recognized European oncology platform involving professionals from all specialties in oncology (medical and radiation oncologists, pathologists, and thoracic surgeons). In particular, the creation of a tissue bank will be a prerequisite for basic research, molecular characterization, translational research, and testing of targeted drugs, which surely represents the most appealing and promising aspect in the recent research in medical oncology.

REFERENCES

1. Engels EA, Pfeiffer RM. Malignant thymoma in the United States: Demographic patterns in incidence and associations with subsequent malignancies. Int J Cancer 2003; 105: 546–51.
2. Maggi G, Casadio C, Cavallo A, et al. Thymoma: results of 241 operated cases. Ann Thorac Surg 1991; 51: 152–6.
3. Regnard JF, Magdeleinat P, Dromer C, et al. Prognostic factors and long-term results after thymoma resection: a series of 307 patients. J Thorac Cardiovasc Surg 1996; 112: 376–84.
4. Kondo K, Monden Y. Thymoma and myasthenia gravis: a clinical study of 1,089 patients from Japan. Ann Thorac Surg 2005; 79: 219–24.
5. Venuta F, Anile M, Diso D, et al. Thymoma and thymic carcinoma. Eur J Cardiothorac Surg 2010; 37: 13–25.
6. Masaoka A, Yamakawa Y, Niwa H, et al. Thymectomy and malignancy. Eur J Cardiothorac Surg 1994; 8: 251–3.
7. Wilkins KB, Sheikh E, Green R, et al. Clinical and pathologic predictors of survival in patients with thymoma. Ann Surg 1999; 230: 562–72.
8. Marom EM, Milito MA, Moran CA, et al. Computed tomography findings predicting invasiveness of thymoma. J Thorac Oncol 2011; 6: 1274–81.
9. Priola AM, Priola SM, Di Franco M, et al. Computed tomography and thymoma: distinctive findings in invasive and noninvasive thymoma and predictive features of recurrence. Radiol Med 2010; 115: 1–21.
10. El Bawab H, Al-Sugair AA, et al. Role of flourine-18 fluorodeoxyglucose positron emission tomography in thymic pathology. Eur J Cardiothorac Surg 2007; 31: 731–6.
11. Endo M, Nakagawa K, Ohde Y, et al. Utility of 18FDG-PET for differentiating the grade of malignancy in thymic epithelial tumors. Lung Cancer 2008; 61: 350–5.
12. Inoue A, Tomiyama N, Tatsumi M, et al. (18)F-FDG PET for the evaluation of thymic epithelial tumors: Correlation with the World Health Organization classification in addition to dual-time-point imaging. Eur J Nucl Med Mol Imaging 2009; 36: 1219–25.
13. Smith CS, Schöder H, Yeung HW. Thymic extension in the superior mediastinum in patients with thymic hyperplasia: potential cause of false-positive findings on 18F-FDG PET/CT. AJR Am J Roentgenol 2007; 188: 1716–21.
14. Puri V, Meyers BF. Utility of positron emission tomography in the mediastinum: moving beyond lung and esophageal cancer staging. Thorac Surg Clin 2009; 19: 7–15.

15. Ruffini E, Van Raemdonck D, Detterbeck F, et al. European Society of Thoracic Surgeons Thymic Questionnaire Working Group. Management of thymic tumors: a survey of current practice among members of the European Society of Thoracic Surgeons. J Thorac Oncol 2011; 6: 614–23.

16. Huang J, Detterbeck FC, Wang Z, Loehrer PJ Sr. Standard outcome measures for thymic malignancies. J Thorac Oncol 2011; 6(7 Suppl 3): S1691–7.

17. Detterbeck FC, Parsons AM. Thymic tumors. Ann Thorac Surg 2004; 77: 1860–9.

18. Moore KH, McKenzie PR, Kennedy CW, McCaughan BC. Thymoma: trends over time. Ann Thorac Surg 2001; 72: 203–7.

19. Herman SJ, Holub RV, Weisbrod GL, Chamberlain DW. Anterior mediastinal masses: utility of transthoracic needle biopsy. Radiology 1991; 180: 167–70.

20. Kattach H, Hasan S, Clelland C, Pillai R. Seeding of stage I thymoma into the chest wall 12 years after needle biopsy. Ann Thorac Surg 2005; 79: 323–4.

21. Detterbeck FC. Does an anecdote substantiate dogma? Ann Thorac Surg 2006; 81: 1182.

22. International Association for the Study of Lung Cancer. Staging Manual in Thoracic Oncology. Orange Park, FL, USA: Rx Press, 2009.

23. Bergh NP, Gatzinsky P, Larsson S, Lundin P, Ridell B. Tumors of the thymus and thymic region: I Clinicopathological studies on thymoma. Ann Thorac Surg 1978; 25: 91–8.

24. Masaoka A, Monden Y, Nakahara K, Tanioka T. Follow-up study of thymomas with special reference to their clinical stages. Cancer 1981; 48: 2485–92.

25. Koga K, Matsuno Y, Noguchi M, et al. A review of 79 thymomas: modification of staging system and reappraisal of conventional division into invasive and non-invasive thymoma. Pathol Int 1994; 44: 359–67.

26. Gamondès JP, Balawi A, Greenland T, et al. Seventeen years of surgical treatment of thymoma: factors influencing survival. Eur J Cardiothorac Surg 1991; 5: 124–31.

27. Yamakawa Y, Masaoka A, Hashimoto T, et al. A tentative tumor-node-metastasis classification of thymoma. Cancer 1991; 68: 1984–7.

28. Tsuchiya R, Koga K, Matsuno Y, Mukai K, Shimosato Y. Thymic carcinoma: proposal for pathological TNM and staging. Pathol Int 1994; 44: 505–12.

29. Bedini AV, Andreani SM, Tavecchio L, et al. Proposal of a novel system for the staging of thymic epithelial tumors. Ann Thorac Surg 2005; 80: 1994–2000.

30. Travis WD, Brambilla E, Muller Hermelink HK, Harris CC. Pathology and genetics of tumours of the lung, pleura, thymus and heart. In: Kleihues P, Sobin LH, eds. WHO Classification of Tumours. 2nd edn. Lyon: IARC Press, 2004: 145–97.

31. Kondo K, Monden Y. Lymphogenous and hematogenous metastasis of thymic epithelial tumors. Ann Thorac Surg 2003; 76: 1859–64.

32. Kondo K, Monden Y. Therapy for thymic epithelial tumors: a clinical study of 1,320 patients from Japan. Ann Thorac Surg 2003; 76: 878–84.

33. Detterbeck F, Nicholson AG, Kondo K, Van Schil P, Moran C. The Masaoka-Koga Stage classification for thymic malignancies: clarification and definition of terms. J Thorac Oncol 2011; 6(7 Suppl 3): S1710–16.

34. Bernatz PE, Harrison EG, Clagett OT. Thymoma: a clinicopathologic study. J Thorac Cardiovasc Surg 1961; 42: 424–44.

35. Levine GD, Rosai J. Thymic hyperplasia and neoplasia: a review of current concepts. Hum Pathol 1978; 9: 495–515.

36. Marino M, Muller-Hermelink HK. Thymoma and thymic carcinoma. Relation of thymoma epithelial cells to the cortical and medullary differentiation of the thymus. Virchows Arch Pathol Anat Histopathol 1985; 407: 119–49.

37. Kirchner T, Marino M, Muller-Hermelink HK. New approaches to the diagnosis of thymic epithelial tumours. Prog Surg pathol 1989; 10: 167–89.

38. Pescarmona E, Rendina EA, Venuta F, et al. Analysis of prognostic factors and clinicopathological staging of thymoma. Ann Thorac Surg 1990; 50: 534–8.

39. Rosai J, Sobin L. Histological typing of tumours of the thymus. In: Rosai J, Sobin L, eds. World Health Organization, International classification of tumours. Berlin: Springer, 1999: 9–14.

40. Okumura M, Ohta M, Tateyama H, et al. The World Health Organization histologic classification system reflects the oncologic behavior of thymoma: a clinical study of 273 patients. Cancer 2002; 94: 624–32.

41. Verghese ET, den Bakker MA, Campbell A, et al. Interobserver variation in the classification of thymic tumours-a multicentre study using the WHO classification system. Histopathology 2008; 53: 218–23.

42. Suster S, Moran CA. Histologic classification of thymoma: the World Health Organization and beyond. Hematol Oncol Clin North Am 2008; 22: 381–9.

43. Muller-Hermelink HK, Engel P, Harris N. Tumours of the thymus. In: Travis W, Brambilla E, Muller-Hermelink H, eds. Tumours of the Lung, Thymus, Heart. Pathology and Genetics. Lyon: IARC Press, 2004.

44. Margaritora S, Cesario A, Cusumano G, et al. Thirty-five-year follow-up analysis of clinical and pathologic outcomes of thymoma surgery. Ann Thorac Surg 2010; 89: 245–52.

45. Lucchi M, Ricciardi R, Melfi F, et al. Association of thymoma and myasthenia gravis: oncological and neurological results of the surgical treatment. Eur J Cardiothorac Surg 2009; 35: 812–16.

46. Ruffini E, Filosso PL, Mossetti C, et al. Thymoma: inter-relationships among World Health Organization histology, Masaoka staging and myasthenia gravis and their independent prognostic significance: a single-centre experience. Eur J Cardiothorac Surg 2011; 40: 146–53.

47. Detterbeck F, Youssef S, Ruffini E, Okumura M. A review of prognostic factors in thymic malignancies. J Thorac Oncol 2011; 6(7 Suppl 3): S1698–704.
48. Wright CD, Wain JC, Wong DR, et al. Predictors of recurrence in thymic tumors: importance of invasion, World Health Organization histology, and size. J Thorac Cardiovasc Surg 2005; 130: 1413–21.
49. Davenport E, Malthaner RA. The role of surgery in the management of thymoma: a systematic review. Ann Thorac Surg 2008; 86: 673–84.
50. Wright CD. Management of thymomas. Crit Rev Oncol Hematol 2008; 65: 109–20.
51. Detterbeck FC, Parsons AM. Management of stage I and II thymoma. Thorac Surg Clin 2011; 21: 59–67.
52. Blumberg D, Port JL, Weksler B, et al. Thymoma: a multivariate analysis of factors predicting survival. Ann Thorac Surg 1995; 60: 908–13.
53. Wright CD, Choi NC, Wain JC, et al. Induction chemoradiotherapy followed by resection for locally advanced Masaoka stage III and IVA thymic tumors. Ann Thorac Surg 2008; 85: 385–9.
54. Ishikawa Y, Matsuguma H, Nakahara R, et al. Multimodality therapy for patients with invasive thymoma disseminated into the pleural cavity: the potential role of extrapleural pneumonectomy. Ann Thorac Surg 2009; 88: 952–7.
55. Lucchi M, Melfi F, Dini P, et al. Neoadjuvant chemotherapy for stage III and IVA thymomas: a single-institution experience with a long follow-up. J Thorac Oncol 2006; 1: 308–13.
56. Bretti S, Berruti A, Loddo C, et al. Piemonte Oncology Network. Multimodal management of stages III–IVa malignant thymoma. Lung Cancer 2004; 44: 69–77.
57. Kunitoh H, Tamura T, Shibata T, et al. JCOG Lung Cancer Study Group. A phase II trial of dose-dense chemotherapy, followed by surgical resection and/or thoracic radiotherapy, in locally advanced thymoma: report of a Japan Clinical Oncology Group trial (JCOG 9606). Br J Cancer 2010; 103: 6–11.
58. Venuta F, Rendina EA, Pescarmona EO, et al. Multimodality treatment of thymoma: a prospective study. Ann Thorac Surg 1997; 64: 1585–91.
59. Kim ES, Putnam JB, Komaki R, et al. Phase II study of a multidisciplinary approach with induction chemotherapy, followed by surgical resection, radiation therapy, and consolidation chemotherapy for unresectable malignant thymomas: final report. Lung Cancer 2004; 44: 369–79.
60. Jacot W, Quantin X, Valette S, Khial F, Pujol JL. Multimodality treatment program in invasive thymic epithelial tumor. Am J Clin Oncol 2005; 28: 5–7.
61. Venuta F, Rendina EA, Klepetko W, Rocco G. Surgical management of stage III thymic tumors. Thorac Surg Clin 2011; 21: 85–91.
62. Dartevelle P, Macchiarini P, Chapelier A. Technique of superior vena cava resection and reconstruction. Chest Surg Clin N Am 1995; 5: 345–58.
63. De Giacomo T, Mazzesi G, Venuta F, Coloni GF. Extended operation for recurrent thymic carcinoma presenting with intracaval growth and intracardiac extension. J Thorac Cardiovasc Surg 2007; 134: 1364–5.
64. Kaiser LR. Surgical treatment of thymic epithelial neoplasms. Hematol Oncol Clin North Am 2008; 22: 475–88.
65. Wright CD. Pleuropneumonectomy for the treatment of Masaoka stage IVA thymoma. Ann Thorac Surg 2006; 82: 1234.
66. Huang J, Rizk NP, Travis WD, et al. Feasibility of multimodality therapy including extended resections in stage IVA thymoma. J Thorac Cardiovasc Surg 2007; 134: 1477–83.
67. Masaoka A, Nagaoka Y, Kotake Y. Distribution of thymic tissue at the anterior mediastinum. Current procedures in thymectomy. J Thorac Cardiovasc Surg 1975; 70: 747–54.
68. Odaka M, Akiba T, Yabe M, et al. Unilateral thoracoscopic subtotal thymectomy for the treatment of stage I and II thymoma. Eur J Cardiothorac Surg 2010; 37: 824–6.
69. Sakamaki Y, Kido T, Yasukawa M. Alternative choices of total and partial thymectomy in video-assisted resection of noninvasive thymomas. Surg Endosc 2008; 22: 1272–7.
70. Johnson SB, Eng TY, Giaccone G, Thomas CR. Thymoma: update for the new millennium. Oncologist 2001; 6: 239–46.
71. Thomas CR, Wright CD, Loehrer PJ. Thymoma: state of the art. J Clin Oncol 1999; 17: 2280–9.
72. Ruffini E, Filosso PL, Oliaro A. The role of surgery in recurrent thymic tumors. Thorac Surg Clin 2009; 19: 121–31.
73. Ruffini E, Mancuso M, Oliaro A, et al. Recurrence of thymoma: analysis of clinicopathologic features, treatment, and outcome. J Thorac Cardiovasc Surg 1997; 113: 55–63.
74. Regnard JF, Zinzindohoue F, Magdeleinat P, et al. Results of re-resection for recurrent thymomas. Ann Thorac Surg 1997; 64: 1593–8.
75. Deeb ME, Brinster CJ, Kucharzuk J, Shrager JB, Kaiser LR. Expanded indications for transcervical thymectomy in the management of anterior mediastinal masses. Ann Thorac Surg 2001; 72: 208–11.
76. Rückert JC, Ismail M, Swierzy M, et al. Thoracoscopic thymectomy with the da Vinci robotic system for myasthenia gravis. Ann NY Acad Sci 2008; 1132: 329–35.
77. Tomaszek S, Wigle DA, Keshavjee S, Fischer S. Thymomas: review of current clinical practice. Ann Thorac Surg 2009; 87: 1973–80.
78. Toker A, Sonett J, Zielinski M, et al. Standard terms, definitions and policies for minimally invasive resection of thymoma. J Thorac Oncol 2011; 6(7 Suppl 3): S1710–16.
79. Cheng YJ, Kao EL, Chou SH. Videothoracoscopic resection of stage II thymoma: prospective comparison of the results between thoracoscopy and open methods. Chest 2005; 128: 3010–12.

80. Cheng YJ. Videothoracoscopic resection of encapsulated thymic carcinoma: retrospective comparison of the results between thoracoscopy and open methods. Ann Surg Oncol 2008; 15: 2235–8.

81. Girard N, Mornex F. The role of radiotherapy in the management of thymic tumors. Thorac Surg Clin 2011; 21: 99–105.

82. Yoshida H, Uematsu M, Itami J, et al. The role of low-dose hemithoracic radiotherapy for thoracic dissemination of thymoma. Radiat Med 1997; 15: 399–403.

83. Gomez D, Komaki R, Yu J, Ikushima H, Bezjak A. Radiation therapy definitions and reporting guidelines for thymic malignancies. J Thorac Oncol 2011; 6(7 Suppl 3): S1743–8.

84. Yagi K, Hirata T, Fukuse T, et al. Surgical treatment for invasive thymoma, especially when the superior vena cava is invaded. Ann Thorac Surg 1996; 61: 521–4.

85. Akaogi E, Ohara K, Mitsui K, et al. Preoperative radiotherapy and surgery for advanced thymoma with invasion to the great vessels. J Surg Oncol 1996; 63: 17–22.

86. Wu KL, Mao JF, Chen GY, et al. Prognostic predictors and long-term outcome of postoperative irradiation in thymoma: a study of 241 patients. Cancer Invest 2009; 27: 1008–15.

87. Kundel Y, Yellin A, Popovtzer A, et al. Adjuvant radiotherapy for thymic epithelial tumor: treatment results and prognostic factors. Am J Clin Oncol 2007; 30: 389–94.

88. Ogawa K, Uno T, Toita T, et al. Postoperative radiotherapy for patients with completely resected thymoma: a multi-institutional, retrospective review of 103 patients. Cancer 2002; 94: 1405–13.

89. Curran WJ Jr, Kornstein MJ, Brooks JJ, Turrisi AT 3rd. Invasive thymoma: the role of mediastinal irradiation following complete or incomplete surgical resection. J Clin Oncol 1988; 6: 1722–7.

90. Monden Y, Nakahara K, Iioka S, et al. Recurrence of thymoma: clinicopathological features, therapy, and prognosis. Ann Thorac Surg 1985; 39: 165–9.

91. Ströbel P, Bauer A, Puppe B, et al. Tumor recurrence and survival in patients treated for thymomas and thymic squamous cell carcinomas: a retrospective analysis. J Clin Oncol 2004; 22: 1501–9.

92. Cesaretti JA. Adjuvant radiation with modern techniques is the standard of care for stage III thymoma. Ann Thorac Surg 2006; 81: 1180–1.

93. Utsumi T, Shiono H, Kadota Y, et al. Postoperative radiation therapy after complete resection of thymoma has little impact on survival. Cancer 2009; 115: 5413–20.

94. Forquer JA, Rong N, Fakiris AJ, Loehrer PJ Sr, Johnstone PA. Postoperative radiotherapy after surgical resection of thymoma: differing roles in localized and regional disease. Int J Radiat Oncol Biol Phys 2010; 76: 440–5.

95. Korst RJ, Kansler AL, Christos PJ, Mandal S. Adjuvant radiotherapy for thymic epithelial tumors: a systematic review and meta-analysis. Ann Thorac Surg 2009; 87: 1641–7.

96. Loehrer PJ Sr, Chen M, Kim K, et al. Cisplatin, doxorubicin, and cyclophosphamide plus thoracic radiation therapy for limited-stage unresectable thymoma: an intergroup trial. J Clin Oncol 1997; 15: 3093–9.

97. Ciernik IF, Meier U, Lütolf UM. Prognostic factors and outcome of incompletely resected invasive thymoma following radiation therapy. J Clin Oncol 1994; 12: 1484–90.

98. Rajan A, Giaccone G. Chemotherapy for thymic tumors: induction, consolidation, palliation. Thorac Surg Clin 2011; 21: 107–14.

99. Girard N, Lal R, Wakelee H, Riely GJ, Lochrer PJ. Chemotherapy definitions and policies for thymic malignancies. J Thorac Oncol 2011; 6(7 Suppl 3): S1749–55.

100. Macchiarini P, Chella A, Ducci F, et al. Neoadjuvant chemotherapy, surgery, and postoperative radiation therapy for invasive thymoma. Cancer 1991; 68: 706–13.

101. Berruti A, Borasio P, Gerbino A, et al. Primary chemotherapy with adriamycin, cisplatin, vincristine and cyclophosphamide in locally advanced thymomas: a single institution experience. Br J Cancer 1999; 81: 841–5.

102. Rea F, Sartori F, Loy M, et al. Chemotherapy and operation for invasive thymoma. J Thorac Cardiovasc Surg 1993; 106: 543–9.

103. Yokoi K, Matsuguma H, Nakahara R, et al. Multidisciplinary treatment for advanced invasive thymoma with cisplatin, doxorubicin, and methylprednisolone. J Thorac Oncol 2007; 2: 73–8.

104. Okumura M, Miyoshi S, Takeuchi Y, et al. Results of surgical treatment of thymomas with special reference to the involved organs. J Thorac Cardiovasc Surg 1999; 117: 605–13.

105. Venuta F, Rendina EA, Coloni GF. Multimodality treatment of thymic tumors. Thorac Surg Clin 2009; 19: 71–8.

106. Lucchi M, Ambrogi MC, Duranti L, et al. Advanced stage thymomas and thymic carcinomas: results of multimodality treatments. Ann Thorac Surg 2005; 79: 1840–4.

107. Cowen D, Richaud P, Mornex F, et al. Thymoma: results of a multicentric retrospective series of 149 non-metastatic irradiated patients and review of the literature. FNCLCC trialists. Fédération Nationale des Centres de Lutte Contre le Cancer. Radiother Oncol 1995; 34: 9–16.

108. Loehrer PJ Sr, Jiroutek M, Aisner S, et al. Combined etoposide, ifosfamide, and cisplatin in the treatment of patients with advanced thymoma and thymic carcinoma: an intergroup trial. Cancer 2001; 91: 2010–15.

109. Fornasiero A, Daniele O, Ghiotto C, et al. Chemotherapy for invasive thymoma. A 13-year experience. Cancer 1991; 68: 30–3.

110. Giaccone G, Wilmink H, Paul MA, van der Valk P. Systemic treatment of malignant thymoma: a decade experience at a single institution. Am J Clin Oncol 2006; 29: 336–44.

111. Giaccone G, Ardizzoni A, Kirkpatrick A, et al. Cisplatin and etoposide combination chemotherapy for locally advanced or metastatic thymoma. A phase II study of the European Organization for Research and Treatment of Cancer Lung Cancer Cooperative Group. J Clin Oncol 1996; 14: 814–20.
112. Loehrer PJ Sr, Wang W, Johnson DH, Aisner SC, Ettinger DS. Eastern Cooperative Oncology Group Phase II Trial. Octreotide alone or with prednisone in patients with advanced thymoma and thymic carcinoma: an Eastern Cooperative Oncology Group Phase II Trial. J Clin Oncol 2004; 22: 293–9.
113. Palmieri G, Montella L, Martignetti A, et al. Somatostatin analogs and prednisone in advanced refractory thymic tumors. Cancer 2002; 94: 1414–12.
114. Rajan A, Giaccone G. Targeted therapy for advanced thymic tumors. J Thorac Oncol 2010; 5(10 Suppl 4): S361–4.
115. Girard N. Targeted therapies for thymic malignancies. Thorac Surg Clin 2011; 21: 115–23.
116. Chau NG, Kim ES, Wistuba I. The multidisciplinary approach to thymoma: combining molecular and clinical approaches. J Thorac Oncol 2010; 5(10 Suppl 4): S313–17.
117. Giaccone G, Rajan A, Berman A, et al. Phase II study of belinostat in patients with recurrent or refractory advanced thymic epithelial tumors. J Clin Oncol 2011; 29: 2052–9.
118. Lucchi M, Davini F, Ricciardi R, et al. Management of pleural recurrence after curative resection of thymoma. J Thorac Cardiovasc Surg 2009; May;137: 1185–9.
119. Ciccone AM, Rendina EA. Treatment of recurrent thymic tumors. Semin Thorac Cardiovasc Surg 2005; 17: 27–31.
120. Haniuda M, Kondo R, Numanami H, et al. Recurrence of thymoma: clinicopathological features, re-operation, and outcome. J Surg Oncol 2001; 78: 183–8.
121. Marulli G, Lucchi M, Margaritora S, et al. Surgical treatment of stage III thymic tumors: a multi-institutional review from four Italian centers. Eur J Cardiothorac Surg 2011; 39: e1–7.2010.
122. Cardillo G, Carleo F, Giunti R, et al. Predictors of survival in patients with locally advanced thymoma and thymic carcinoma (Masaoka stages III and IVa). Eur J Cardiothorac Surg 2010; 37: 819–23.
123. Liu HC, Hsu WH, Chen YJ, et al. Primary thymic carcinoma. Ann Thorac Surg 2002; 73: 1076–81.
124. Suster S, Rosai J. Thymic carcinoma. A clinicopathologic study of 60 cases. Cancer 1991; 67: 1025–32.
125. Ruffini E, Oliaro A, Novero D, Campisi P, Filosso PL. Neuroendocrine tumors of the thymus. Thorac Surg Clin 2011; 21: 13–23.
126. Marx A, Shimosato Y, Kuo TT, et al. Thymic neuroendocrine tumours. In: Travis WD, Brambilla E, Muller-Hermelink HK, et al., eds. WHO Classification of Tumours. Pathology and Genetics of Tumours of the Lung, Pleura, Thymus and Heart. Lyon: IARC Press, 2004: 188–95.
127. Moran CA, Suster S. Neuroendocrine carcinomas (carcinoid tumor) of the thymus. A clinicopathologic analysis of 80 cases. Am J Clin Pathol 2000; 114: 100–10.
128. Girard N, Mornex F, Van Houtte P, Cordier JF, van Schil P. Thymoma: a focus on current therapeutic management. J Thorac Oncol 2009; 4: 119–26.
129. Detterbeck F. International Thymic Malignancies Interest Group. J Thorac Oncol 2010; 5: S365–70.
130. Detterbeck F. International thymic malignancies interest group: a way forward. J Thorac Oncol 2010; 5(10 Suppl 4): S365–70.

Index